Public Health, Disease and Development: Social Perspectives

Public Health, Disease and Development: Social Perspectives

Reyna Escobar

AMERICAN
MEDICAL PUBLISHERS
www.americanmedicalpublishers.com

AMERICAN
MEDICAL PUBLISHERS
www.americanmedicalpublishers.com

Cataloging-in-publication Data

Public health, disease and development : social perspectives / Reyna Escobar.
p. cm.
Includes bibliographical references and index.
ISBN 979-8-88740-411-0
1. Public health--Social aspects. 2. Social medicine. 3. Diseases. 4. Public health--Economic aspects.
5. Health planning. 6. Medical care. 7. Medical care--Economic aspects. I. Escobar, Reyna.
RA418 .P83 2023
362.1--dc23

American Medical Publishers,
41 Flatbush Avenue,
1st Floor, New York,
NY 11217, USA

ISBN 979-8-88740-411-0 (Hardback)

Contents

Preface

Over the recent decade, advancements and applications have progressed exponentially. This has led to the increased interest in this field and projects are being conducted to enhance knowledge. The main objective of this book is to present some of the critical challenges and provide insights into possible solutions. This book will answer the varied questions that arise in the field and also provide an increased scope for furthering studies.

Health is a state where a person has complete emotional, physical and mental wellbeing and it is dependent upon a stable mind and healthy environment. Public health refers to the science of preventing disease, prolonging life and encouraging health through the organized efforts and informed decisions of society, organizations, communities and individuals. The foundation of public health is the examination of a population's health and the challenges it faces. The social perspectives of public health and disease take into account the interaction between health and society. It encompasses all the aspects of life, including modern and historical influences, which have affected and transformed the wellbeing and heath of people. The status of health in a society is directly interlinked with its value system, cultural traditions and its political, economic and social organization. According to the social perspective, disease and its development is considered a result of poverty, which is measured through per capita income along with malnutrition, poor health, sanitation, clothing and shelter. This book contains some path-breaking studies in the field of public health as well as its relation to disease and development. It will provide comprehensive knowledge to the readers.

I hope that this book, with its visionary approach, will be a valuable addition and will promote interest among readers. Each of the authors has provided their extraordinary competence in their specific fields by providing different perspectives as they come from diverse nations and regions. I thank them for their contributions.

Reyna Escobar

Chronic Diseases and Epidemiological Change in Africa

Megan Vaughan and
Kafui Adjaye-Gbewonyo

On a Wednesday morning the primary healthcare clinic in a small rural South African town is busy.[1] A line of caregivers, mostly women, wait with babies and small children for routine check-ups and immunisations. In the adjacent waiting room patients sit or stand outside a door marked 'Chronic Clinic'. A nurse is taking blood pressure readings and recording the numbers in the notebooks that patients have brought with them. When her turn comes, Agnes, a woman in her late forties, enters the consulting room and, helped by the woman doctor in charge, cautiously lowers herself onto a seat. A domestic worker, some weeks ago Agnes slipped while washing a floor and fractured her ankle, which is in a cast. She was treated for this medical emergency in the town's hospital and has returned there for check-ups. She's not here for her ankle, but her broken ankle is relevant to her health story, as the doctor is well aware. Agnes is her complex family's main breadwinner. She was diagnosed as a type 2 diabetic five years ago. The doctor is concerned that her latest blood sugar readings indicate that the condition is not under control. Agnes explains that, although she is receiving government disability benefit, this amounts to much less than her usual wages and so she has had to economise on the household's food budget. This means cutting out the more expensive items, including fresh vegetables, and relying heavily on the refined carbohydrates which form the staple of most working-class diets in this region – refined maize flour and white bread – supplemented with cheap cuts of meat. She looks anxious as she explains that her living situation is stressful. She's worried about her finances and what will happen if, for some reason, her broken ankle turns into a more permanent disability. It's hard to make ends meet and, to add to that, her brother, an alcoholic with mental health problems, has arrived back, unannounced, to stay with her. He is a disruptive presence and on occasions is violent.

Elements of Agnes's story will be familiar to anyone who has tracked what is frequently described as an 'epidemic' of chronic non-communicable conditions in lower- and middle-income countries, but there are also aspects of it that are specific to her small town location in a largely rural region of South Africa. Though there is no typical story, Agnes might well agree that this is an 'epidemic'. Type 2 diabetes, along with a number of other conditions including hypertension, are widely viewed by both patients and medical professionals as 'new' diseases, but now they seem to have taken an intractable hold. Agnes knows of many other people in her community, and her extended family, with these conditions but they were rare, if not completely unheard of, in her grandparents' generation. Agnes's 'sugar' condition requires long-term monitoring and self-management, particularly in relation to her diet. Managing her diet in the context of a constrained budget and a food system in which processed energy-dense but nutritionally poor foods are cheaper to buy than a healthier, fresher, more diverse array of foodstuffs makes it hard for her to follow the doctor's advice. Elsewhere on the continent this element of Agnes's story might be present but less significant, although it is becoming more common. Agnes is overweight. More women than men in Southern Africa are defined as 'overweight' or 'obese' so, in this respect, Agnes is far from unusual. You could say that Agnes is fortunate in some ways. She is being paid a disability benefit by the South African government and the provincial health care system has instituted a special clinic for patients with chronic conditions like hers, as well as a reasonably efficient system to ensure that, should she move elsewhere, her treatment would be continued. She's fortunate that she is being seen by a caring doctor who is committed to helping her manage this long-term condition, who has access to a good supply of medications and who can refer her on to a specialist diabetes clinic should she develop complications. Few or none of these favourable conditions are common in many other parts of the continent for diabetes patients unable to pay for private treatment. Agnes is also not unusual in finding her situation stressful. In fact, she wonders if stress is what brought on her diabetes in the first place. She knows for certain that, now she has diabetes, it is adding to her stress. She worries about her future and about the grandchildren who depend on her.

Also worried are a group of men in urban Ghana brought together by a researcher for a 'focus group discussion' on stroke.[2] They are puzzled that in their community it is not only middle-aged and older men who are stricken but, increasingly, younger, apparently healthy men too. Most of them know about hypertension and how dangerous this 'hidden' condition can be. The blood pressure monitor is a familiar sight in local clinics and on advertising billboards. Some of the group are taking anti-hypertensive medications themselves. As the group discussion progresses, a diverse range of issues are discussed and disputed, from the economic to the spiritual, the moral to the biological, often intertwined. An older man suggests that moral lassitude, particularly sexual promiscuity, is the cause of stroke in young men; another group member thinks that the strong alcoholic bitters widely marketed in Ghana are at the root of the problem. There is a discussion about the difference between 'right-side' and 'left-side' strokes and the role of spiritual forces in producing them. Another man, who has been diagnosed with hypertension himself, points to a more mundane fact: the country's national health insurance scheme does not pay for the full cost of the medications he needs. Without money, how do you avoid the danger of a stroke? The other men nod in agreement. They have all seen the devastating consequences of stroke in their community – the men and women now seriously disabled, unable to work or function normally, cared for by hard-pressed relatives, sometimes hidden away inside housing compounds. These are the patients who don't even make it into the country's stroke statistics – they literally do not count.

At the end of a long day in a rural hospital in Zimbabwe a newly qualified doctor is struggling to provide the statistics being requested by an international non-governmental organisation that helps fund medical services in the district. They want figures on the incidence of non-communicable diseases (NCDs) in the area (as these conditions are known by the experts), which represent a growing threat to the health of populations in sub-Saharan Africa. The doctor dutifully works through the outpatient and inpatient statistics, filling in the spreadsheets as best she can. But she is slightly puzzled, and a little irritated. Maybe these conditions are regularly seen in the private clinics of Harare, frequented by the country's elite, but they certainly do not occupy her working days. The cholera epidemic that overran medical facilities six months ago is thankfully over. But the clinics are still full of undernourished children with diarrhoea and malaria, the poorly resourced maternity ward still struggles to manage the large number of women who arrive here, late in labour, with birth complications. The HIV/AIDS clinic, fortunately well funded by an international NGO, remains busy with both newly diagnosed cases and patients on long-term medication who are living with AIDS as a chronic disease. The hospital's buildings are in desperately poor repair, the generator frequently runs out of fuel and, perhaps most worrying of all, there is a chronic shortage of medical staff.

Transition, temporalities and the epidemiological imagination

As these opening examples indicate, patterns of disease are intimately connected with the social, economic and political conditions of life, but also with the biopolitics of disease categorisation and data collection and with epidemiological imaginaries. The door through which Agnes walks in South Africa is labelled Chronic Clinic, implying that her medical issues will require long-term management and care. As has been noted more generally, this 'chronicity' comes with its own set of assumptions and imperatives, and its own temporalities.[3] Agnes's Chronic Clinic is run and managed by the South African state, which has recognised that diabetes, hypertension and other long-term conditions are placing an increasing burden on communities, on the health system, and potentially on the economic future of the country. The Chronic Clinic is, however, a rarity in sub-Saharan African healthcare systems, with their focus on infectious diseases, immunisation and infant, child and maternal health. As the men in the Ghana focus group are well aware, many serious 'chronic' conditions are invisible – unacknowledged and uncounted by institutions and, sometimes, consciously hidden away by communities themselves. Meanwhile the young doctor in rural Zimbabwe may be feeling not only that this category of diseases labelled 'NCDs' is a luxury of sorts in a setting experiencing ongoing infectious disease emergencies, but also that it is just the latest preoccupation of the international funders on which so much Zimbabwean healthcare depends.

In this volume we argue that a particularly powerful way of thinking about the changing epidemiology of African societies in the late twentieth and twenty-first centuries has been one of 'transition', and its accompanying categorisation of 'stages'. From a variety of disciplinary and methodological standpoints, our contributors trace the effects of this form of epidemiological imagination and its relationship to lives, social relations and experiences of health and disease. Many criticisms have been made of transition theories as applied to historical epidemiology and the larger framing of modernisation theory of which they are a part. However, they continue to exert a hold in part because they allow for global comparisons and projections and because they acknowledge the degree to which the whole of humanity is subject to many of the same forces.[4] Given that, in so much colonial and postcolonial discourse on 'Africa', disease has played such an important role in marking the continent and its inhabitants as intrinsically 'different' and indeed, intrinsically diseased, it is easy to see the attraction of models which (in theory at least) put the emphasis not on difference but on comparability and commensurability.[5] In parts of the continent most marked by historical racial thinking, especially Southern Africa, this is important to remember. Many of those arguing within a framework of 'transition' in the twentieth century were in a minority and were self-consciously distinguishing themselves from the dominant modes of racial thinking in which African biologies and pathologies were figured as *incommensurable* with 'white' ones. But the polarisation between universalising and racialisation theorisation is often more apparent than real, as difference, and sometimes 'race', find their way back into transition theory, often through marked associations between groups of people and 'stages of development'. Urbanising Africans, in particular, were often pathologised in these accounts. In this framework the health problems associated with urbanisation and migration could be attributed not to the social, economic and political conditions that produced them, but to the 'maladjustment' of 'tribal' rural Africans to the conditions of modern life.[6]

By the 1960s, the more obviously 'colonial' accounts of these processes were sidelined, but the era of 'development' was in full swing, with its own versions of modernisation and transition from 'under-developed' to 'developed'.[7] Demography and epidemiology were central to these understandings of how societies would move through the transition to 'modernity'. In this volume we focus on the theory of 'epidemiologic transition', which we argue has had a lasting impact on the ways in which the changing epidemiologies of African societies have been imagined, conceptualised and counted. Moving away from transition as the dominant framework for understanding change allows for other temporalities and realities to be recognised and for a more nuanced and realistic understanding of the challenges faced by communities and healthcare systems in sub-Saharan Africa.

Medical students the world over are taught that the increasing incidence of chronic non-communicable disease is intrinsic to a much larger set of demographic and epidemiological patterns known as the 'epidemiologic' (or 'epidemiological') transition.[8] The idea of the epidemiologic transition, though critiqued and tweaked (sometimes almost beyond recognition) since its first articulation by demographer Abdul Omran in 1971, remains the dominant meta-narrative of changes in disease patterns in sub-Saharan Africa. This is an evolutionist account and a version of a broader modernisation theory which informed policy in the post-war world. As Weisz and Olszynko-Gryn have shown, it was not immediately influential, but began to be very widely cited in the 1980s and 1990s, just as the World Health Organization was beginning to recognise 'NCDs' as a growing problem in the 'developing world'.[9] Omran's starting point was that mortality was the major driving force of population change. This allowed him to identify three 'Ages' or successive historical stages in modern human societies: firstly, the 'Age of Pestilence', when mortality was dominated by epidemic disease and famine; second, the 'Age of Receding Pandemics' when mortality declines progressively and epidemics become less frequent or disappear and third, the 'Age of Degenerative and Man-Made Disease' when, with ageing populations, mortality and morbidity are both dominated by what we would now call chronic non-communicable diseases. Omran proposed that societies would 'transition' between these three successive stages. To illustrate how this might happen, he used the example of England and Wales from around the beginning of the eighteenth century to the mid-twentieth century, which he labelled the 'Classical or Western Model', in which the 'Age of Receding Pandemics' was long and drawn out.

Omran's theory, once it reached a wider audience in the 1980s and 1990s, was subject to much commentary and revision, including an auto-critique by Omran himself.[10] Additional 'stages' have been proposed to his original three, as well as a range of 'transitions' reflecting new developments since Omran first proposed his theory, as well as some recognition of regional variations. The linear notion of 'transition' itself, however, remains largely intact in these revisions, implying that the path to the 'Age of Degenerative and Man-Made Disease' might be a little rocky, but everyone will get there in the end. However, there have been more thoroughgoing critiques of Omran's theory and its successors. Some of these have come from historians of the 'west' who dispute the accuracy of Omran's account of his foundational, classical model, particularly the case of Britain. Simon Szreter (in this volume and in other publications) points to the fundamental importance of state interventions in reducing mortality from epidemic disease and famine, and the reversibility of those processes. Historians of medicine have indicated that Omran's account greatly underestimates the importance of chronic disease in the 'Age of Pandemics'. More radically, Alexander Mercer, drawing on contemporary work in the global south (of which more below) to reassess the European historical record, has argued that the distinction between infectious and non-communicable disease, intrinsic to the theory, is misleading.[11]

Faced with inadequate data and great diversity, analysts of change in African populations since the 1980s have come up with a variety of adaptations of Omran's model. In eastern and southern Africa in particular, the massive impact of the HIV/AIDS epidemic, coming as it did after a period in which epidemic disease had appeared to be receding, seemed to call for a rethink. Even in parts of Africa where HIV/AIDS had not radically upset the anticipated transition in mortality and morbidity, the observed changes in demography and epidemiology over the last century do not fit neatly into Omran's transitional framework.[12] This probably comes as little surprise to most historians of the region, who have long argued that 'modernisation' is an inadequate frame through which to view the complex economic and social changes brought by colonialism, uneven economic development and the enduring importance of social institutions such as kinship.[13] From the 1950s to the mid-1970s it may have looked to some external observers as if African societies were, indeed, on a largely predictable path of 'modernisation', but the economic crisis of the 1980s, the subsequent imposition of austerity measures and (in some parts of the continent at least) the recurrence of political instability, conflict and famine marked an end to this scenario. In recognition that the 'epidemiological transition' was too restricted a framework to account for changes in population health, Frenk and others proposed the broader concept of a 'health transition' that would incorporate a wider array of factors including health systems themselves and responses to them as well as educational levels.[14] In a comprehensive review of the African evidence in relation to transition theory (including the more inclusive 'health transition' theory), Defo has convincingly argued for their inadequacy and for the need for new conceptual frameworks and a better evidence base.[15] However, the recurring theme of 'transition' in much literature on health in Africa is striking, with many scholarly articles beginning with some variant of the phrase 'Africa is undergoing the epidemiologic transition…'.[16] For example, for Agyei-Mensah and de-Graft Aikins the 'protracted-polarised' variant of the epidemiological transition appears to describe the history of population health in Accra, Ghana.[17]

Even where the notion of transition remains intact there is a widespread acknowledgement that the burden of disease has not simply shifted from that constituted by infectious conditions to that imposed by non-communicable ones. A 'protracted' transition seems to entail a 'double burden of disease' in which non-communicable diseases increase but infectious diseases remain a significant health problem. Two sets of health problems which, in Omran's theory, belonged to separate 'eras' were existing simultaneously. Some argued that this was more accurately characterised as a 'triple burden of disease' consisting of malnutrition, infectious disease and NCDs. In 2011, Julio Frenk and Octavio Gomez-Dantes also proposed that developing nations were suffering a 'triple burden' of disease. Their definition of this was rather different, consisting of, firstly, the 'backlog' of common infections, undernutrition and maternal mortality; secondly the 'emerging challenges' of NCDs and, thirdly, 'problems directly related to globalisation, like pandemics, and the health consequences of climate change'.[18] Other analyses propose that injuries should constitute a discrete element of the 'triple burden', and in South Africa a 'quadruple burden' of disease was delineated as consisting of communicable disease (including HIV and TB), maternal and child mortality, NCDs and, finally, injury and trauma.

Accounts of double, triple and quadruple burdens are essentially descriptive. However, other theories point to interactions and mechanisms of causation which further blur the boundaries of the disease categories employed by Omran, and introduce temporalities other than the evolutionary stages envisioned by him. At the level of the individual, the recognition that two or more conditions ('co-morbidity' or 'multi-morbidities') might co-exist and interact has long been recognised. That these co-morbidities or multi-morbidities might belong to apparently different disease categories, such as communicable and non-communicable, also points to a complexity of causation unanticipated by a model of 'stages' such as Omran's. In particular, the role of inflammatory responses to infections in precipitating or predisposing an individual to a range of NCDs has become very clear in research on the African continent as well as in other locations where infectious diseases are widespread.[19] That there might be multiple aetiological pathways to any one NCD is recognised in much research, and appears to exist in tension with approaches and public health policies which continue to position 'communicable' and 'non-communicable' diseases in distinct categories.[20] In southern and eastern Africa, the HIV/AIDS epidemic was probably the single most important factor in producing research that highlighted not only the co-infections commonly experienced by people living with AIDS but also a range of other co- and multi-morbidities. These included conditions such a hypertension, type 2 diabetes and chronic kidney disease.[21] Such complex interactions almost certainly existed in other contexts and other times, as Alexander Mercer's recent historical research indicates, as did the pioneering research on infection and cancer carried out in East Africa in the 1960s.[22]

At the population level, much recent literature refers to the theory of syndemics, first put forward by anthropologist Merrill Singer in the mid-1990s. Singer and his colleagues are at pains to point out that the theory of syndemics is not simply an account of co-morbidity writ large, though it clearly rests in part on the recognition of the importance of co- and multi-morbidities at the individual level.[23] At its simplest, a syndemic describes the aggregation of two or more concurrent or sequential epidemics, or clusters of disease, in a population in such a way as to aggravate the burden of disease. In their Introduction to a *Lancet* special issue in 2015, Singer and colleagues put the case for this approach:

> Specifically, a syndemics approach examines why certain diseases cluster (i.e. multiple diseases affecting individuals and groups), the pathways through which they interact biologically in the individual and within populations, and thereby multiply their overall disease burden and the ways in which social environments, especially conditions of social inequality and injustice, contribute to disease clustering and interaction, as well as to vulnerability.[24]

As this description makes clear, the theory of syndemics draws attention not only to the population-level interaction between diseases, but also to the social, political, economic and environmental factors at work which multiply the disease burden for certain groups. In this respect it can be said to reflect pre-existing approaches to the political economy and social determinants of health and illness.[25] Recently the syndemics approach has been taken up by researchers in South Africa (and to a lesser extent in other parts of the continent) to account for the cumulative effects of inequalities on both physical and mental health, and the multiplying effects of disease interactions, particularly in relation to NCDs.[26] Increasingly, the impact of global environmental factors is seen as intrinsic to the syndemics approach, highlighting, for example, the impact of climate change on re-emergent infections, on zoonotics and on nutrition. This is evident, for example, in the recent *Lancet* Commission on the 'Global Syndemic of Obesity, Undernutrition and Climate Change'.[27] Though the syndemics approach implies a very different kind of approach to historical change than that proposed by Omran's 'stages' and 'transitions', nevertheless the language of 'transition' still seems to exercise a hold. For example, in their account of the syndemic of poverty, depression and diabetes, Mendenhall and their colleagues refer to 'transitioning populations' as the subject of their analysis.[28]

While the syndemics approach emphasises disease interactions at the population level and their wider social, political and economic context, the 'developmental origins of health and disease' (DOHAD) theory focuses on the individual life course. These approaches are not necessarily mutually exclusive, but their different foci and implicit time frames are nevertheless significant (see Pentecost in this volume).

First put forward by David Barker and his colleagues in the late 1980s, the theory drew on epidemiological data for England and Wales to hypothesise that certain adult diseases, particularly cardiovascular disease, could be traced to foetal origins, especially undernutrition in gestation.[29] As Moffat Nyirenda and others have argued, this approach appears to have particular relevance to some contexts in sub-Saharan Africa where 'lifestyle' factors alone do not seem to provide a sufficient explanation for the occurrence of NCDs and where undernutrition and childhood infections remain significant factors.[30] As Michelle Pentecost has shown, this approach has been widely adopted in South Africa and reformulated as 'The First Thousand Days'. In the process, as she argues, it has focused attention again on reproductive health but sometimes, and problematically, is narrowly concerned with the mother/child dyad rather than the larger context in which reproduction occurs.[31] With advances in epigenetics, the developmental origins hypothesis has in some versions now been extended to account for health outcomes across more than one generation, popularised in the phrase 'You are what your grandmothers ate'. For some critics, in this version it has resonances of discredited theories of 'race' and disease; for others it is a significant and positive advance in biosocial thinking, enabling us to understand more fully the mechanisms by which health inequalities are reproduced.[32]

Taken together, these alternative conceptions of the histories of disease and accounts of epidemiological change appear to provide a more productive way of approaching the multiple and varying health challenges facing populations in sub-Saharan Africa than the limited epidemiological imagination implied by transition theory. The fact that, despite these theoretical advances, the idea of transition appears to remain so attractive is however not merely a function of disciplinary blind-spots, though those undoubtedly exist. In so far as epidemiological transition theory gestures to the importance of history and of comparative perspectives and acknowledges forces that operate at a global level, it contains some useful elements. Most of us would agree that there might be something to be gained from studying the experience of social and economic change in contexts other than our immediate environments. Many of the factors influencing our health are global in reach – including environmental factors, global food systems and global pharmacologies, as well as infectious diseases that know no borders. The reassuring simplicity of the historical trajectory proposed by epidemiological transition theory implied that by looking at the past we could know the future – and presumably prepare for it – and hence its undoubted attraction to health policy makers. Complexities in the relationship between bodies and environments, overlapping temporalities, stalled or reversed 'transitions', political ideologies and radical inequalities both within and between societies may look hard to factor into a public health policy. However, we would suggest that these perspectives ultimately have more to offer than a reductive evolutionist account.

Numbers and categories

The evolutionist conception of 'stages' and 'transition' which has been so influential in the conceptualisation of epidemiological change has inevitably influenced the collection of the statistics on which further knowledge is built. Everyone in the 'global health' world is agreed that we need better statistics for health conditions in sub-Saharan Africa, and not the substitute estimates that so often fill the gaps. But we also need a critical approach to the collection of those statistics and particularly to the framing of the categories employed. This is nowhere more evident than in the case of the category 'non-communicable disease'.[33] Though not co-terminous with the concept of chronic disease, the category of NCDs shares some of the same roots, as George Weisz has shown.[34] By the 1970s the NCD category was being employed by the World Health Organization and a decade later was beginning to be applied to the analysis of epidemiological change in low- and middle-income countries (LMICs). From its inception, the category was closely allied to the evolutionist model of 'epidemiologic transition' but was also linked to the development of new statistical techniques which gave rise to the Global Burden of Disease studies that have informed much global health policy and planning since the mid-1990s.[35] Simply put, as societies 'develop' economically (development being measured largely by GDP), so their mortality rates from infectious (communicable) disease are assumed to fall, their fertility rates decline and their populations age. Increasingly, then, both morbidity and mortality become dominated by chronic non-communicable diseases – including cancer, cardiovascular disease, chronic respiratory disease and diabetes. Often long-term conditions, the scale of their burden on societies was illuminated by the construction of another (much disputed) statistic, that of the disability adjusted life year (DALYs).[36] Though sometimes conceived of as diseases of ageing populations, NCDs were also framed initially as 'diseases of civilisation', linked to increased affluence and the lifestyles of highly industrialised regions, as the famous Framingham Study on heart disease had shown.[37] Once framed as 'lifestyle' diseases, it was possible to identify the major 'modifiable risk factors', which today are named as the 'big four': smoking, poor diet, inadequate physical activity and excessive alcohol consumption.

Many commentators have noted that, in theory, NCDs – as a category of diseases – are clearly linked not only to changing demographies and patterns of mortality, but also to inequality and to exposure to environmental conditions over which the individual has little control. They have also noted that the 'lifestyle drift' inherent in many analyses tends to direct attention away from political economy and environment towards individual responsibility.[38] Directing attention to 'modifiable risk factors' is, of course, important for public health, but it has limits and can lead to the invisibilisation of other conditions (and risk factors) that do not neatly fit this reductive definition of non-communicable disease. Mental health, for example, though arguably a large contributor to NCD morbidity, frequently gets left out of the category (and hence the data collection).[39] This is true of a number of other conditions – either because they are hard to diagnose or measure, or because their 'risk factors' so evidently operate at a societal or even global level – and air pollution would be one example. In addition, as several authors in this volume argue, the apparently hard and fast distinction between infectious and non-communicable disease is itself questionable, particularly given what we now know about the role of infection in producing non-communicable conditions.[40] Indeed, observations in the 1950s/60s in East Africa on the role of infection in some cancers were at the forefront of this research, which now identifies inflammatory responses to infection as an important factor in a number of conditions.[41]

As many of the contributors to our volume point out, the framing of the category of NCDs in Africa contains assumptions about the continent's social and economic development, and also ideas about 'race', ethnicity and difference which are inherited from colonial thinking and reconfigured in the postcolonial period. As we know, preconceptions that have no basis in scientific fact can directly influence the practice of data collection. Put simply, there are some so-called facts about the epidemiology of sub-Saharan African societies in the last hundred years which we will probably never know because it was assumed that Africans were immune to certain conditions owing to their 'stage of development' or inherent 'racial' characteristics. In other cases, where data was collected, assumptions were built into the selection of statistics that constrained the possibilities for interpretation and analysis.

More mundanely, in the case of much of sub-Saharan Africa, the collection of health data for conditions such as cancer, heart disease or diabetes barely existed in any consistent form until the 1980s, and in some places much later than that. Throughout much of the twentieth century, concerns about fertility and population control, particularly of non-white populations, largely informed the focus of demography, international health, and population studies. As Sivaramakrishnan discusses in her chapter on demographic ageing in the global south, theories of demographic transition became prominent in the post-World-War-II era. These demographic theories suggested that, as societies progressed and modernised, mortality would decline as infection and epidemics were controlled. These reductions in mortality, in particular child mortality, would be followed by and spur reductions in fertility and together these changes would further drive and improve economic prosperity. Economic growth and development were contingent on population control, and therefore family planning to reduce fertility was necessary for development.[42] These ideas meant that international health in this period focused largely on studying fertility patterns, child mortality and maternal mortality, and much of the health data that have been routinely sponsored and collected in Africa have therefore been demographic in nature. Since 1984, for example, the US Agency for International Development (USAID) has sponsored the Demographic and Health Surveys (DHS), collecting nationally representative data on fertility and family planning, nutrition and maternal and child health in LMICs roughly every five years.[43] The DHS programme developed out of the World Fertility Surveys and Contraceptive Prevalence Surveys and focused primarily on children and women of childbearing age,[44] reflecting the international development sphere's anxieties about reducing fertility, including by improving child survival. Similarly, the UNICEF-sponsored Multiple Indicator Cluster Surveys (MICS), which began in the mid-1990s, collect standardised data from LMICs to monitor indicators of fertility, immunisation, water and sanitation, diarrhoea and breastfeeding, among other topics relevant to child survival and maternal health.[45] With the advent of the HIV/AIDS epidemic, and given the infectious disease and poverty-focused Millennium Development Goals (MDGs), these surveys expanded to include data on issues such as HIV/AIDS, malaria and gender. The DHS programme and MICS have become dominant sources of nationally representative health information in many LMICs, including on the African continent.

Similarly, health and demographic information has been a central focus of the establishment of the demographic surveillance system (DSS) sites, now health and demographic surveillance system (HDSS) sites. These sprung up in Asia and Africa primarily to monitor population dynamics through routine longitudinal data collection on demographic events such as births, deaths and migration using censuses of largely rural communities. For instance, the first HDSS site was established in Matlab, Bangladesh in 1966 in order to provide population estimates to support epidemiological and public health research at the diarrhoeal disease hospital established in the area.[46] While there has been an increasing emphasis on monitoring morbidity with regard to ageing and NCDs at the HDSSs, the initial focus of their health surveillance largely revolved around communicable diseases, including HIV/AIDS and malaria, with some exceptions noted below.[47] The Karonga HDSS in Malawi, for example, developed out of a decades-long history of cohort studies in the area examining infectious diseases such as leprosy, TB and HIV, with an aim to provide a platform for such studies. Since 2012, however, the site has been involved in significant efforts in the area of NCDs.[48]

Thus, much of the routine population health data that has been collected in African countries has often been backed by foreign entities and was initially informed by either colonial concerns about endemic infectious disease, maternal/child health and depopulation[49] or Malthusian concerns about overpopulation, economic development programmes and ideas of demographic transition coupled with epidemiological transition.

The assumption that chronic diseases were not relevant to and did not affect 'poor' people such as Africans, a belief David Reubi also discusses in his chapter on the smoking epidemic, perhaps led to missed opportunities to study such conditions in the African context. Data relating to chronic NCDs historically were most likely to be found in hospital or clinic reports rather than in population- or community-based samples. Sanuade touches on some of these sources with respect to Ghana in his chapter. While some HDSS sites have been collecting cause-of-death data using verbal autopsy for several decades, including NCD-related mortality,[50] morbidity data were not traditionally part of this surveillance. Thus, given the focus on nutritional and infectious diseases and maternal and child health in the DHS and MICS surveys, as well as the demographic and communicable disease focus of the HDSS sites, population-based NCD morbidity data has been limited on the African continent outside of hospital and clinical settings.

South Africa is one of the few African countries that has been collecting national population-based data on NCD morbidity since at least the 1990s. As Sivaramakrishnan notes in her paper, even from the 1960s, South Africa was viewed by some demographers and social scientists as being ahead on the path to modernisation compared to other countries. Therefore, given this fact as well as the high prevalence of some of the recognised risk factors for NCDs such as overweight and obesity, it may not be surprising that the 'diseases of development' have been considered in national data collection and incorporated into South Africa's DHS surveys since 1998. South Africa also implemented a National Health and Nutrition Examination Survey (SANHANES) in 2012, similar to the comprehensive NHANES surveys that have been implemented in the US since the 1960s which include a clinician-facilitated physical examination component. By contrast, apart from BMI data which have been collected as part of the nutritional component of the DHSs for several years (often to measure undernutrition), many other African countries have only begun incorporating questions relating to chronic NCDs into national surveys since the late 2000s and early 2010s. For example, as Sanuade highlights in his chapter, Ghana only added blood pressure collection and a few other NCD measures into its DHS in 2014.

Not only has national health data collection in South Africa had a longer history of attention to NCDs, local data collection at the HDSS sites also reflects this interest. The Dikgale and Agincourt HDSSs were established largely to provide a sampling frame for population monitoring of NCDs and their risk factors, with the establishment of the Agincourt HDSS also intended to provide data to inform the decentralisation of healthcare in South Africa.[51] Thus, these sites differ from many of the other African HDSSs in terms of their motivations and initial attention to NCDs.

It is clear that assumptions about the health issues that are of importance and relevance in Africa have shaped what data have been collected and what conditions have been measured on the continent, with a heavy focus on maternal and child health and communicable disease. It becomes difficult then to paint an accurate picture of disease burden and construct comprehensive statistics when whole classes of disease have not been measured regularly in a population setting.

In addition to *what* is being measured, the issue of *how* conditions are being measured creates another complication. Kafui Adjaye-Gbewonyo reflects on these issues in her chapter on the validity of chronic disease measures in African settings. She notes that many of the instruments used to measure disease symptoms, including questionnaires for depression and ischaemic heart disease, were developed in and for European or North American populations and were subsequently adapted for global use. However, questions about whether these instruments, when applied to various African populations, are actually measuring what was intended to be measured and whether the constructs themselves translate accurately across cultures deserve further attention.

Aside from the issues of what types of diseases and conditions are being recorded and how, another complication with statistics is the scale at which they are calculated and the areas which they represent. As Shane Doyle notes in his chapter on 'Maternal health, epidemiology and transition theory in Africa', national averages often obscure regional and local variation in health outcomes and often do not represent the true values for any area of a country. In many African countries, where colonial activities shaped who received access to global networks, formal education and allopathic medicine, there is often wide variation in health outcomes within countries. Doyle's examples from Kenya and Uganda provide evidence of this.

Many national health surveys such as the DHS are designed to take nationally representative samples and often to be representative at the first administrative level as well – for example at the regional level in Ghana or provincial level in South Africa. These surveys, therefore, can produce estimates representing national averages as well as regional/provincial averages and sometimes averages for urban areas and rural areas separately.[52] However, even within a single metropolitan area, health and social outcomes can be vastly different for some neighbourhoods compared to others – for instance comparing the wealthy suburb of Sandton to Alexandra Township in Johannesburg, or comparing Agbobloshie to East Legon in Accra. Therefore, even averages at the first administrative level (region or province) or for urban versus rural can obscure many differences. Local surveillance, such as through DSS sites or health facilities, can provide more relevant statistics for these specific localities, but these are often limited to a few select locations with large areas of countries not covered by health and demographic surveillance. David Reubi's chapter on smoking highlights some of the pitfalls of using data from select locations and populations to estimate statistics for entire nations or regions. Thus, a critical issue in health and data statistics is the lack of national data that can produce estimates for small areas.

Furthermore, as is hinted at by the above discussion, there is a particular lack of longitudinal data on chronic disease. While the HDSSs have been collecting longitudinal data, their focus until recently has primarily been on demographic statistics and communicable disease.[53] Ground-breaking cohort studies that have identified major risk factors for chronic NCDs in Europe and the US, such as the Framingham Heart

Study and Nurses' Health Study, have not had counterparts in Africa. NCD risk factor surveillance such as the NHANES and Behavioral Risk Factor Surveilllance System (BRFSS) are also not common on the continent. Currently, a major hindrance to such work is funding.[54] In the US and in many European countries, cohort studies and longitudinal surveys are often government-funded. Many African governments have not prioritised and devoted significant resources to this type of research, no doubt in part because of its expense.

Large-scale statistical studies provide one kind of necessary evidence. But, as many of our contributors show, contextualised knowledge is vitally important, both in its own right, but also to inform the collection of large-scale data. Fine-grained ethnography and historical studies, we argue, are not an optional extra, but are central to producing new knowledge, new ways of understanding the dynamics of health and disease, and better ways of formulating health policies.

Radical contextualisation

Many of the chapters in this volume speak to the importance of a 'radical contextualisation' of health in Africa. We take this term from Chapman and Berggren's account of racial/ethnic disparities in health in the US context, in which they argue that ethnography can be used as a tool for formulating 'alternative models of biosocial pathogenesis'.[55] Employing a radical, historically informed ethnographic method allows researchers to better understand the multiple and multiplying effects of the changing environment, broadly conceived, and its complex interactions with individual and social bodies. Much well-intentioned qualitative research on non-communicable disease in Africa employs ethnography with a view to understanding how 'local' perspectives on disease might be at odds with biomedical theories and act as an impediment to effective preventative health education. For example, it is frequently observed that there is a 'cultural' preference for large bodies in many African societies and that this preference acts as an impediment to health education on the increasing problem of overweight and obesity, particularly for women. But female overweight and obesity, where they exist, need to be understood at a number of different levels and in context. A cultural preference might be imposed by one group in society over another; a community with a history of nutritional precarity and infectious disease might view body fat as a useful 'reservoir'; adult central obesity might in fact be the sequel of undernutrition earlier in life; the entire environment might be obesogenic, with limited food choices and levels of personal insecurity that make physical exercise difficult. Or, it might be the case that a 'cultural preference' is in fact an act of resistance against the imposition of yet another 'western' norm: in this case the (historically recent) 'cultural preference' for the slim female form.

Many of the locations studied in this volume are layered sites of colonial and postcolonial biomedical research and intervention, meaning that local experiences are already in a deep sense global. Community histories of both past intervention and neglect by biomedical agencies inform current understandings of newly visible conditions such as hypertension and diabetes, as well as of HIV/AIDS, TB and Ebola. Susan Reynolds-Whyte's rich ethnographic research on NCDs in Uganda illuminates both the specific temporalities associated with hypertension and diabetes, and also how understandings of these conditions and their treatability has been informed by the experience of HIV/AIDS.[56]

Theories, though they might derive from very different sources, are not always radically incompatible. For example, the idea of the cross-generational transmission of certain diseases or susceptibilities is not unique to genetics or epigenetics, but common to many non-biomedical theories. Indeed, in some parts of the world, environmental epigenetics has been adopted by indigenous groups for whom it appears to offer a useful account of the effects of structural violence on their communities' health.[57]

Establishing that a condition might be related to an early episode of oxidative stress certainly involves a different set of technologies to those used to diagnose the spiritual source of, for example, stroke, but both seek to uncover an underlying imbalance that operates at a level some way removed from the individual's control over their 'risk factors'. As we observed at the beginning of this Introduction, Agnes's experience of a broken ankle and diabetes has to be understood in the context of South Africa's long history of structural oppression, racism, the destruction of rural livelihoods and the workings of a globalised food system. It is also of course relevant to note that she has access to a functioning healthcare system and one that she has not had to pay for, as well as to some basic income support. Despite this, Agnes's overwhelming sense is that it is stress, manifested mainly through her family relationships, that has brought on the diabetes and that diabetes in its turn is causing her further stress. The apparently random accident that gave her a broken ankle (itself of course related to her overall health and working conditions) is what turned a manageable 'chronic' condition into something of a health and personal crisis.

The importance of the social context of illness and of its social meanings is a feature of human experience everywhere, but no more so than in circumstances in which the work and responsibility of care falls heavily on family members, particularly women. In many of the locations described in this volume, the challenges of care associated with long-term conditions (including HIV/AIDs) raise profound moral and ethical issues for individuals and their communities, sometimes challenging strongly held principles of social connection and obligation. As what are known to some as NCDs become more common, sometimes rapidly spreading within families and communities, it is perhaps unsurprising that people may regard them as 'communicable' (see Moran-Thomas in this volume). This is not to imply that there is a confusion between infectious and non-infectious conditions, but rather that the notion of 'non-communicable' has little meaning in these circumstances. It points not only to the fact that all illness communicates something, but also that some conditions are patterned and spread in ways that reflect the social, historical and economic conditions in which they arise. As Moran-Thomas shows in her work on Belize, many patients with diabetes, viewing the widespread and devastating consequences of 'sugar' in their communities, feel that they have been 'caught' by the disease (Moran-Thomas, this volume). These patients have arrived at a critique of the communicable/non-communicable binary by a somewhat different route to that taken by some public health professionals, but the conclusion is similar: understanding an epidemic of a non-communicable disease is not helped by the binary models of causation, but requires more holistic thinking and a radical contextualisation.

The contributions of this volume

Bringing together historians, social epidemiologists and anthropologists, our aim in this volume has been both to provide a critical history of the epidemiological models that have informed knowledge and policy-making towards NCDs in sub-Saharan Africa, and to draw on the lessons of lived experience to indicate alternative histories and understandings. To be clear, we do not intend to oppose the local and the global, and nor do we propose that there is anything exceptional about experiences on the African continent. We do, however, argue that only by appreciating the complexities of the relationships illuminated by cross- and interdisciplinary approaches can we hope to arrive at a better understanding of epidemiological changes in present-day sub-Saharan Africa.

Some of our contributors focus on the history of the epidemiological models that have dominated knowledge production on African health from the mid-twentieth century and point to their intellectual origins and policy manifestations. Simon Szreter dissects Omran's evolutionary model of the epidemiological transition and tests it against the historical record for England and Wales (the classical model) for the period from c.1600 to 1914. Szreter points out that Omran's model owed much to the work of Thomas McKeown and others who saw economic growth as the essential motor of a modernisation process which was unidirectional. This process would result in marked decreases in mortality from infectious disease and famine (the 'Age of Pestilence') and a transition, first to the 'Age of Receding Pandemics' and finally to the 'Age of Degenerative and Man-Made Diseases'. Szreter's chapter focuses on the first of these 'transitions', and his analysis is a political one. Re-examining the evidence for the decline of both plague mortality and famine, Szreter points to the critical role played by government intervention. The British historical record for the eighteenth and nineteenth centuries indicates that plague mortality fell, not because of factors that could be attributed to 'economic development', but because of aggressive anti-plague state policies which actually inhibited the free movement of trade. The historical record for famine further demonstrates what Szreter characterises as an 'opposite' set of patterns to those proposed by Omran. Famine, supposedly eliminated by the end of Omran's 'Age of Pestilence', returned in the deadly Great Irish Famine (1845–48) caused at least in part by free-trade policies and by British policy and attitudes to the Irish poor. Szreter sees a close connection between the historical analysis which underpinned Omran's theory and western postwar economic development policies directed towards African countries, particularly after the oil shocks of the 1970s. He identifies an underlying assumption that improvements in the health status of the populations of sub-Saharan Africa would follow from economic growth, and that economic growth would itself depend on less rather than more government intervention. Neither of these assumptions seems to be supported by the record of the 'classic case' of England and Wales, and neither do they appear to be supported by much of the evidence emerging from sub-Saharan Africa since the 1980s.

David Reubi's chapter on constructions of the 'smoking epidemic' in postcolonial Africa also addresses the assumptions of modernisation theory, although in this instance with a focus on one of the 'dark sides' of economic development. Theories of modernisation have always acknowledged that there is a human cost to the process of economic development, though precisely how this cost has been understood has of course depended on political perspective. Increased tobacco consumption was predicted to be one of the less desirable and certainly unhealthy consequences of rising incomes and urbanisation. The theory of epidemiological transition was ambitiously universalising, predicting that low- and middle- income countries would follow the patterns identified for Europe and North America. As many other chapters in this volume also argue (though in differing ways), epidemiological theories and the quantification techniques associated with them are underpinned by powerful political and social theories. For the experts whose work is examined in Reubi's paper, the adoption of 'modern western' lifestyles would inevitably follow from economic development and urbanisation in Africa, with tobacco smoking being one of the 'pathologies' tied to this process. Smoking habits would follow a trajectory that mirrored the anticipated stages of economic development, and so could be easily predicted and potentially prevented. As Reubi shows, despite the considerable attention paid to this issue in the 1970s and 1980s, the data remained unreliable and difficult to interpret. The figure of the 'African smoker' produced by this research appears to have been somewhat elusive in reality, but the hold of the modernisation imaginary was firm. In the process attention was directed less at the operations of the powerful international tobacco companies, which saw Africa as a site of both production and consumption, and more towards the 'lifestyle' choices of urbanising Africans. As Reubi argues in the final part of his chapter, many of the arguments linking tobacco consumption to modernisation are reflected in the larger literature and policy framework for NCDs.

While David Reubi argues for the powerful hold of a US and European-centric modernisation theory on postwar epidemiology, in her chapter Kavita Sivaramakrishnan sees less uniformity and a strong element of ambivalence towards transition models amongst experts on demographic ageing. Focusing on the work of the American demographer Kingsley Davis, the Indian demographer Sripati Chandrasekar, and the writings of social activists in both South Asia and Southern Africa from the 1960s, Sivaramakrishnan shows that transition theories were continually challenged by the research which captured a more complex and contingent reality on the ground and that this evidence was often used to argue for the need for interventions of various sorts. In the view of these researchers and activists, demographic and epidemiological 'transitions' were 'changeable and contingent' and should not be viewed as 'transformative generalisations'. Economic and political transformations do not take place in a political or social vacuum, as Sivaramakrishnan's examples show. In Zimbabwe in the 1980s, just emerging from a long war of liberation, the experience of ageing amongst poorer communities did not appear to be conforming to the normative western model predicted by modernisation theorists. Many elderly people were faced less by the social isolation characteristic of ageing in the 'west' and more by the double burden of caring both for themselves and for grandchildren. In India, researchers at the Indian Social Institute reported that amongst poorer sections of communities, many elderly people experienced extreme economic precarity: dying of 'old age' was, in fact, frequently a euphemism for dying of starvation. The experience of ageing, here as elsewhere, is fundamentally affected by social inequalities and mediated by social expectations, neither of which are visible in transition models.

The ageing of populations was central to Omran's theory of epidemiological transition. But Omran had little to say about an important and intractable problem for many African societies – maternal mortality. In his chapter on maternal health, epidemiology and transition theory in eastern Africa, Shane Doyle examines the historical record and draws on contemporary observations to argue that maternal mortality sits awkwardly within epidemiological transition theory. His complex and multi-layered account compares the maternal health histories of two eastern African societies: the Buganda region of Uganda and the Kisumu area of western Kenya. In the process, Doyle reflects on an issue that features in many of the chapters of this volume: that of data collection and its interpretation. Statistics on the decline of maternal mortality in Buganda, Doyle suggests, may have been distorted by the fact that, over time, the population of mothers experiencing institutionalised delivery widened beyond those referred for 'problem' births. Appropriate interventions can have rapid effects on mortality and morbidity in the area of maternal health, supporting the larger argument made by Szreter and others. However, as Doyle shows, there may be widely divergent trends between neighbouring societies, reflecting not only the availability and quality of health services, but also the accumulated experience and knowledge of cross-generational communities of women. Much health literature, Doyle argues, tends to assume that critical health decisions are made by individuals but, in the socially and morally charged area of childbirth, this assumption is particularly questionable. Doyle's chapter also draws attention to another issue that appears at many points in this volume – the category of 'non-communicable diseases'.

Researchers based on the African continent in the 1950s–80s played an important part in the evolution of this concept. What are now referred to as NCDs were previously known as 'diseases of civilisation' and then as 'diseases of affluence'. Africans, along with other 'non-European' peoples, were assumed to experience very low rates of these conditions, because of their relatively low life expectancies, but also because their largely agricultural lives did not expose them to the industrialised diets, urban stresses and physical inactivity which were increasingly viewed as responsible. But as rates of urbanisation and migration increased in many parts of Africa, particularly after the Second World War, some researchers began to document the increasing visibility of conditions previously unknown, or at least unremarked upon. In South Africa a racial political economy had produced large-scale industrialisation and urbanisation, with damaging results for the health of African communities, both rural and urban. A dominant strand in colonial medical discourse, particularly evident in South Africa, argued that Africans were inherently poorly 'adjusted' to urban life, and that this accounted for their vulnerability to certain conditions. This victim-blaming account, which presented urbanisation as a pathological process for African peoples was, of course, politically expedient for a government which, from 1948, began formally enacting 'apartheid'. Yet African urbanisation continued apace, particularly after the Second World War and, as many South African medical commentators pointed out, urban Africans began to show signs of vulnerability to conditions that had been thought of as 'white', including hypertension, certain psychological disorders, obesity and type 2 diabetes. Megan Vaughan's chapter discusses the work of one South African medical doctor and researcher, George D. Campbell, from the late 1950s to the 1970s, who was one of the first to draw attention to the growing problem of diabetes in urban African communities. Campbell's pioneering diabetes clinic in Durban was soon overwhelmed with African patients. Initially most of these were better-off, educated middle-aged men who had adopted sedentary lifestyles and urban eating habits, inspiring Campbell's description of type 2 diabetes as the 'disease of the briefcase'. But, increasingly, the clinic saw patients from lower socio-economic sections of the community. Campbell began to suspect that diabetes was not an inevitable consequence of urbanisation and rising living standards, nor straightforwardly of 'lifestyle' choice, but rather the outcome of a South African food industry, and particularly a sugar industry, which was targeting African consumers and deliberately creating a desire for sugary and processed food. On the basis of his research and clinical experience, Campbell became an early and vocal critic of the sugar industry and its advertising strategies.

As Catherine Burns's paper on the history of breastfeeding also shows, in the postwar period South Africa was the site of much prescient in-depth and sensitive research on the social and economic determinants of health. Her paper examines how 'expert' breastfeeding knowledge and advice in the time of HIV/AIDs, and more recently in discussions over NCDs, appear to have lost the 'radical contextualisation' of these earlier studies. Breastfeeding is a fascinating and revealing case of the ways in which scientific research (into HIV transmission for example) and international expertise become enmeshed in the lives of women and their babies in low- and middle-income countries such as South Africa. Nutrition, infection and the 'developmental origins' of disease are all implicated in breastfeeding practices which have also, of course, been the target of an unscrupulous global infant formula industry. Expert advice (and admonitions) directed at mothers have not been consistent and, as Burns shows, do not take into account the multiple meanings of the practice(s) beyond infant nutrition. Just as Shane Doyle's chapter points to the important influence of social context and the advice of older women in decision making over childbirth, so Burns's chapter shows how the feeding of babies is enmeshed in ideas about inter-generational harm, sexuality, infection and blame, in ways that are likely to make adherence to the latest policy advice complicated, at the very least.

The case of type 2 diabetes in South Africa shows clearly that NCDs did not suddenly appear in Africa with globalisation in the 1980s, as is sometimes implied, but that they have longer histories, not least in relation to both infectious diseases and 'developmental origins' as proposed in the DOHAD theory. However, the absence of longitudinal data for much of sub-Saharan Africa makes it extremely difficult to say anything definitive about long-term trends. Both Kafui Adjaye-Gbewonyo and Olutobi Sanuade deal directly with the problems of data in their respective chapters. In the field of NCD research and policy in low- and middle-income countries, the statistics and projections produced by the Global Burden of Disease studies coming from the Institute for Health Metrics and Evaluation at the University of Washington in the US loom very large. Sanuade looks behind the Global Burden of Disease (GBD) figures for Ghana to examine the data which underpins them. Ghana, like most countries in Africa, does not have a comprehensive epidemiological surveillance system. Policymakers in the field of health in Ghana rely on a range of sources of evidence for NCDs and their risk factors, which Sanuade examines in his chapter. These range from the one national survey which is the WHO SAGE survey (Study on global AGEing and adult health), to the five-yearly Demographic and Health

Survey, to the hospital- and community-level surveys carried out by a range of organisations. Sanuade points to the inadequacies of the hospital records system and, drawing on his own research, points out the ways in which community-based surveys may produce misleading results. The delays in the reporting of the SAGE survey findings, and the patchiness of other data on NCDs, means that the reliance on GBD estimates and projections is likely to remain for the foreseeable future. In her paper, social epidemiologist Adjaye-Gbewonyo examines the validity of the measures used for chronic diseases in Africa. Self-reported, symptom-based measures play an important part in the production of knowledge of NCDs and chronic conditions, but their applicability across different settings is the subject of a large literature. In comparing two such measures – one for depression and the other for angina – Adjaye-Gbewonyo makes the important point that, while psychological conditions might seem particularly vulnerable to misinterpretation and inaccuracy, this is also the case for the reporting of symptoms for the apparently less problematic case of physical illness. This observation reflects a wider trend in the syndemics literature (see above) pointing to the complex interactions between conditions normally confined to different categories. In her chapter, Adjaye-Gbewonyo digs below the data into instruments measuring both depression and angina: the Center for Epidemiologic Studies of Depression (CES-D) Scale and the Rose Angina Questionnaire (RAQ). Acknowledging that there is a large literature on the question of whether the concept of 'depression' has any validity when applied to communities outside the North American and European contexts in which it was first applied, Adjaye-Gbewonyo turns to assess the evaluation of the CES-D scale and its application to the South African context. Clearly, paying attention to locally derived measures and to the context in which symptoms of distress occur is centrally important, but Adjaye-Gbewonyo concludes that it is also important not to completely dismiss instruments such as CES-D, which does sometimes produce useful results, and sheds light on issues previously unrecognised. Examining the evidence for the validity of the Rose Angina Questionnaire in African contexts also produces more questions than answers. In particular, the inconsistent results seem to point to the need for further research into the development and presentation of ischaemic heart disease in these settings. So, whilst the instrument may not always produce the reliable results it was designed for, it nevertheless appears to be suggestive of important questions. Adjaye-Gbewonyo concludes with the more general point that there is always going to be some trade-off between generating measures which will allow for comparison across time and place, and generating results that are context specific, possibly more meaningful, but less immediately useful for large-scale comparative or longitudinal analysis.

The final section of the book consists of chapters that are context-specific, their authors employing these ethnographic studies to speak not only to experience, but also to the larger themes of this volume: temporalities, causalities, categories. Importantly, all of these chapters also point to the way in which socio-economic, political and policy contexts impact directly on the experience of chronic conditions in a variety of settings, including the impact of inequalities, funding regimes and the policies of both national governments and international actors in the global health field.

In her chapter on the concept of the 'para-communicable', Moran-Thomas draws on ethnographic research in two very different locations, Northern Ghana and Belize, to trace the trajectories of what is considered by some to be a global epidemic of type 2 diabetes. Reflecting on the analyses made by both communities, Moran-Thomas points to the grounded perception that this disease can be 'caught', not only disrupting the distinction between 'infectious' and 'non-communicable' diseases, but also raising important questions about causality and generalisability. Moran-Thomas also points to the ways in which policy interventions or their absence can actually transform the disease itself, producing biological multiple variants of diabetes both at the level of the individual and that of the population. For example, the implication of horizontal gene transfer in the development of drug-resistant diabetic ulcers raises a number of troubling issues, as well as pointing to the possible transmissibility of one widely experienced 'symptom' of diabetes.

Michelle Pentecost's chapter on 'The First Thousand Days' in South Africa similarly draws attention to the direct impacts of categorisation and conceptualisation of disease, and to the underpinning imaginaries that inform policymaking. Pentecost's chapter traces the history of 'transition' theories in the context of South Africa, where 'transition' has a particular political as well as demographic and health resonance. Reflecting back on the debates on epidemiological transition theory, Pentecost shows how particular versions of this – the 'protracted-polarised' model, and the 'protracted complex' model – took hold as a way of framing both the radical inequalities in the burden of disease within South Africa, and the co-existence of different kinds of 'burden' (infectious disease, non-communicable disease, infant and child mortality, violence and injuries). She goes on to describe how the Developmental

Origins of Health and Disease (DOHaD) first formulated by Barker drew attention to a different kind of temporality – that of the life course – and focused attention again on early life experiences. By a different logic to that described by Moran-Thomas, DOHaD approaches also blur the distinction between communicable and non-communicable disease. Yet, as Pentecost argues, much DOHaD research and policy formulation still takes place within an imaginary of 'transition' at the population level. Pentecost discusses one consortium of cohort studies working with a DOHaD framework that has been formed from studies conducted in Guatemala, India, Brazil, Philippines and South Africa. These sites are conceived of as 'transitioning societies' of the 'global south' – 'transition' standing in for a number of socioeconomic and cultural factors, foregrounding assumed similarities in context and assuming a particular direction of travel. These 'DOHaD geographies', argues Pentecost, demonstrate clear continuities with 'past logics of intervention'.

The 'logics of intervention' both past and present are also under examination in the final two chapters by anthropologists Betsey Brada and Ruth Prince. Inherent to these logics are not only the epidemiological concepts and imaginaries which inform them, but also the often brutal realities of economics and inequality. Chronic conditions, whether 'non-communicable' like heart disease or infectious like HIV/AIDS, require long-term care and money which, in the context of scarce and fractured provision, most often falls on family members. The 'burden' of disease, as both of these chapters so graphically demonstrate, is emotional as well as economic. Ruth Prince traces the pursuit of diagnosis and care followed by cancer patients in Kisumu, western Kenya. Cancer has risen to public prominence in Kenya in the last decade and is a highly charged and politicised condition, exposing the deepening health inequalities in the country in painful ways. Access to diagnosis and treatment within the public health care system is scarce and fractured, often involving patients in long delays, long-distance travel, deep uncertainty and the extensive and often frustrating pursuit of elusive treatment and care. Therapeutic inequalities are writ large in the case of cancer treatment. It is widely known that treatments (and therefore hope) exist for cancer patients, but accessing them depends ultimately on a family's economic resources as well as their willingness to dedicate themselves to their pursuit. While wealthy Kenyans travel abroad for treatment, even their middle-class compatriots with some degree of health insurance often find their resources quickly depleted. Despite the extraordinary efforts of some health workers, the prospect for most poorer patients is bleak. Layered onto an epidemiological landscape of the HIV/AIDS epidemic and other infectious and non-communicable conditions, cancer, argues Prince, does not always stand out as a discrete disease. Yet it is hard to read her chapter without coming away with a profound sense of the disjuncture between hope and disappointment which characterises the cancer experience in Kisumu, as well as the huge inequities of access to health in Kenya – a situation all too familiar from other locations across the world.

The burden of care is also a focus of Betsey Brada's study from Botswana, which draws on her fieldwork in an externally funded paediatric HIV clinic. Here, as elsewhere in the region, older women are typically the main carers for young children with HIV. The exclusive focus of the clinic on children with HIV obscures the fact that the success of paediatric HIV treatment depends heavily on the willingness and ability of this older generation of women to carry out the not inconsiderable duties of the primary carer. Here the temporality of a chronic but 'communicable' HIV epidemic collides with that of a chronic 'non-communicable' one and an ageing population. Brada's carefully contextualised research illuminates how fractured health systems, funding regimes and the conceptualisation of disease categories fail to take into account the social realities of care, on which, ultimately, the success or failure of health policies depend. As Brada shows, a syndemics approach is useful here, but must be extended to encompass 'multiple bodies and generations'. Here she draws our attention to the Tswana diagnostic category of *dikgaba*, an illness manifested in a child, but the causes of which lie within the network of related kin, living and dead. As Batswana are well aware, the health and well-being of each of us are fundamentally contingent on the health and well-being of those connected to us, both near and far, from our most intimate relationships to our distant ancestors, our immediate neighbours and more remote yet connected kin. As Brada and many of our other contributors also suggest, we have much to learn from this instantiation of the 'epidemiological imagination'.

A COVID-19 coda

As we complete this volume a pandemic of a new coronavirus, COVID-19, is sweeping across the world. Such a global pandemic has been predicted for some time. We could not have known that this particular virus would emerge as the culprit, but 'new and emerging' infectious diseases, particularly those arising from non-human hosts, have long been on the agenda. Yet, as we watch this highly infectious disease devastate populations in the 'global north', it appears that those of us who live in these locations have become unaccustomed to the realities of infectious disease prevention and management, in a way that would perhaps surprise our friends and colleagues in sub-Saharan Africa who are more accustomed to the necessity for basic public health messaging ('wash your hands!') if not to the misleadingly named 'social distancing' now required of us. It would appear that the 'era of infectious disease' is far from over. Still in shock that this could be happening to 'us' rather than 'them', those of us who live in Europe and North America may feel that history has gone into reverse – popular 'lockdown' reading includes accounts of the medieval Black Death and Samuel Pepys' 1665 London plague diary.

It is too soon to draw any conclusions from this dramatic global event, but we can offer a few reflections on the different ways in which it resonates with the themes of this volume.

Firstly, COVID-19 offers an important lesson in common human vulnerability to lethal pathogens, and to our fundamental interconnectedness. This may sound trite and obvious, but it is, we think, worth reflecting on. It is also offers an important lesson to those in political and policymaking positions, in national and global health bodies, that contemporary biomedicine, for its sophistication, requires political and social institutions to be effective and that sophisticated modelling is useless in the absence of basic public health.

Countries with older populations have (so far) been hardest hit with high mortality rates, reminding us again of the confounding of supposed 'stages' at a societal level with individual life cycles. It is too soon to say whether the apparently low current rates of infection in most African countries will persist – we hope so.

Striking, and perhaps most relevant for this volume, is the heightened susceptibility of individuals with 'underlying conditions', by which, in most cases, is meant 'non-communicable' diseases such as diabetes, heart disease and hypertension. As this pandemic progresses, we can see clearly how these conditions in turn map onto social and economic inequalities, affecting poorer communities disproportionately and, in some instances, black and 'ethnic minority' groups in particular. If we ever needed a reminder of the colliding syndemic of poverty, infectious disease and chronic conditions, this is it. As deaths go uncounted in our care homes, we are reminded of the shadow economy of ageing societies, the outsourcing of care to low-paid workers (often from the global south, including many carers from Africa). It seems that not every death counts. We are reminded that dealing with a rapidly spreading infectious disease also has costs – economic, social and more immediate health costs. In the UK, we are told that the death toll from cancers gone undetected or untreated in this period may eventually exceed that from the virus itself. On the day of writing this, South Africa is reporting a *reduction* in overall mortality rates over the past month, due to a decrease in road accident fatalities and (reported) homicides. If nothing else, epidemics and pandemics lay bare the fault lines in our societies. Though a pandemic of this nature was not unpredicted, it seems that our 'epidemiological imaginations' could not stretch far enough to prepare for it.

Notes

1 This case study draws on fieldwork carried out for the 'Chronic Disease in Africa' project, Dr Beth Vale, Eastern Cape of South Africa, April 2018.
2 This case study draws on research carried out by Sanuade, 'Understanding the Cultural Meanings of Stroke'.
3 Manderson and Smith-Morris (eds.), *Chronic Conditions, Fluid States.*
4 Debate on historical scholarship and the question of 'modernity' in *American Historical Review*.
5 Lock and Nguyen, *An Anthropology of Biomedicine.*
6 Vaughan, *Curing Their Ills.*
7 Cooper, *Colonialism in Question.*
8 See Szreter in this volume. For the original statement of the theory: Omran, 'The Epidemiologic Transition: A Theory of the Epidemiology of Population Change'. On the theory, its influence and afterlives: Weisz and Olszynko-Gryn, 'The Theory of Epidemiologic Transition: The Origins of a Citation Classic'; Mooney, 'Historical Demography and Epidemiology'.
9 Szreter, this volume; Weisz and Olszynko-Grin, 'The Theory of Epidemiologic Transition'.
10 Mooney, 'Historical Demography'; Szreter, this volume; Omran, 'The Epidemiologic Transition Theory Revisited Thirty Years Later'; Omran, 'The Epidemiologic Transition Theory: A Preliminary Update'.
11 Mercer, *Infections, Chronic Disease, and the Epidemiological Transition*.
12 See Defo, 'Demographic, Epidemiological and Health Transitions'; National Research Council, *The Continuing Epidemiological Transition in Sub-Saharan Africa*.
13 For the clearest articulation of this critique see Cooper, *Colonialism in Question.*
14 Frenk et al., 'Elements for a Theory of the Health Transition'; Defo, 'Demographic, Epidemiological and Health Transitions'.
15 Defo, 'Demographic, Epidemiological and Health Transitions'.
16 One example: 'Kenya like many other LMICs is undergoing an epidemiological transition – from infectious diseases to NCDs…', Onyango and Onyango, 'The Rise of NCDs in Kenya'.
17 Agyei-Mensah and de-Graft Aikins, 'Epidemiological Transition and the Double Burden of Disease in Accra'.
18 Frenk and Gomez-Dantes, 'The Triple Burden'.
19 Ogoina and Onyemelukwe, 'The Role of Infections in the Emergence of Noncommunicable Diseases'; Nyirenda, 'NCDs in Sub-Saharan Africa'.
20 Vaughan, 'Conceptualising Metabolic Disorder'; Oni and Unwin, 'Why the Communicable/Non-Communicable Disease Dichotomy is Problematic for Public Health Control Strategies'.
21 Engelman and Kehr, 'Double Trouble? Towards an Epistemology of Co-Infection'.
22 Mercer, *Infections, Chronic Disease, and the Epidemiological Transition*; Walusansa, Okuku and Orem, 'Burkitt Lymphoma in Uganda'.

23 On the difference between 'co-morbidity' and syndemics see Singer, *Introduction to Syndemics*; Nichter, 'Co-Morbidity: Reconsidering the Unit of Analysis'.
24 Singer et al., 'Syndemics and the Biosocial Conception of Health'; Mendenhall et al., 'Non-Communicable Disease Syndemics'; Singer, *Introduction to Syndemics*; Adjaye-Gbewonyo and Vaughan, 'Reframing NCDs?'.
25 Krieger (ed.), *Embodying Inequality*; Farmer, *Infections and Inequalities*; Farmer, *Pathologies of Power*; Marmot, *The Health Gap*.
26 Mendenhall et al., 'Non-Communicable Disease Syndemics'; Mendenhall et al., 'Stress, Diabetes and Infection'; Mendenhall and Norris, 'When HIV is Ordinary and Diabetes New'.
27 *Lancet* Commission on Global Syndemic of Obesity, Undernutrition and Climate Change.
28 Mendenhall et al., 'Non-Communicable Disease Syndemics'.
29 Barker, 'The Origins of Developmental Origins Theory'.
30 Nyirenda, 'NCDs in Sub-Saharan Africa'; Vaughan, 'Conceptualising Metabolic Disorder'.
31 Pentecost and Ross, 'The First Thousand Days: Motherhood, Scientific Knowledge and Local Histories'; Pentecost, 'The First Thousand Days: Epigenetics in the Age of Global Health'.
32 Meloni, 'Epigenetics for the Social Sciences'; Lock, 'Comprehending the Body in the Era of the Epigenome'.
33 Adjaye-Gbewonyo and Vaughan, 'Reframing NCDs?'; Herrick, 'NCDs: Names, Sums and Parts'; Allen and Feigl, 'What's in a Name?'; Rigby, 'Renaming Noncommunicable Disease'; Vaughan, 'Conceptualising Metabolic Disorder in Southern Africa'; Reubi, Herrick, and Brown, 'The Politics of Noncommunicable Disease in the Global South'.
34 Weisz, *Chronic Disease in the Twentieth Century*; Weisz and Vignola-Gagne, 'The World Health Organization and the Globalization of Chronic Noncommunicable Disease'.
35 Murray and Lopez, 'The Global Burden of Disease'.
36 Adams, 'Metrics of the Global Sovereign'; Arneson and Nord, 'The Value of DALY Life'.
37 Kannel et al., 'Factors of Risk in the Development of Coronary Heart Disease'.
38 Vaughan, 'Conceptualising Metabolic Disorder'; Glasgow and Schrecker, 'The Double Burden of Neoliberalism?'; Stuckler and Siegel, *Sick Societies*.
39 Saxena et al., 'Countdown Global Mental Health 2030'; Stein et al., 'Integrating Mental Health with Other Non-Communicable Diseases'.
40 Mercer, *Infections, Chronic Disease, and the Epidemiological Transition*; Blundell and Hine, 'Non-Communicable Diseases'; Moran-Thomas in this volume.
41 Mika, 'Fifty Years of Creativity, Crisis, and Cancer in Uganda'; see also below.
42 Omran, 'The Epidemiologic Transition: A Theory of the Epidemiology of Population Change'; Szreter, 'The Idea of Demographic Transition and the Study of Fertility Change'.
43 ICF, 'The DHS Program: Who We Are'.
44 Corsi et al., 'Demographic and Health Surveys'; Fisher and Way, 'The Demographic and Health Surveys Program'; Kendall, 'The World Fertility Survey'.
45 Khan and Hancioglu, 'Multiple Indicator Cluster Surveys'.
46 Alam et al., 'Health and Demographic Surveillance System (HDSS) in Matlab, Bangladesh'.
47 Ng et al., 'Using the INDEPTH HDSS to Build Capacity'; Akuze et al., 'Do Different HDSS Surveillance Systems Result in Different Quality of Pregnancy Outcome Data?'.
48 Crampin et al., 'Profile: The Karonga Health and Demographic Surveillance System'; Malawi Epidemiology and Intervention Research Unit, 'Non-Communicable Diseases'.
49 Samuel, 'Tensions of Colonial Demography'.
50 Streatfield et al., 'Cause-Specific Mortality in Africa and Asia'; Streatfield et al., 'Adult Non-Communicable Disease Mortality in Africa and Asia'; Sankoh and Byass, 'Cause-Specific Mortality at INDEPTH Health and Demographic Surveillance System Sites in Africa and Asia'; Fottrell and Byass, 'Verbal Autopsy'.
51 Alberts et al., 'Health & Demographic Surveillance System Profile'; Kahn et al., 'Profile: Agincourt Health and Socio-Demographic Surveillance System'.
52 National Department of Health, Statistics South Africa, South African Medical Research Council and ICF, *South Africa Demographic and Health Survey 2016*; Ghana Statistical Service, Ghana Health Service, and ICF International, *Ghana Demographic and Health Survey 2014*.
53 Ng et al., 'Using the INDEPTH HDSS'.
54 Holmes et al., 'Non-Communicable Diseases in Sub-Saharan Africa'.
55 Chapman and Berggren, 'Radical Contextualisation'. Our thanks to Michelle Pentecost for this reference.

56 Whyte, 'Chronicity and Control'; Whyte, 'Knowing Hypertension and Diabetes'; Whyte, 'Timeliness and Chronic Medication'.

57 Warin, Kowai, and Meloni, 'Indigenous Knowledge in a Postgenomic Landscape'.

Bibliography

Adams, Vincanne. 'Metrics of the Global Sovereign: Numbers and Stories in Global Health'. In *Metrics: What Counts in Global Health*, edited by Vincanne Adams. Durham, NC: Duke University Press, 2016: 19–57.

Adjaye-Gbewonyo, Kafui and Megan Vaughan. 'Reframing NCDs? An Analysis of Current Debates', *Global Health Action*, 12 (2019), doi: 10.1080/16549716.2019.1641043.

Agyei-Mensah, Samuel and Ama de-Graft Aikins. 'Epidemiological Transition and the Double Burden of Disease in Accra', *Journal of Urban Health*, 87 (2010): 879–97.

Akuze, Joseph et al. on behalf of the INDEPTH Network–ENAP metrics study team. 'Do Different HDSS Surveillance Systems Result in Different Quality of Pregnancy Outcome Data?'. In *The 28th International Population Conference of the International Union for the Scientific Study of Population (IUSSP)*. Cape Town, 2017.

Alam, Nurul et al. 'Health and Demographic Surveillance System (HDSS) in Matlab, Bangladesh', *International Journal of Epidemiology*, 46 (2017): 809–16.

Alberts, Marianne et al. 'Health & Demographic Surveillance System Profile: The Dikgale Health and Demographic Surveillance System', *International Journal of Epidemiology*, 44 (2015): 1565–71.

Allen, Luke and Andrea Feigl. 'What's in a Name? A Call to Reframe Noncommunicable Diseases', *Lancet Global Health*, 5 (2) (2017): e129–30.

American Historical Review Roundtable, 'Historians and the Question of "Modernity"', *American Historical Review*, 116 (2011): 631–751.

Arneson, Trude and Erik Nord. 'The Value of DALY Life: Problems with Ethics and Validity of Disability Adjusted Life Years', *BMJ*, 319 (7222) (1999): 1423–5.

Barker, David. 'The Origins of Developmental Origins Theory', *Journal of Internal Medicine*, 261 (2007): 412–17.

Blundell, Harriet J. and Paul Hine. 'Non-Communicable Diseases: Ditch the Label and Recapture Public Awareness', *International Health* (2018): 5–6, doi:10.1093/inthealth/ihy063.

Chapman, Rachel R. and Jean R. Berggren. 'Radical Contextualisation: Contributions to an Anthropology of Racial/Ethnic Disparities', *Health: An Interdisciplinary Journal for the Social Study of Health, Illness and Medicine*, 9 (2005): 145–67.

Coghe, Samuel. 'Tensions of Colonial Demography: Depopulation Anxieties and Population Statistics in Interwar Angola', *Contemporanea*, 18 (3) (2015): 472–8.

Cooper, Frederick. *Colonialism in Question: Theory, Knowledge, History*. Berkeley, CA: University of California Press, 2005.

Corsi, Daniel J. et al. 'Demographic and Health Surveys: A Profile', *International Journal of Epidemiology*, 41 (2012): 1602–13.

Crampin, Amelia C. et al. 'Profile: The Karonga Health and Demographic Surveillance System', *International Journal of Epidemiology*, 41 (2012): 676–85.

Defo, Barthelemy K. 'Demographic, Epidemiological and Health Transitions: Are They Relevant to Population Health Patterns in Africa?', *Global Health Action*, 7 (2014), doi:10.3402/gha.v7.2243.

Engelman, Lukas and Janina Kehr. 'Double Trouble? Towards an Epistemology of Co-Infection', *Medical Anthropology Theory*, 2 (2015): 1–13.

Farmer, Paul. *Infections and Inequalities: The Modern Plagues*. Berkeley, CA: University of California Press, 1999.

Farmer, Paul. *Pathologies of Power: Health, Human Rights and the New War on the Poor*. Berkeley, CA: University of California Press, 2003.

Fisher, Andrew A. and Ann A. Way. 'The Demographic and Health Surveys Program: An Overview', *International Family Planning Perspectives*, 14 (1988): 15.

Fottrell, Edward and Peter Byass. 'Verbal Autopsy: Methods in Transition', *Epidemiologic Reviews*, 32 (2010): 38–55.

Frenk, Julio et al. 'Elements for a Theory of the Health Transition', *Health Transition Review*, 1 (1991): 21–38.

Frenk, Julio and Octavio Gomez-Dantes. 'The Triple Burden: Disease in Developing Nations', *Harvard International Review*, 33 (2011): 36.

Ghana Statistical Service (GSS), Ghana Health Service (GHS) and ICF International. *Ghana Demographic and Health Survey, 2014*. Rockville, MD: GSS, GHS and ICF International, 2015.

Glasgow, Sara and Ted Schrecker. 'The Double Burden of Neoliberalism? Noncommunicable Disease Policies and the Global Political Economy of Risk', *Health and Place*, 34 (2015): 279–86.

Herrick, Clare. 'NCDs: Names, Sums and Parts', *Medical Anthropology Today*, 6 (2019), doi/org/10.17157/mat.6.1.689.

Holmes, Michelle D. et al. 'Non-Communicable Diseases in Sub-Saharan Africa: The Case for Cohort Studies', *PLoS Med*, 7 (2010): e1000244.

ICF. 'The DHS Program: Who We Are', U.S. Agency for International Development, https://www.dhsprogram.com/Who-We-Are/About-Us.cfm.

Kannel, William et al. 'Factors of Risk in the Development of Coronary Heart Disease – Six-Year Follow-up Experience: The Framingham Study.' *Annals of Internal Medicine*, 55(1) (1961): 33–50.

Kendall, Maurice. 'The World Fertility Survey: Current Status and Findings', *Population Reports*, 7 (4) (1979): M-73–M-104.

Kahn, Kathleen et al. 'Profile: Agincourt Health and Socio-demographic Surveillance System', *International Journal of Epidemiology*, 41 (2012): 988–1001.

Khan, Shane and Attila Hancioglu. 'Multiple Indicator Cluster Surveys: Delivering Robust Data on Children and Women across the Globe', *Studies in Family Planning*, 50 (2019): 279–86.

Krieger, Nancy (ed.). *Embodying Inequality: Epidemiologic Perspectives*. Abingdon: Routledge, 2011.

Lancet Commission on Global Syndemic of Obesity, Undernutrition and Climate Change, *Lancet Commissions*, 393 (2019): 791–846.

Lock, Margaret. 'Comprehending the Body in the Era of the Epigenome', *Current Anthropology*, 56 (2015): 151–77.

Lock, Margaret and Vinh-Kim Nguyen. *An Anthropology of Biomedicine*. Chichester: Wiley-Blackwell, 2010.

Malawi Epidemiology and Intervention Research Unit. 'Non-Communicable Diseases', London School of Hygiene and Tropical Medicine, https://meiru.lshtm.ac.uk/non-communicable-diseases.

Manderson, Leonore and Carolyn Smith-Morris (eds.). *Chronic Conditions, Fluid States: Chronicity and the Anthropology of Illness*. New Brunswick, NJ: Rutgers University Press, 2010.

Marmot, Michael. *The Health Gap: the Challenge of an Unequal World*. London: Bloomsbury, 2016.

Meloni, Maurizio. 'Epigenetics for the Social Sciences: Justice, Embodiment and Inheritance in the Postgenomic Age', *New Genetics and Society*, 34 (2015): 121–51.

Mendenhall, Emily et al. 'Non-Communicable Disease Syndemics: Poverty, Depression and Diabetes in Low Income Populations', *Lancet*, 389 (2017): 951–62.

Mendenhall, Emily et al. 'Stress, Diabetes and Infection: Syndemic Suffering at an Urban Kenyan Hospital', *Social Science and Medicine*, 146 (2015): 11–20.

Mendenhall, Emily and Shane A. Norris. 'When HIV is Ordinary and Diabetes New: Remaking Suffering in a South African Township', *Global Public Health*, 10 (2015): 449–62.

Mercer, Alex. *Infections, Chronic Disease, and the Epidemiological Transition: A New Perspective*. Rochester, NY: University of Rochester Press, 2014.

Mika, Marissa. 'Fifty Years of Creativity, Crisis, and Cancer in Uganda', *Canadian Journal of African Studies / Revue canadienne des études africaines*, 50 (2017): 395–413.

Mooney, Graham. 'Historical Demography and Epidemiology: The Meta-Narrative Challenge'. In *The Oxford Handbook of the History of Medicine*, edited by Mark Jackson. Oxford: Oxford University Press, 2012.

Murray, Christopher J. L. and Alan D. Lopez. *The Global Burden of Disease: A Comprehensive Assessment of Mortality And Disability from Diseases, Injuries, and Risk Factors in 1990 and Projected to 2020: Summary*. Boston, MA: World Health Organization, Harvard School of Public Health, 1996.

National Department of Health (NDoH), Statistics South Africa (Stats SA), South African Medical Research Council (SAMRC) and ICF. *South Africa Demographic and Health Survey, 2016*. Pretoria and Rockville, MD: NDoH, Stats SA, SAMRC and ICF, 2019.

National Research Council. *The Continuing Epidemiological Transition in Sub-Saharan Africa: A Workshop Summary*. Washington, DC: National Academies Press, 2012, doi.org/10.17226/13533.

Ng, Nawi et al. 'Using the INDEPTH HDSS to Build Capacity for Chronic Non-Communicable Disease Risk Factor Surveillance in Low And Middle-Income Countries', *Global Health Action*, 2 (1) (2009): 1984.

Nichter, Mark. 'Co-Morbidity: Reconsidering the Unit of Analysis', *Medical Anthropology Quarterly*, 30 (2016): 536–44.

Nyirenda, Moffat. 'NCDs in Sub-Saharan Africa: Understanding the Drivers of the Epidemic to Inform Intervention Strategies', *Journal of International Health*, 8 (2016): 157–8.

Ogoina, Dimie and Geoffrey C. Onyemelukwe. 'The Role of Infections in the Emergence of Noncommunicable Diseases (NCDs): Compelling Needs for Novel Strategies in the Developing World', *Journal of International Health*, 2 (2009): 14–29.

Omran, Abdel R. 'The Epidemiologic Transition: A Theory of the Epidemiology of Population Change', *Milbank Memorial Fund Quarterly*, 49 (1971): 509–38.

Omran, Abdel R. 'The Epidemiologic Transition Theory: A Preliminary Update', *Journal of Tropical Paediatrics*, 29 (1983): 305–16.

Omran, Abdul R. 'The Epidemiologic Transition Theory Revisited Thirty Years Later', *World Health Statistics Quarterly*, 51 (1998): 99–119.

Omran, Abdul R. 'The Epidemiologic Transition: A Theory of the Epidemiology of Population Change', *Milbank Quarterly*, 83 (2005): 731–57.

Oni, Tollulah and Nigel Unwin. 'Why the Communicable/Non-Communicable Disease Dichotomy is Problematic for Public Health Control Strategies: Implications of Multimorbidity for Health Systems in the Context of Health Transition', *International Health*, 7 (2015): 390–9.

Onyango, Edward M. and Benjamin M. Onyango. 'The Rise of NCDs in Kenya: An Examination of Time Trends and the Contribution of Changes in Diet and Physical Inactivity', *Journal of Epidemiology and Global Health*, 8 (2018): 1.

Pentecost, Michelle. 'The First Thousand Days: Epigenetics in the Age of Global Health'. In *The Palgrave Handbook of Biology and Society,* edited by Maurizio Meloni, 269–94. London: Palgrave Macmillan, 2018.

Pentecost, Michelle and Fiona Ross. 'The First Thousand Days: Motherhood, Scientific Knowledge and Local Histories', *Medical Anthropology* (2019): 1–14.

Reubi, David, Clare Herrick, and Tim Brown. 'The Politics of Noncommunicable Disease in the Global South', *Health and Place*, 39 (2016): 179–87.

Rigby, Michael. 'Renaming Noncommunicable Disease', *Lancet Global Health*, 5(7) (2017): e653.

Sankoh, Osman and Peter Byass. 'Cause-Specific Mortality at INDEPTH Health and Demographic Surveillance System Sites in Africa and Asia: Concluding Synthesis', *Global Health Action*, 7 (2014): 25590.

Sanuade, Olutobi. 'Understanding the Cultural Meanings of Stroke in the Ghanaian Setting: A Qualitative Study Exploring the Perspective of Local Community Residents', *Wellcome Open Research* (2018), doi.org/10.12688/wellcomeopenres.14674.2.

Saxena, Shekhar et al. 'Countdown Global Mental Health 2030', *Lancet*, 393 (2019): 858–9.

Singer, Merrill. *Introduction to Syndemics: A Critical Systems Approach to Public and Community Health*. San Francisco, CA: John Wiley and Sons, 2009.

Singer, Merill et al. 'Syndemics and the Biosocial Conception of Health', *Lancet*, 389 (2017): 941.

Stein, Dan J. et al. 'Integrating Mental Health with Other Non-Communicable Diseases', *BMJ*, 364 (2019): L295.

Streatfield, P. Kim et al. 'Cause-Specific Mortality in Africa and Asia: Evidence from INDEPTH Health and Demographic Surveillance System Sites', *Global Health Action*, 7 (2014): 25362.

Streatfield, P. Kim et al. 'Adult Non-Communicable Disease Mortality in Africa and Asia: Evidence from INDEPTH Health and Demographic Surveillance System sites', *Global Health Action*, 7 (2014): 25365.

Stuckler, David and Karen Siegel. *Sick Societies: Responding to the Global Challenge of Chronic Disease*. Oxford and New York: Oxford University Press, 2011.

Szreter, Simon. 'The Idea of Demographic Transition and the Study of Fertility Change: A Critical Intellectual History', *Population and Development Review*, 19 (1993): 659.

Vaughan, Megan, *Curing Their Ills: Colonial Power and African Illness*. Stanford, CA: Stanford University Press, 1991.

Vaughan, Megan. 'Conceptualising Metabolic Disorder in Southern Africa: Biology, History and Global Health', *BioSocieties*, 14 (2018): 123–42.

Walusansa, Victoria, Fred Okuku, and Jackson Orem. 'Burkitt Lymphoma in Uganda, the Legacy of Denis Burkitt and an Update on the Disease Status', *British Journal of Haematology*, 156 (2012): 757–60.

Warin, Megan, Emma Kowai, and Maurizio Meloni. 'Indigenous Knowledge in a Postgenomic Landscape: The Politics of Epigenetic Hope and Reparation in Australia', *Science, Technology and Human Values* (2019), doi.org/10.1177/0162243919831077.

Weisz, George. *Chronic Disease in the Twentieth Century: A History*. Baltimore, MD: Johns Hopkins University Press, 2014.

Weisz, George and Jesse Olszynko-Gryn. 'The Theory of Epidemiologic Transition: The Origins of a Citation Classic', *Journal of the History of Medicine and Allied Sciences*, 65 (2010): 287–326.

Weisz, George and Etienne Vignola-Gagne. 'The World Health Organization and the Globalization of Chronic Noncommunicable Disease', *Population Development Review*, 41 (2015): 507–32.

Whyte, Susan R. 'Chronicity and Control: Framing 'Noncommunicable Diseases' in Africa', *Anthropology and Medicine*, 19 (2012): 63–74.

Whyte, Susan R. 'Timeliness and Chronic Medication: Knowledge about Hypertension and Diabetes in Uganda', Working Paper No.7, *GFR: Adaptation and Creativity in Africa: Significations in the Making of Order and Disorder*. Leipzig and Halle, 2014.

Whyte, Susan R. 'Knowing Hypertension and Diabetes: Conditions of Treatability in Uganda', *Health Place*, 39 (2016): 219–25.

Part 1

1

Epidemiologic Transition Model: From Britain to Africa

Simon Szreter

Introduction

This chapter offers a revisionist appraisal of the classic 1971 version of the epidemiologic transition model, which was much cited throughout the 1980s and 1990s when the World Bank was imposing structural adjustment plans and conditional loans on many countries in Africa and across the world. This was a general historical model that relied principally on evidence about British history for its empirical plausibility. Despite its wide currency and subsequent influence, it was not a model historians of Britain have ever signed up to. This chapter points out that, in fact, demographic historians' reconstruction of England's epidemiological history is greatly at variance with the transition model. The policy options which British history indicate as being most important for Africa today are extremely different from those suggested by the still-influential notion of history as a process of epidemiologic transition. Instead the chapter demonstrates the importance of politics and ideology and whether or not states adopt universalist principles of welfare and health provision.

The epidemiologic transition model

Abdel R. Omran's 1971 theory of 'epidemiologic transition' was an evolutionary model of epidemiological change, which complemented the postwar liberal social science orthodoxies of demographic transition and modernisation theory.[1] Like them, it envisaged economic growth as the prime mover in history, which enabled human society to move on from a long-existing 'Age of Pestilence and Famine' when mortality was high and wildly fluctuating, striking fear and uncertainty into all. The modern economic growth of the industrial revolution appeared as a knight in shining armour, which enabled populations, starting with Britain's, at last to transit into a second epidemiological phase, an 'Age of Receding Pandemics' – when epidemic peaks became less frequent and the overall burden of infectious disease mortality declined. Finally, a third era of epidemiological modernity was reached, 'the Age of Degenerative and Man-Made Diseases', when mortality stabilised, the threat of death became a more predictable function of ageing, and its incidence was at a relatively low level, allowing the biblical aspiration of three-score and ten years to become the expected norm for everybody's duration of life.

Omran started from the premise (his 'Proposition One'), bequeathed to him by the orthodoxy of demographic transition theory, that mortality was clearly the most important factor driving population dynamics throughout most of history: 'No secular downward trend in mortality is apparent before the middle of the eighteenth century, about the time that population growth began to demonstrate an exponential curve.'[2] He distinguished three major successive stages of the epidemiologic transition:

i) The Age of Pestilence [that is, epidemics] and Famine when mortality is high and fluctuating.
ii) The Age of Receding Pandemics when mortality declines progressively and the rate of decline accelerates as epidemic peaks become less frequent or disappear.
iii) The Age of Degenerative and Man-Made Diseases when mortality continues to decline and eventually approaches stability at a relatively low level.

This model of three successive stages was designed to illustrate 'Proposition Two', which has generally been seen as the key original aspect of his theory:

> During the transition a long-term shift occurs in mortality and disease patterns whereby the pandemics and infections are gradually displaced by degenerative and man-made diseases as the chief form of morbidity and primary cause of death.[3]

Omran accompanied his presentation with a graphical depiction (his Figure 2, p.515) of available data on the course of population growth, birth and death rates in England and Wales from 1700 to 1970.

On this empirical basis he envisaged that in Britain:

i) The Age of Pestilence and Famine had come to an end between about 1650 and 1790, probably from about 1750 onwards.
ii) The Age of Receding Pandemics encompassed the whole period from about 1750 to 1920.
iii) The Age of Degenerative and Man-Made Diseases finally emerged in the course of the twentieth century after the Great War.

Although Omran also presented data for Sweden, England and Wales was the principal national example that Omran discussed in detail to illustrate the nature of this 'Classical or Western Model' of epidemiologic transition, featuring a long drawn-out stage ii). This was because only England and Wales had an extensive historical series of cause of death data, recently analysed by Thomas McKeown, which Omran could draw on for his epidemiological exposition. He was clear that, in England and Wales during the many decades between 1750 and 1920, there had been a 'gradual shift in disease patterns' encompassing 'steady decline of infectious diseases (including tuberculosis and diarrhoea)'.[4]

Omran recognised that some other countries, like Japan, which had industrialised a century after Britain, had experienced an 'Accelerated Transition Model', while yet others, such as Chile or Ceylon (now Sri Lanka), were experiencing a 'Contemporary or Delayed Model'.[5] In his subsequent publications, Omran added a fourth and even a possible fifth stage to his transition model, while other authors have also suggested a further range of types of possible epidemiological transitions focusing on the differences and novel developments that have been emerging in the later twentieth and twenty-first centuries.[6] But in this chapter, I want to focus solely on the more historical aspects of Omran's original Epidemiologic Transition (ET) theory; in particular the posited shift from the first to the second stage in the model. I will reassess Omran's certainty that the Age of Pestilence and Famine had come to an end in Britain between 1650 and 1790, and also that the whole period 1750–1920 can be accurately characterised as one of gradually receding pandemics and epidemics, featuring steady decline in a range of communicable diseases like tuberculosis and diarrhoea. I will propose that these summary descriptions are close to the opposite of the truth regarding Britain's epidemiological history during these three centuries.

By paying careful attention to the true and rather more extraordinary chronology of the British population's relationship with famines, pandemics and epidemics in the centuries from 1600 until 1920, we can approach an understanding of the causation involved that is far more informative than ET theory. It is also an understanding which relates much more closely to the experience of many less developed countries, such as African populations during the last one hundred years or so. During this time they, too, have been progressively and ever more intensely exposed to the forces of expansionary capitalism and the long-distance movement of goods and microbes, just as the British population was over those three centuries.

Both Omran's chronology for Britain and his theory of causation were derivative from orthodox demographic transition and modernisation theory, and more specifically from Thomas McKeown's pioneering epidemiological research on British mortality in the eighteenth and nineteenth centuries. Omran ascribed the reduction of mortality in Britain in stage ii) from about 1750 to 1920 as being due to, firstly, 'ecobiologic determinants' and, secondly, 'socioeconomic factors'. By contrast, he thought medicine had played little role: 'the influence of medical factors was largely inadvertent until the twentieth century.'[7]

Precisely what Omran meant by 'ecobiologic factors' was actually surprisingly vague. He gave just one example. This was the disappearance of plague, which never reappeared in western Europe after the final Marseilles outbreak of 1720–1. However, he offered no reason for this, apart from speculating that 'the mysterious disappearance of the black rat… 'may have been a contributing factor'.[8] He went on to define his second category of causation, 'socioeconomic, political and cultural determinants' as, firstly, improved 'standards of living' and, secondly, 'hygiene and nutrition', which, he spelled out, 'are included here, rather than under medical determinants because their improvement in western countries was a by-product of social change rather than a result of medical design'. Thirdly, he also was sure that 'medical and public health determinants', which 'include improved public sanitation, immunization and development of decisive therapies' only 'came into play late in the western transition' (but, he conceded, 'have an influence' in accelerated and contemporary transitions).[9] This ranking of the importance of these three factors in the British historical case – rising living standards first, medical and public health contributions last – directly repeats Thomas McKeown's conclusions first published in his innovative research article of 1962,[10] and then disseminated in his widely influential 1976 best-seller, *The Modern Rise of Population*.

McKeown's emphasis, in his interpretation of Britain's historical epidemiology, on a direct transmission mechanism between economic growth, rising living standards and declining mortality, while minimising the role of public health medicine or politics, was an historical model which suited down to the ground those who wished during the 1980s to promote the then-new, neoliberal 'development' policies for less developed countries. This occurred even though McKeown, a Professor of Social Medicine, was not himself an advocate of a narrowly economic approach to the world's contemporary health problems.[11] These neoliberal policies focused primarily on opening those economies to free trade, assuming that health improvements would then follow automatically on the economic growth that was supposed to be thereby generated. The utility of epidemiologic transition theory to the neoliberal programme, which was vigorously promoted by the World Bank from 1982 onwards (see below), is reflected in Weisz and Olszynko-Gryn's bibliometric finding that, while Omran's 1971 theory remained on the sidelines for a whole decade in the 1970s, it was specifically during the 1980s and 1990s that his theory of epidemiologic transition experienced a citations explosion among health and development policy professionals and epidemiological researchers.[12]

There is much that is never explicitly discussed in Omran's 1971 theory of epidemiologic transition: government policies, ideas and ideologies, politics and culture.[13] Nor, indeed, is economic growth and urbanisation explored. It is simply invoked as a benign influence, via supposedly automatically generated 'rising standards of living'. There is nothing here about the causal role in this of worker protest, labour organisations, collective bargaining and the long, complex history of trade-union struggles for initial recognition and then for improved pay and conditions.[14] There is no acknowledgement of the possibility that economic growth might be a source not only of economic, but also of epidemiological, destruction as well as 'creation' (to adapt Schumpeter's celebrated description of the processes of growth and the functions of entrepreneurs in a market economy as those of creative destruction).

In the rest of this chapter I will review Britain's longer-term epidemiological history c.1600–1914, focusing on those aspects which are key features of Omran's enunciated transition theory of 1971. I will use this review to argue that the British historical record indicates almost the opposite set of patterns to those which Omran's model propounds, concerning the historical relationship between economic growth and both epidemics and famines in British history.

In fact, the principal historical research studies of British epidemiological and demographic history from the sixteenth through to the nineteenth centuries, published since 1971, hardly refer to Omran or the epidemiologic transition theory at all.[15] The main exception is an important recent volume which is radically critical of the theory of epidemiologic transition on the grounds that its fundamental distinction between infectious and chronic diseases is no longer valid or helpful, consequent on recent immunological research on the diverse sequelae of inflammatory reactions.[16]

However, there has certainly been continuing critical engagement with Omran's transition theory more broadly among epidemiological, public health, anthropological and other social science scholars.[17] Indeed, a recent volume dedicated to *Revisiting the Second Epidemiologic Transition* contains an impressive range of methodologically diverse contributions from leading scholars.[18] The reference in the subtitle of this recent volume to the 'second epidemiologic transition' derives from an important revisionist article arguing that Omran's epidemiologic transition needs to be relocated within an historical or 'evolutionary' framing of much longer duration, which would envisage it as the second of three epidemiologic transitions.[19] The first related to the Neolithic era's innovation of settled agriculture and denser populations 10,000 years ago, and the third to 'emerging and re-emerging' infectious disease from the late twentieth century onwards.[20] However, this expanded timescale for epidemiologic transition theory does not appear to address Omran's transition from his stage i) to his stage ii) as a distinct subject of research at all. Instead, the second transition of the book's title appears to be conceptualised as a single phase, comprising transition from Omran's stage i) through his stage ii) to arrive at his stage iii). As a result of this concatenation of the first two of Omran's original stages (and the transition between them), the recent volume does not mention either plague or famines. Instead, it concentrates mainly on decline in a range of other infectious, parasitic, malnutrition, sanitary, environmental and hygiene diseases, dated approximately from 1850 to 1970 (depending on which country's population is studied), and the rise, in their place, of chronic, degenerative, psychological and, lately, allergenic diseases (according to the recently proposed 'hygiene hypothesis').[21]

Yet famine mortality is a subject which it is impossible to avoid if we are giving serious, critical attention both to the most significant epidemiological factors that threatened all settled human societies after the Neolithic revolution, and also to Omran's theory of epidemiologic transition as a whole and the validity of its historico-theoretic framing. Famine also, sadly, continues to be a central feature of the epidemiology of war-torn Africa and the Middle East to the present day. As is well known, most of the deaths that occur during and after famines are not due to starvation but to a wide range of infectious, hygiene, sanitation and malnutrition diseases, often occurring in epidemic fashion. The abandonment of interest in examining the relationship between the first and second of Omran's transitions in this latest approach to epidemiologic transition incurs a significant analytic loss. There is much to be learned, at least from Britain's relatively well-documented history, in contextualising study from the mid-nineteenth century onwards within a perspective that fully comprehends the several hundred preceding years. Peter Kitson's chapter in this recent volume provided a valuable, precise historical demographic study of Sedgley, an industrialising community in England, across the whole period 1580–1837. As such it was the only chapter which did interrogate the period embracing Omran's stages i) and ii) in England's history. Kitson concluded that, 'The evidence presented here makes the notion of a straightforward transition in the epidemiologic environment during the eighteenth and nineteenth centuries problematic.'[22]

It will be argued here that an understanding of the complex long-term relationship between economic growth and both famine-related and epidemic mortality in British history – embracing and distinguishing between Orman's stages i) and ii) and once cleared of the uni-directional myths of transition theory – can provide illuminating, historically based insights into some of the principal causes of the recent, distressing trends in African mortality during the last half-century.

Plague: the greatest epidemic of all and its disappearance from Britain and Europe

Let us begin with plague, since that is the one concrete example of a stage i) epidemic disease which Omran chose to discuss. The plague of Justinian in 451–2 CE left documentary evidence attesting to the terrifying power of this particular epidemic disease. As is well known, as recently as 1347– 9, bubonic plague, in the form of the Black Death, probably wiped out a third or more of Europe's population and this included a third of Britain's population. Next to this, most other pandemics in recorded history, including the virulent influenza of 1919–20, which killed many more people worldwide than the First World

War, have had relatively limited capacity to disrupt whole societies and cause their economies to falter. Only HIV/AIDS has proven to have similar, terrible powers in some communities of today's poorest countries in sub-Saharan Africa although, as we go to press, the COVID-19 pandemic of 2020 is also inflicting an extraordinary degree of economic disruption on the highly interconnected global free-trade economy of the twenty-first century.

How then does the history of the decline of plague in Britain and western Europe measure up to the epidemiologic transition theory's original emphasis by Omran on non-medical, non-governmental, ecobiological changes and general rising living standards?

In fact, bubonic plague never reappeared as an epidemic in the British Isles after the final London outbreak of 1665–6 (which finished in the heroically self-immured community of Eyam, Derbyshire in October 1666, where it had killed 259 out of 350 people over a 13-month period). However, it remained an affliction in eastern Europe and especially within the Ottoman Empire for the next two centuries. Furthermore, the salient fact that there was even one small and contained outbreak in Suffolk coastal villages as late as 1906–18 indicates that plague didn't just disappear from the Eurasian landmass. There was something actively keeping plague out of Britain during the centuries after 1665–6.[23] The key to Britain's successful avoidance of plague lay, in fact, in the hands of other national governments.

We now have a good deal of detailed research, which has documented exactly how and why Britain after 1666, and indeed the whole of western Europe after the 1720s, became free from this most dreaded of scourges.[24] It is a very different story from that of Omran's vague invocation of ecobiologic or socioeconomic factors. It is primarily a story of political and administrative mobilisation and intervention by sovereign states on a massive scale to create *cordons sanitaires* to prevent the geographical movement of those who might be infected. Plague visitations came to western Europe from the east, where it was almost an endemic affliction. It arrived on merchant boats and wagons carrying rats and their fleas alongside the traded goods. Britain benefited primarily from the quarantining, surveillance and detention systems to monitor – and, if necessary, stop – this traffic, which were set up by organised national governments in central and southern Europe, notably by the Spanish, the French and the Habsburg Austro-Hungarians. Quarantine measures, and the isolation in lazarettos of those suspected of infection, had a long history in the Italian city states, dating from the Black Death. However, the scale of the state interventions organised during the late seventeenth and eighteenth centuries was something quite new.

To contain the final outbreak of plague in Marseilles in 1720–1, large parts of France were effectively fenced off for months at a time.[25] Walls up to 60 miles long were rapidly built at great expense by the French government, which mobilised one-third of its cavalry and one-third of its infantry to man thousands of guard posts to prevent movement from infected areas. Furthermore, on Europe's eastern border between 1728 and 1780, through the *Pestpatente* decrees, the Habsburgs turned the whole of their land border with the Ottoman Empire (1,900 kilometres) into a gigantic permanent cordon sanitaire, the *Militärgrenze*. Permanently manned by 4,000 soldiers, this force was doubled as soon as there was any intelligence of plague appearing in any part of the Ottoman Empire to the east and tripled if plague was known to be present in the territories neighbouring the *Militärgrenze*.[26] This first-ever 'iron curtain' between west and east in Europe was thus built to protect against disease and it was effectively maintained for over a century until 1873, by which time the Turks themselves had finally – and vigorously – adopted anti-plague regulations and successfully eliminated the disease from the Ottoman territories. Although the exact etiology and science of plague was not known and the microbe itself, *Pasteurella pestis*, was not identified until 1894 by Alexandre Yersin, who named it after his great teacher, Louis Pasteur, the strategy worked well. It simply maintained a strict physical separation between those possibly infected and those presumed still healthy. Although they didn't have the science to know how it worked, it did so because plague has quite a long and therefore vulnerable chain of infection. (Infection with plague micro-organisms occurs when the carrier – a flea – bites a human host to get blood. However the flea first has to acquire the bacteria from an infected rat before the rat itself dies; and the flea has to transfer itself from the rat to a sufficiently nearby human host before the flea dies of cold, having lost its rat host.)

Thus, in relation to the most significant epidemic disease of all time, the plague, its impact ceased long before the general rise in living standards associated with modern economic growth. Neither were vague ecobiologic factors involved but, rather, quite specific, well-documented, determined political and administrative interventions. Primarily this action was taken by sovereign states other than Britain – to protect the health of their own populations: Britain's freedom from plague after 1666 was a beneficial by-product.

The early disappearance of famine in pre-industrial England

What of famine and its supposed gradual disappearance in Britain before 1790?

The periodic occurrence of food shortages, typically due to climatic fluctuations, was of course a fact of life for medieval and early modern European populations. Both sovereigns and local communities had evolved a range of laws and practices to attempt to insure against the worst consequences of harvest failure. Such failure could result in the price of grain doubling or more, causing difficulty for the poor and the possible outbreak of social disorder. However, given the relatively poor state of communications between many regions and the possibility of repeated harvest failure in more than one year, these provisions were far from foolproof. Consequently, as a distinguished tradition of historiography has demonstrated through correlating evidence on food prices with burial records from parish registers, national populations throughout Europe were continuing to experience lethal subsistence crises from the sixteenth century until the late eighteenth century.[27] However, it has also been shown that England (though not Scotland or Ireland) had – more or less uniquely in Europe – become free from famine-related national subsistence crisis mortality after the first quarter of the seventeenth century. The last definite famine crisis mortality to affect English communities was that of 1623–4, which mainly impacted the more remote upland zones of the Pennines and Cumbria. Even the high prices caused by the triple harvest failure of 1647–50 and the 'hungry nineties' of 1697–9 produced no significant impact on the Cambridge Group's national sample of parish death rates, quite unlike France, for instance.[28] Although individual parishes still suffered occasionally, there was no general crisis relationship between food shortages and mortality in England after the 1620s, as there continued to be in the rest of Europe well into the next century.

To explain this remarkable difference between England and the continent, it is not adequate simply to focus on narrowly economic factors, such as the relative productivity and efficiency of English agriculture, or improvements in transport and communications. England was, if anything, behind parts of Europe in this respect in the mid-seventeenth century, notably the agriculturally and commercially advanced Holland during its Golden Age. As Amartya Sen has argued, lack of entitlements among certain sections of the population is the key problem in times of dearth.[29] When harvests fail, the subsistence poor have little return from their plots and must sell whatever assets they have to buy food. Even those with modest wage or commercial incomes may find them inadequate when faced with higher food prices.

Bearing this in mind, while the existence of an increasingly efficient agricultural economy and transport system were no doubt necessary preconditions, the key to the English population's early emancipation from famine mortality most probably lies in certain crucial legislative actions taken by the powerful Elizabethan state to transform the entitlement of all subjects. A national social security system, unique in Europe at that time, was created by the newly Protestant state and overseen by the resilient and reliable institutions of local civil society, notably the magistracy or JPs, which the state relied on to implement its policies locally.

In order specifically to address crises due to harvest failure, the so-called Book of Orders was codified in 1586–7 so as to ensure sufficient stocks of grain were maintained, to which the poor were to be given priority access and financial assistance if necessary.[30] However, this was only the emergency relief version of a much more important and more all-encompassing, genuine social security system, created by two statutes 'For the Relief of the Poor' in 1598 and 1601 at the end of Elizabeth I's reign. By these acts, every one of the 10,000 or more parishes in England and Wales was mandated to create a parish fund, financed by a local tax on property, in order to support the local poor – orphans, widows, the old and disabled and the unemployed. The crucial practical question of defining who counted as the local poor, with a legitimate claim on the funds of any parish, was managed through a subsequent series of so-called Settlement Acts from 1662 through to 1795. The whole system was policed and adjudicated by the local magistrates sitting in their local courts of petty session – they held their office at the pleasure of the Crown, not the local taxpayers.[31] The economic historian Peter Solar, in an important article in 1995, emphasised how unique this English social security system was.[32] Solar was particularly impressed that the English state was sufficiently powerful and its JPs sufficiently conscientious that the system functioned fully even in the countryside, as all primary historical research has confirmed.[33] On the continent Poor Laws, or their equivalents, only existed in cities and towns. Consequently, in times of harvest failure, the bedraggled rural poor often sought refuge in the towns, creating crowding problems and frequently bringing disease with them. In England there was no need for the hungry poor to leave their rural parishes when harvests failed, hence the absence of a correlation in

England between high grain prices and famine mortality – most of the latter was due to epidemic disease.[34]

The resurgence of epidemics in nineteenth-century England

In addition to general concerns to preserve social order during times of threat, it was the justifying ideology and *raison d'état* of mercantilist economic doctrine that lay behind both the French and Austro-Hungarian states' vigorous actions to protect their populations from the spread of plague.[35] Mercantilism was the dominant theory of economics and statecraft in western Europe from the seventeenth to the eighteenth centuries, first formalised in the writings of various seventeenth-century Englishmen.[36] It held that there was a relatively fixed amount of wealth in the world and that sovereign states were in direct competition with each other for their share of it. Population was seen as a form of national wealth to be protected and, if possible, increased.

Firstly, this was because mercantilist theory held that the principal peaceful way to enhance national wealth was through a positive balance of trade with other nations, always exporting more manufactures than were imported, resulting in an inward flow of gold from other countries to pay for the surplus of exports. Larger populations were seen as providing a larger labour supply capable of producing more manufactures (the cost of food – all assumed to be domestically produced – was entirely discounted and hence the extra consumption costs of a larger population did not feature in mercantilist analysis). These policies meant that Europe's mostly absolutist sovereigns were quite accustomed to a regime of protectionist trade measures trying to restrict imports through high tariffs while also attempting to protect and encourage the output of their own nation's industries. Quarantine measures to halt, if necessary, all movement across borders, like the *Militärgrenze*, were a logical extension of this policy. Secondly, another method for increasing national wealth was conquest of the territory and populations of competitors. A larger population meant a more powerful army both for defence and for expansionist competition for the available markets, which increasingly included overseas and imperial competition, as well as wars in Europe. Thus the dictum of Frederick II (Frederick the Great) of Prussia that 'the number of the people makes the wealth of states.' This fundamental political principle of 'wealth in people' has not been uncommon in history and is not at all alien to students of indigenous pre-colonial African political history.[37]

However, this overarching ideology of mercantilism came under fundamental reassessment and challenge during the last quarter of the eighteenth century with the rise of the liberal free-trade and free-market theories of the followers of Adam Smith, including of course Thomas Malthus. Smith's *Wealth of Nations* was published in 1776, decrying tariffs and protections and extolling the economic benefits for all of free trade, with each nation exporting only what it could genuinely produce more efficiently and competitively than others. In 1798 Malthus's *Essay on Population* undermined the naively pro-populationist assumptions of mercantilism. By the 1830s and 40s, as Hilton, Mandler and others have shown, the new laissez-faire ideology of political economy had become a powerful new political orthodoxy, especially in Britain.[38] Given a moral inflection by evangelical divines, such as Thomas Chalmers, the ideology had become acceptable among influential sections of the Anglican church and the ruling landed and commercial elite. This new ideology had direct implications for precisely those kinds of government policies which we have identified as having been so important for minimising famine mortality in England for the previous two centuries and also in preventing even that most deadly of epidemics, plague, from spreading across Europe. The classical political economy of Smith, Malthus and Ricardo was against any barriers to free trade (such barriers being a direct consequence of the quarantine method of disease prevention) and it was also against the Poor Law. This law was seen by Smith as an impediment to the free movement of labour in the economy, by Malthus as an inducement to overpopulation and by others as encouraging a dependency culture or 'pauperism' as the Victorians called it.

The primary method to prevent epidemics, which had worked so well in defeating plague, was the absolute interdiction of mobility of persons between territories by national governments. This strategy was at loggerheads with the new principles of free trade and individual liberty championed by Smith and his successors. The restrictions on trade represented by this heavy-handed deployment of state power, all having to be paid for out of taxes on the private individuals whose economic activity was being so restricted, were an anathema to the new, liberal political economy. An alternative theory of disease causation, implying very different practical methods of prevention, was therefore most welcome to those concerned to preserve and expand free trade above all else. This alternative was the theory of miasma or filth as the principal cause of lethal diseases, including epidemics. As a theory which was turned into official government policy it is intimately associated with the name of Edwin Chadwick, the most formidable *éminence grise* in British government during the two crucial decades of the 1830s and 40s, a man who has been justifiably called 'a civil servant genius', more powerful and influential than most of the politicians of the time.[39]

The miasma theory argued that epidemics of diseases occurred because individuals ingested through their pores, their noses and their mouths the rotting effluvia of decaying organic matter, which effectively poisoned them – a different kind of poison for each of the different recognised diseases. People fell victim to diseases in clusters and at the same time. This was not because they were infected by other individuals – the opposed contagionist theory (which has subsequently been vindicated but which remained unprovable before microscopy permitted the science of bacteriology to develop from the 1860s) – but because they were all co-victims of the same insanitary environment. The Chadwickian solution to early Victorian Britain's health problems, therefore, was primarily to clean up the environment and remove miasmas, so as to avoid outbreaks of epidemics, with the added extra precaution of mandatory hospitalisation in special fever hospitals for those individuals who were actually sick and suffering from the disease when an outbreak occurred (because their exhalations were deemed to be miasmatic and poisonous). The attraction of this approach for laissez-faire economics was that there was no proposal for quarantines and general restrictions on trade or the mobility of non-sick persons from places which were trading partners, even if disease was rife there and even where epidemics might be currently raging.[40] From the late 1860s the English port sanitary authorities had powers to inspect boats before arrival, to place infected individuals in fever hospitals and to require disinfection of ships and even destruction of merchandise, but there was no absolute interdiction on trade and movement under 'the English system'.[41]

It was Chadwick's ideas which informed the nation's first Public Health Act of 1848 and he was appointed to head the new General Board of Health. The implementation of Chadwick's great 'Sanitary Idea' was not, however, a cheap one. It ideally required all towns and cities to invest in both a clean water supply to all streets and homes and a corresponding mains-sewered network to remove continually all insanitary household wastes. Unpopular because of the enormous expenses that his scheme implied for local ratepayers, Chadwick himself fell from his high perch in 1853, just five years after his landmark Public Health Act, and was never to work in government again. The Royal Commission on Sanitation of

1869–71 found over 20 years later that no cities, apart from London, had yet created an integrated sewering system. Furthermore, none, including London, had achieved domiciliary water supply to all inhabitants, something that was to take many further decades of tightening building regulations and inspections to achieve.[42]

The nation's trading activities and economic prosperity may have been promoted by the retreat from a strict quarantining approach to the prevention of epidemic disease. However, the endorsement by government of the miasmatic approach, combined with the failure of either central or local government to follow through on the full costs of the expensive sanitarian strategy for disease prevention, had the consequence that in health terms the mid-nineteenth century in Britain became a period in which epidemics almost became an endemic experience. One could say that endemics struck repeatedly in epidemic form. Britain's rapidly expanding industrial cities were full of rural migrants, made redundant by both enclosure and the mechanisation of different branches of industry, and their infants and young children. These were dislocated persons searching for work in an alien and new environment where they had to crowd into the cheapest rooms available, such as the notorious dormitories of common lodging-houses, whose notoriety earned them the first regulatory attention from the state through the Shaftesbury Acts from 1851 onwards.[43] Meanwhile, hard-pressed families regularly doubled up in multiple family occupation of a single room to economise on rent;[44] a common situation today in Africa as I have seen for myself in Khayelitsha, an informal township on the Cape Flats near Cape Town. Under-regulated capitalism exerted then, as now, very similar pressures on the living spaces and on the basic hygiene facilities of the urban poor, a pressure that is conducive to the spread of all forms of communicable diseases.[45] The poor Irish in Liverpool, Manchester or the other mill towns like Preston were at the bottom of the pile. Many of the poor were virtually refugees at the mercy of rack-renting landlords and employers seeking the cheapest possible labour.[46] It was the personal observation of the desperate living conditions and opportunities of the wage-earning poor in cities such as Manchester, where his father owned a cotton mill, which radicalised the young German, Friedrich Engels, Marx's later patron and key collaborator, recorded in his *The Condition of the Working Class in England* in 1844.

An important part of the reason for the desperate condition of so many of the wage-earning families, which Engels observed, was that the Poor Law no longer provided the kind of wide-ranging social security and welfare provision, extending even to domestic care for the aged and health care for the ill, which the English populace had come to enjoy during the previous two centuries.[47] The belief in the divinely ordered and also rational virtues of the principle of free trade and free markets included the price of labour. Allied to Malthus's strictures on the dangers of overpopulation, which he argued was inherent in the out-dated and misguided mercantilist system of the Poor Laws, this led to calls for its abolition. In 1834 the Poor Law was not abolished but it was radically overhauled to render it a deterrent system.[48] The workhouse test was supposed to end cash handouts to people in their homes and to ensure that the poor would rather work for any wage offered by the free market, no matter how low, than seek public assistance. If truly desperate, they would now have to endure institutionalisation, under strictly regulated and sex-segregated conditions, performing tedious chores in return for being kept alive in the workhouse. The proportion of GDP spending on the Poor Laws was savagely cut from 2 per cent to 1 per cent in just a few years after 1834.

In this context these decades also saw much social unrest, such as anti-Poor-Law and anti-policing protests and of course Chartism, the campaign for manhood suffrage. Thus, during the 1830s and 40s in particular, with the social security system having been semi-dismantled and open political antagonism between middle and working classes, Britain's urban population was subject to absolutely devastating mortality rates. As symbolised by the rebellion of the urban ratepayers against Chadwick's 1848 Public Health Act, public administration in Britain's new cities was apathetic and self-serving. It was no longer necessarily prepared to fund through local taxes the measures for preservation of the local populace's health offered to them by the Westminster government. Life expectancy in most industrial cities and towns, from Liverpool, Manchester and Glasgow to much smaller places like Carlisle, Wigan and West Bromwich, fell, in places, to below 30 years, in both these decades.[49]

Epidemic waves included attacks of Asiatic cholera, never seen before in Britain, in 1830–1 and again in 1847–9, 1853–4 and 1866; also of typhoid and typhus, measles, scarlet fever, diphtheria and whooping cough. These epidemics were occurring in the context of relentless, massively high rates of diarrhoea and dysentery – particularly fatal to infants – and all the respiratory diseases of 'flu, bronchitis, pneumonia and, of course, that 'Captain of all the Men of Death', pulmonary tuberculosis. After these two devastating decades, water supply in most of these cities did at least improve somewhat after the 1848

Public Health Act, while there was also a long period of relatively full employment and rising real wages from 1850 to 1873, the so-called mid-Victorian boom. During the 1850s and 60s, death rates in the industrial towns abated from the ferocious levels seen in the 1830s and 40s, although the expectation of life in all these cities was in fact no higher by 1870 than it had been in the 1820s.[50] Even though the British national economy had experienced the most extraordinary accumulation of wealth ever seen in human history across that half-century, the average health of the country's urban working class was no better in 1870 than it had been in the 1820s. It was only in the subsequent four decades after 1870, down to 1914, that the devastation of the lives of urban workers and their families began to be redressed. This was not simply due to higher wages but to an entirely new ideology and administrative practice taking hold, first in Birmingham and Glasgow and then in the other major provincial cities, as they pioneered municipal loans to buy up local monopoly services of gas, water and transport, in order to generate revenues to fund urban preventive health services.[51] Infant mortality and diarrhoea rates did not fall steadily as Omran supposed they had, but remained stubbornly high until 1900 when they, too, finally succumbed to the intensive municipal sanitary and hygiene efforts being directed at the poorest neighbourhoods and homes.[52]

Thus, quite contrary to the epidemiologic transition model, British history in both the eighteenth and nineteenth centuries indicates that a decline in the most important pandemic – plague – actually preceded (and perhaps partly facilitated) the world's first ever episode of economic development. Rather than being a consequence of ecobiologic change or socioeconomic improvement, the defeat of plague was due to an aggressive political ideology, mercantilism, which nevertheless had the domestically benign consequence that sovereign powers saw themselves as having stewardship over the health and size of their populations and were therefore motivated to deploy very considerable resources to protect these populations from such evident threats. Paradoxically, however, the process of modernising economic change itself – and its accompanying new ideology of laissez-faire and changed government priorities and policies – initially resulted in a massive resurgence of epidemics, not their gradual decline and petering out. Examination of the reasons for this – and for its eventual reversal after 1870 – clearly indicates the importance of ideology, politics, government policy and state–society relationships, rather than 'ecobiologic' or general socioeconomic forces.

The return of famine to the United Kingdom: The Great Irish Famine, 1845–9

We now return to the subject of famine in modern British history.[53] Here, there is a close – and, indeed, related – parallel to that of the history of epidemics. Again, the chronology claimed by epidemiologic transition theory is the reverse of the truth. England had been the first country in Europe to achieve freedom from famine mortality from as early as the second quarter of the seventeenth century, as we have seen. Yet, well over 200 years later, when the United Kingdom was the most advanced, powerful and prosperous country in the world, with a global empire at its command, it experienced one of the most awful and prolonged episodes of mass starvation in modern history.

The great Irish famine of 1845–9 occurred during the middle of a 120-year period when the whole of Ireland was an integral part of the United Kingdom, with its elected representative government in Westminster, London.[54] The Irish famine's originating cause was the mysterious *Phytophthora infestans* fungus, which reached Ireland's potato crop in August 1845 (the antidote of copper sulphate solution was only finally devised in 1882). There was a 50 per cent crop loss in 1845. 1846 saw almost 100 per cent failure. In 1847 there were high yields per acre but a greatly reduced acreage. 1848 was a final hammer blow when once again there was almost 100 per cent crop failure.

How bad was the Irish famine? At one million dead, its toll was smaller than many other major famines in the nineteenth century, such as several of those in China and India. But the Irish famine actually exceeded any of these as a proportionate death rate of Ireland's population total (8.2 million at the 1841 census). Furthermore, unlike India or China, the Irish population continued to decline after the famine for another half-century and also failed to increase afterwards. Even in 2011, 170 years later, the population of Ireland and Northern Ireland combined was still only 6.4 million, way below its 1841 total.[55]

Why didn't the wealthiest society and the strongest imperial state in the world, the London government in Westminster, act effectively to prevent the loss of life that occurred in one of its own provinces? There is a complex context that needs to be taken into account and there is also a complex narrative of how events unfolded from 1845 through to 1849. There was the long-standing problem that relations between Protestant landlords and Catholic tenants were lacking in mutual trust and there was no effective law of contractual relations. This resulted in tenant insecurity and no right of compensation for improvements, with landholders reciprocally complaining of tenant negligence and their lack of proprietorship rights. Such non-improving behaviour (in fact rational in the circumstances) was interpreted through religiously and racially biased lenses as an intransigent backwardness in the Catholic Irish peasant, which could only be cured by something akin to economic 'shock-therapy' (the term applied to the policies embarked on in post-Communist eastern Europe after 1989). On top of this, Ireland's backwardness was considered to leave her vulnerable to overpopulation and famines. There had been famine crises in 1740–1 and 1744–5 and a narrowly averted one in 1799–1801.

Malthus could not blame the Poor Law as the cause of overpopulation in Ireland as there was not a Poor Law in Ireland in his lifetime (he died in 1834). His diagnosis of Ireland's problems was that the fragmented system of land occupancy had allowed the poor to multiply to dangerous levels, while sustaining them with a diet of cheap potatoes, the wonder food imported originally from South America. Therefore, the solution was consolidation of holdings and conversion of all small, subsistence cottiers into wage-labourers as had happened in England with the Enclosure movement. This would impose a deterrent on 'improvident' marriages. Denied his traditional subsistence potato plot, the Irish labourer would have new incentives to search for more productive work, enabling the expansion of manufacturing in Ireland.

Quite opposed to Malthus, and associated orthodox economists like Nassau Senior, other contemporaries like George Cornewall Lewis and Poulett Scrope argued in the early nineteenth century that only a Poor Law could stop the vicious circle of underemployment and undercapitalisation in the Irish countryside, due to chronic insecurity created by (Protestant) landlord exploitative rack-renting. The imposition of a Poor Law relief system, supported by rates levied on the landlords, would provide an indolent Protestant landowning class with reasons to invest and to improve the productivity of the land and so enable their tenants – the Irish poor – to become more economically productive.[56] In 1838 an Irish Poor Law Act was duly passed but not the Poor Law which Lewis and Scrope envisaged. It was modelled on England's radically reformed New Poor Law of 1834 with its detested workhouses, 130 of which were duly built in Ireland by 1845.[57] The New Poor Law of less eligibility and the deterrent workhouse test was, thus, the new social security system for Ireland, which had just been put in place by the British state when the famine struck.

The British government response to the Irish potato failures occurred in two distinct phases. The initial emergency policy was to set up in March 1846 a Board of Public Works. By March 1847 a peak of 750,000 were employed on such schemes.[58] However, the Public Works policy was fatally flawed because of its 'less eligibility principles' of deliberately paying no more than a normal minimum wage because such relief schemes should not discourage any workers from returning to the free market in labour, even though such a labour market patently did not exist. In times of abnormally high prices, what was on offer was literally a starvation wage to an Irish worker's family in return for his day's work; hence crimes against property trebled.[59]

In early 1847 this first phase response concluded when the government, acknowledging that its public works policy was not working in the way it wanted, switched to a second strategy of providing soup kitchens. This is generally considered to have been the most practically successful anti-famine intervention. This switch was largely due to the English state's fetishisation of the eradication of abuses. Administrators were concerned that the public works approach was a charter for proliferating moral corruption, with government money being dispensed all over Ireland for so-called schemes, which either didn't exist or mainly benefited intermediaries. The fight against moral corruption had a higher priority than saving lives for this ideology, though it did inadvertently have the result of saving lives when it shifted from public works policies to direct feeding by soup kitchens. This resulted in the effective delivery of relief entitlements to those in most need. It is estimated that the soup kitchens were dispensing 3 million meals daily at their peak in July 1847.

But there was then another fateful change in government policy, with the passing in June 1847 of the Irish Poor Law Extension Act. This marked the second phase in government response and it placed the main burden of relief back on the Irish Poor Law and Ireland's landlords.[60] It amounted to a declaration by Westminster that the famine and the emergency measures to combat it were over, apparently discounting entirely the possibility that there might be another catastrophic potato failure, as there was in the following year, 1848. The new policy to place all responsibility back in Ireland was accompanied by a Bill to extend the Irish 1838 Poor Law to create a separate Irish Poor Law Commission, with the power (unlike in England) to allow outdoor relief (beyond the workhouse) to the able-bodied.[61] This had strong support from British domestic public opinion, resentful of Irish landowners transferring their deserved burdens for 'their' poor onto British taxpayers (in fact mainly onto the citizens of Liverpool, whose municipal institutions bore the brunt of the costs of coping with the mass flight of the starving Irish poor across the Irish Sea to Britain). The 1847 Bill was seen as re-moralising Irish landowners, 'a class without social humanity, without legal obligation, without natural shame', according to *The Times*.[62]

The determined opposition of the Irish landlords and their representatives in Parliament, however, produced the surprise Lords amendment, the infamous Gregory Clause (proposed by William Gregory): that small tenants owning more than a quarter acre and all their dependants should be excluded from outdoor relief. Gregory claimed it was these smallholders of a few acres who were the most usual fraudsters, getting relief even though they were not bankrupt. They should be excluded from relief unless they gave up their land, which it was claimed they did not cultivate at all efficiently anyway. The amendment was accepted in face of critics like Poulett Scrope, who warned it would presage a complete clearance of small farmers in Ireland. In fact this was one of the chief objects of the large Irish landholders, because they believed the repeated failure of the potato showed that the small cottier population had no future. Irish agriculture should turn in future to large-scale beef and dairy production and the surplus cottiers be encouraged to emigrate to avoid them becoming a permanent burden on Irish landlords, the Poor Law rate-payers.[63]

When the blight returned to destroy the 1848 harvest the Irish Poor Law simply couldn't cope with the size of the burden now placed on it. Consequently, by July 1849, all Irish workhouses were full to bursting, containing 200,000 persons. In addition there were another 800,000 persons on outdoor relief, despite the hated Gregory Clauses, which meant that many of these were composed of families whose parents had given up their small family plots, rather than starve to death – as the policy intended.[64] The result, as predicted by the opponents of Gregory's Clause, was that 200,000 smallholdings disappeared during the famine.[65]

It was quite clearly within the technical capacity of the British state to have avoided the disaster in 1840s Ireland. Had the UK state maintained the exchange entitlements of the starving poor directly by continuing the soup kitchens and reexpanding them in 1848 when the crop failed again, that would have prevented most of the excess deaths of 1848–9. The fact that the soup system appeared to work (with relatively low mortality during summer 1847) by delivering 3 million meals per day is important in demonstrating that the bureaucratic apparatus of the British state in Ireland was sufficiently effective to have stopped famine mortality.[66] Given the political will and (quite modest) funding, there was no problem of technical capacity. Overall the English Treasury spent £8m on famine relief in 1845–50, half in un-repaid loans and the other half on soup kitchens and public works. This represents about

0.3 per cent of UK GNP or 2–3 per cent of public expenditure at that time. Through Poor Rates, the Irish themselves paid £7m and landlords borrowed £1m.[67] To put this expenditure in context, the English state had recently spent £20m in compensation to owners of freed slaves and was about to spend £60m in the 1850s to fight the Crimean War.

The potato blight returned in less severe form several times between 1850 and 1900, usually in the far west of Ireland (in 1860–2, in particular, it caused serious damage to the value of farmers' output). But never again was it permitted by the Westminster government to cause excess mortality because it always thereafter elicited unstinting poor relief from the UK state (for example, 1879–84 £2.6m spent, with workhouse inmates up from 1.1m 1874–8 to 1.7m 1879–83). This reflected the fact that Westminster had learned that the workhouse test should never again be applied in times of crisis and, in February 1880, the infamous Gregory Clause was dropped when the government agreed to authorise relief for all the destitute. Also public works paying realistic wages became the norm and was used in 1890–2, 1897–8 and 1904–5.[68] Hence Peter Gray's summing up:

> the inescapable conclusion remains that the state failed to make optimum use of its resources to contain the number of deaths, especially in later stages of the Famine from the autumn of 1847.[69]

Partly this was due to resistance from local elites and others, but primarily:

> This policy failure was due in large part to the success of the dominant faction in the government prioritizing another ideologically-driven agenda – that of grasping the heaven-sent 'opportunity' of famine to deconstruct Irish society and rebuild it anew. Liberal moralists were prepared to play a deadly game of brinkmanship in their campaign to impose a capitalist cultural revolution on the Irish.[70]

This:

> was the fruit of a powerful social [Evangelical] ideology that combined a providentialist theodicy of 'natural laws' with a radicalized and 'optimistic' version of liberal political economy. According to this theology, God and nature had combined to force Ireland from diseased backwardness into healthy modernity; any

> unnecessary suffering incurred in the transition was the result of human folly and obstruction, and could not be attributed to the will of God or to those who understood his purposes and acted accordingly.[71]

The mass destruction of lives of Irish peasants living within the United Kingdom during the 1840s was the first modern mass famine in the sense that Stephen Devereux and others have so designated the famines seen during the second half of the twentieth century in Africa.[72] These are famines occurring in a situation where it is absolutely certain that there exist both sufficient supplies of food and the transport and administrative infrastructure to deliver it; such that famine need not occur. Yet famine mortality occurs because of ideologies (which in Africa have frequently been expressed in open political conflicts, both inter- and intra-state), which cast those afflicted with severe food shortages as 'others', whose institutionalised socioeconomic regimes supposedly require ideological reconstruction. Their 'conversion' to accept a new cultural or economic regime is seen as a higher priority than keeping the human inhabitants of that 'other' regime alive. Though never again in Ireland, the British imperial ruling elite continued to preside over such modern famines after 1849.[73] In British India the sub-continent's agriculture was re-oriented towards exports for imperial needs which in some regions, Berar for instance, again resulted in the dangers seen in Ireland of widespread mono-cropping – in this case cotton, not potatoes. A poor law for the backward peasantry of India was deemed an unconscionably expensive and misguided policy, which would only discourage the work ethic. So, when the crop failed across a region, deaths ensued in a population whose meagre wages disappeared with the lack of cotton to harvest. This occurred in Berar in 1877 and again in 1899, when fully 8.5 per cent of the populace perished in the subsequent famine of 1900.[74]

Development ideologies and policies in Africa since c.1940: economic growth and health

The colony-acquiring, 'advanced' nations of the North themselves only became fully democratic polities extremely recently – between 1918 and 1950 in most cases. With the exception of undemocratic Portugal, and in response to the acknowledged nationalist pressure of the African continent's independence movements, these democratising colonial powers did make rather more of an effort to organise, if not fully fund, the rudiments of more widely diffused basic social, economic and health infrastructure in their last decades of colonial rule. These efforts were continued and redoubled by the new governments of national independence emerging in the late 1950s and 1960s, who were encouraged by western governments and the World Bank, under the prevailing international Keynesian growth orthodoxy, to borrow liberally for such productive purposes as building and staffing schools, hospitals, roads and all the other infrastructure necessary for modernising economic transformation.[75]

For Africa the key empirical point about this period, c.1940–75, is that the growth and development 'bottom lines' both show that, in general, the investments and resources being deployed in most of these newly emerging sub-Saharan democracies were delivering strong, if gradual, positive effects. Per capita income was rising, life expectancy was rising, institutional infant and maternal mortality rates were falling, literacy rates and school enrolment rates for both sexes were rising, some universities beyond South Africa – such as Makerere in Kampala and Dar es Salaam in Tanzania – were acquiring regional – and even global – reputations.[76]

As is well known, the 1970s proved to be a decade of dislocation and difficulty for the world's wealthier liberal democracies. Firstly, the Bretton Woods international currency exchange controls system was undermined by financiers in London and New York.[77] Secondly, the Arab-dominated OPEC cartel imposed sudden and steep oil price rises twice during the decade. This precipitated industrial and social turmoil and relatively slow and patchy economic growth in the west, whose economies and democracies struggled to readjust to such changes. The Keynesian economic consensus – which had legitimated the postwar economic model of governments' commitment to full employment, countercyclical demand management and public investment, relatively high taxes and consequent growing civic equality – was de-throned. In its place arose a new policy orthodoxy, termed neoliberalism in acknowledgment of its policy principles that have much in common with the ideology discussed above, the classical economic and political liberalism of laissez-faire Victorian Britain. Neoliberalism lauded the virtues of competition, 'the private sector', free markets, and 'free trade', advocating dramatic reductions in taxes and cuts to 'inefficient' publicly funded services. It accepted, and even justified, rising inequality as simply a by-product of successful competitive individualism, which supposedly carries no serious downsides, provided that some part of the wealth generated by the successful somehow 'trickles down' to everybody else. Extended to the international arena as a new development policy orthodoxy, implemented during the 1980s and 90s both by the IMF and the World Bank and from 1995 the WTO, this has come to be known as 'the Washington consensus'.

The disruptions to world trade in the 1970s also left most African countries with debt problems, which were no longer viewed from within a Keynesian perspective.[78] Consequently they were now instructed by the west, notably through the conditions attaching to the structural adjustment loans made by the IMF and the World Bank, to cut dramatically their commitments to public-financed infrastructure and any aspirations they may have had to universal provision of public services for their citizens, so that 'user-fees' were brought in even for basic health services.[79] The new consensus held that the private sector would rise up and flood in to fill these gaps once the inefficient public sector had been cleared out of their way. Given that this never happened in most countries, the new 'development' policy was, in effect, one of state disinvestment in much-needed infrastructure, such as road maintenance, hospital staffing, teachers and doctors, resulting in deteriorating healthcare, particularly for the most vulnerable.[80] The most grievous and unfair policy myth of all grew up at this time, which was that HIV/AIDS spread so widely and became such a killer in Africa because of 'African culture'. The HIV/AIDS epidemic was so devastating in Africa only in part because of aspects of sexual culture, but mainly for two other reasons. Firstly, because the epidemic had been stealthily spreading unnoticed probably since the early decades of the twentieth century.[81] The disease was only recognised in the 1980s, when HIV/AIDS finally reached the west.[82] Secondly, by the 1980s most African nations were busy dismantling their nascent, publicly funded healthcare systems at the instruction of their creditors in the west. A process of rebuilding such systems has only belatedly begun during the last decade or so since the early 2000s, following the absolutely devastating protracted period of non-development and associated HIV/AIDS deaths in most of sub-Saharan Africa, c.1980–2005.

Of course, individual countries each have their own tale to tell; and in some cases national governments, their internal disputes and various forms of corruption were also part of the story. However, it is difficult to escape the conclusion that it was the imposition of the novel Washington consensus policies that accounted for the general and widespread pattern of reversal of previously positive socioeconomic and epidemiological trends, c.1945–75, during the following three decades across so many different regimes in Africa. This untold collateral human damage occurred all across Africa due to the reversal of support for a range of national public service policies, which had previously been expanding free health and welfare services among the world's poorest populations.[83] The disinvestment coincided with the decline in international support for the WHO, which, as a multilateral organisation with equal voting rights among its members, had enjoyed competitive funding from both sides in the Cold War in pursuing its founding objective to lead international efforts to improve health.[84] Its leading funding role was replaced by the World Bank, also nominally a UN institution but one with a majority of voting rights accorded to its funders and with the nomination of its President in the hands of the White House.[85] As an institution focused primarily not on health, but on promoting economic development, it was only prepared to fund health policies on the basis of arguments that they would promote productivity. The reference point for most of its US-trained economists was the US privatised healthcare system. Hence, 'selective' primary healthcare came to be adopted as the Bank's preferred policy, an approach which was in fact fundamentally subversive of the universalist principles of the 1978 Alma Ata declaration, internationally endorsed by WHO.[86]

When, in 1981, President Reagan began his two terms in the White House, thus marking the arrival of the new, neoliberal economic policy at the apex of government in the US, this was also rapidly translated into the policies pursued by the World Bank. Robert McNamara and Hollis Chenery, as President and Chief Economist, were replaced by Alden Clausen (1981) and Anne Krueger (1982).[87] Krueger cleared out almost 80 per cent of the Development Research Department's economists to replace them with true believers in the Chicago school of free enterprise, tax cuts and free trade.[88] Armed with a new model for economic growth, including the Berg plan for Africa, the Bank's priorities quickly shifted towards structural adjustment conditional loans, aimed at forcing less developed countries to create the 'right environment' – privatised and deregulated – for free enterprise to flourish.[89] The belief was that maximising their trading potential with the rest of the world would grow these less developed economies more effectively than any other policy prescription, despite long-standing evidence to the contrary.[90] Cutting taxes and cutting publicly provided services was all part of opening up these economies for free enterprise: healthcare was to be a commercial opportunity, as it already was in the US, with user-fees.

However, by 1987, with the scale of the impact of HIV/AIDS becoming evident, open criticism of the excessive 'social costs' of the

Bank's policies from another UN organisation, UNICEF, coincided with the departures of Clausen (1986) and Krueger (1987).[91] The Bank rediscovered a need to address poverty and poor health, both now rapidly growing. This move, building on its long-standing policies of selective primary healthcare, culminated in the Bank's highly influential 1993 Word Development Report, *Investing in Health*. Selective primary healthcare had long been the Bank's preferred policy to offer residual coverage so as not to stymie the hoped-for growth of a medical market place. The health policies now proposed in 1993 were simply more of the same: user-fees, privatisation and the increased use of the voluntary sector remained central, with a place for risk-pooling insurance for those who could afford it. With HIV/AIDS ripping through African communities and devastating the capacities of families to support themselves, this was analogous to the Liberal government's 1847 Irish Poor Law Extension Act in response to the needs of the Irish rural poor, ravaged by famine.[92] Just as then in Westminster, there was a continuing belief at the World Bank in Washington in the over-riding need to promote a free-market economic model for the supposed future benefit of the economy. Consequently, there was to be no significant relaxation of the 'laws of the market' to indulge in a universalist provision of social support and healthcare, called for by the Alma Ata Declaration of 1978. This was regardless of the fact that the populace of much of Africa now needed this more than ever.[93]

Throughout the 1990s, however, alongside the promotion of selective primary healthcare and user fees, the World Bank's programme of structural adjustment loans also continued unabated.[94] In terms of health provision for the poor of Africa, structural adjustment was taking away gouges of public funding with one hand, while *Investing In Health* was replacing it with a single finger's worth of aid with the other hand.

Thus, many sub-Saharan African populations in the course of the last 70 years or so, since 1940, have first benefited from, but then suffered from, a similar switchback in the governing class's ideology and its associated policies to that which played out in Britain's past. The long-standing mercantilist and paternalist economic and moral principles adhered to by its leaders, privileging wealth in people, came to be replaced as dominant government policy in Britain between 1830 and 1850 by a strongly evangelical and self-confident brand of individualist, free-market political economy. So, too, the African poor have been subjected to the policy consequences of the reactionary reprise of a similar ideology since the late 1970s.

Africa since c.1940 in the mirror of British history: the unhelpful telescope of epidemiologic transition

Omran noted in 1971 that some countries like Japan experienced an 'accelerated epidemiologic transition' due to 'the availability to these countries of modern, scientific sanitation, vaccine/immunization and antibiotic technologies effective against many infectious diseases'. But this modern medicine was also 'available' to all other countries after the Second World War. Yet most of India's enormous population, for instance, did not seem to benefit much for many decades.[95] On the other hand, the equally massive, poor peasant society of China did benefit, as also did two of federal India's southernmost provinces, Tamil Nadu and Kerala. The reason was that, unlike India in general, these two states, along with Sri Lanka, China and Japan, were governed with ideologies which prioritised and funded free and universal provision of these preventive, public health and sanitary technologies; and they effectively implemented the policies, even among a relatively poor rural populace.[96] This represented the recognition of the practical importance of a policy which applied this principle of universal primary healthcare provision as a 'human right', which was encapsulated in the famous WHO/UNICEF sponsored Alma Ata Declaration of 1978.

Without knowing it, these states and the Alma Ata declaration were following the spirit of England's precociously universalist Old Poor Law, insisting on making life-saving resources available to absolutely everybody in the realm, even women and children in the most remote, rural settlements.[97] The Alma Ata Declaration, if it had been subsequently fully operationalised as a policy, would, in effect, have seen this rolled out to the whole of Africa during the course of the 1980s.[98] That never happened. All the wonderful medical science and health-saving technology, which in theory placed the world in such a different position to save lives and to promote health than had been the case in seventeenth- or eighteenth-century England, remained underused and ineffective for much of the poor of Africa. Neither the World Bank nor many African national governments were prepared to implement the most important lesson of Britain's early modern history. This was the enormous value to its population of the universalist provision principle of its precocious social security, welfare and health system, the Elizabethan Poor Laws. Why this did not happen is the key question and the answer has been summarised in the previous section. This returns us to the causal centrality of politics and ideologies in accounting for most of the epidemiological trends during the centuries addressed by Omran's theory; and the need to locate politics and ideology centrally in our epidemiological imagination.

What, then, are the possible, helpful lessons or analogies from Britain's pre-twentieth-century past, which can inform a more critical understanding of the modern epidemiological history of Africa in the course of the late twentieth and twenty-first centuries? Obviously, there has been much diversity in the experience of different nations and communities across this vast continent, but nevertheless there are some commonalities in the kinds of policies that have been deployed to promote economic growth and to address health and social security concerns.

It has been shown that the epidemiological history of Britain during its protracted centuries of industrialising modernisation is in fact close to the opposite of that described by Omran's 1971 model. Epidemiologic transition theory assumed economic growth could only ever have a beneficial effect on 'living standards'. The long term was deemed identical to the short term. It therefore ignored the importance of politics and ideology in accounting for the *changing* health fortunes of populations during epochs of economic change, often initially suffering disruption, deprivation, disease and death in the historical record and only subsequently converting wealth into health through intrinsically political, negotiated processes.[99] Such a politics-free view suited the neoliberal approach so dominant in the 1980s and 1990s.

But Africa's epidemiologic history since 1945 also shows, like Britain's long-term history, that economic growth, per se, does not necessarily result in a benign epidemiological transition. As long ago as 1991 Julio Frenk et al., in their seminal statement of the theory of health transition, critiqued epidemiological transition theory on the grounds that:

> it seems incorrect to assume that change must always occur smoothly and in one direction. In fact, a reversal of trends may occur. The most outstanding example is the emergence of AIDS, a viral disease. ... small or large 'counter-transitions' may take place.[100]

However, the main generalisable message of the interpretation offered here, regarding long-term British mortality history, is that counter-trends are not simply unfortunate and possible anomalies as economies grow. Their existence is more ubiquitous and they are in fact evidence that the term 'transition' itself is unhelpful and inhibitory for the imagination.

It is misleading in its failure to recognise the intrinsically disruptive nature of economic growth in relation to population health. Economic growth and the accompanying transformation in the relationship between a population and its environment offers no guarantee of a transition from anywhere to anywhere, least of all from a generally higher to a generally lower morbidity and mortality regime. To deploy the notion of transition as a framing device is to avoid addressing directly the question of governing ideologies and politics as the key to whether such economic growth wreaks havoc or not in any specific population.[101] The most outstanding example of the importance of these political forces was not, in fact, Frenk's identification of the postwar policy world's surprise at the outbreak of HIV/AIDS. It was the well-documented much earlier history of the UK's own epidemiological history throughout the period in which it provided the world with the first ever case-study of sustained, modern economic growth and urbanisation, c.1600–1870. The late twentieth-century 'surprise' of AIDS was created by a teleological misreading of British history through the telescopic and monocular vision of linear transition thinking, applied both by Omran and, earlier, by Thomas McKeown as well as, before him, by demographic transition and modernisation theory.

Economic prosperity can be conceptualised as something primarily measured through healthy productive people, as mercantilists like Elizabeth I and Frederick II did, or as ethical, social democrats like Amartya Sen might today. However, maximisation of capitalist profit rates became the new orthodoxy in Britain in the early nineteenth century. Just over a century later this ideology and its policies were temporarily superseded by the need to fight a world war of national survival against fascism and by the Keynesian welfare state consensus of the period 1945–73. However, within a further generation, the capitalist ideology once again returned to dominance with the mantras of maximising growth rates in national per capita GDP and shareholder value.[102] With these measures as the ultimate arbiters, the political and moral ideology which informs the government policies that are supposed to promote or sustain such economic growth can, it seems, be excused for exerting devastating effects on the health and even the mortality of the poorer sections of the world's populations. Such costs borne by the poor are justified by the greater goal of attending instead to the competitive 'health' of the nation's economy.[103] These depredations can even extend to the more vulnerable sections of the world's wealthiest societies, as happened in mid-Victorian Britain with its incarceral workhouses and is clearly again the case in foodbank Britain today.[104] In the contemporary US, too, poor white males have seen an epidemic of suicides on such a scale that working-age life expectancy has seen recent declines,[105] while large proportions of the young black male population are incarcerated.[106]

Life expectancy reversals have happened even more extensively in many countries of sub-Saharan Africa from the 1980s until the 2000s, as the most developed nations and commercial corporations of the world's increasingly global and financialised economies have jointly pursued a set of policies which they believed would best sustain their own national GDP rates and their shareholder value and profits. Africa has also of course witnessed a number of major and minor famines during this period since the 1970s, considerably more so than during the period 1930–70. Given both this and the HIV/AIDS pandemic, it is extremely hard to give credence to the benign linearity of the epidemiologic transition theory as a helpful guide for the epidemiological imagination in thinking about the relationship between economic growth, disease and death in Africa's recent history, any more so than in Britain's history.

It would seem to be much more accurate and helpful to approach economic growth as a fundamentally disruptive force, where the health of populations is concerned. Although economic growth can certainly provide the flow of resources in the longer run, to fund improvements in health, the crucial point is that there is nothing but ideology and politics which can guarantee the equitable distribution of that growth. Furthermore, ideological commitments to unregulated free markets and minimalist public services are quite certainly a political recipe to ensure that such wider distribution of the benefits does not happen. The rising inequality globally, led by the US and UK during the last four decades, demonstrates this.[107] This directs us to examine the reasons for such disruption and the ways in which the social deprivations and diseases caused by these aspects of economic growth are either permitted to run their course, resulting in premature deaths for many, or else are addressed and actively redressed. This in turn leads us to study carefully the nature and relative effectiveness, not simply of medical technology or even of healthcare systems per se, but of government policies and the national – or even international – political economy and accompanying ideologies. These either justify or refute the value of the universal provision of the necessarily expensive and resource-demanding policies required to preserve and promote human welfare and health under conditions of capitalist economic expansion.[108]

In a recent article generally critical of the value of the notion of epidemiologic transition, the leading Cameroonian and African demographer Barthelemy Kuate Defo has concluded:

> Its various criticisms suggest that it is relevant as a way of describing and understanding to some extent the relation among disease and mortality patterns in the course of population change in Western societies until the 1950s, rather than as a universal description or prediction regarding population health patterns enlightening to the formulation of health policies in contemporary societies or in developing countries. The historical and contemporary demography and epidemiology of these countries are quite distinct from historical experiences of the Western societies. Moreover, they are faced with enormous and unprecedented disease burdens in tandem with ill-equipped, poorly funded and often dysfunctional health care systems in social contexts where the family largely remains the sole source of social security and health insurance for the majority of people faced with disease and risks of premature death.[109]

While agreeing with Defo in his reflections on the predicaments of African society and families today, the burden of this chapter is to show that, in fact, once it is realised how misleading the epidemiologic transition model is as a guide to disease and mortality patterns in the past, including notably Britain's past, there may be rather more to learn from that past than is suspected.

Defo's final sentence, describing the predicament many African communities have been facing for the last several decades, closely resembles that which was facing the British labouring poor in the brave new world of the workhouse and urban epidemics, when Queen Victoria ascended the throne in 1837. I concur with Defo and, indeed, with Alexander Mercer, that it is high time to move on from the limits imposed by 'transition thinking'. But I would advise that history can offer much more helpful and richer imaginative resources than the epidemiologic transition model suggests.[110] Rwanda, for instance, presents the example of a society in Africa which has truly revolutionised the health and welfare of its population since the catastrophe of the genocide against the Tutsi. The improvement in maternal mortality rates is absolutely exceptional and is proof that its healthcare policies are reaching the most vulnerable: rural women.[111] It has done so through committing to a universalist system aimed at regional and social equity as part of the nation's unifying healing process. This is ideology and politics and agency in action.[112]

Conclusion: time is history, not transitions

The development policy world of discourse is full of 'transitions'. They come in many shapes and sizes and degrees of complexity, sometimes called models, sometimes called theories. The intellectual work that all 'transitions' do is to deal ahistorically with the problem of time. They are handy translation devices between past, present and future. They enable social scientists and policy practitioners, trained in all the multitude of important biomedical, engineering, planning and socioeconomic disciplines involved in development and public policy work, to appear to acknowledge that they live and work in historical time. However, they do this without having to engage with the complexity of the history, which historians research and write, involving the contingencies of ideological, cultural and political conflict. Defenders of epidemiologic transition may choose to ignore plague, famines and the theory's limitations in summarising pre-twentieth-century history. They will point to the widespread decline in most childhood infectious diseases as evidence that 'an epidemiological transition' has occurred across the world. It has, but this has been brought about not as the automatic application of science through the diffusion of economic growth, but through an intensely politically mediated process, as Mary Brazelton's new study of mass vaccination in the People's Republic of China makes abundantly clear.[113]

The epidemiologic transition takes the history and the agency out of epidemiological change and renders it into a reassuringly easily grasped linear sequence of stages. You can't escape from history but you can radically simplify it, so that you have the illusion of control over it and so that you no longer need to call on professional historians, with all their confusing 'noise' and detail from the past. The cost, however, is that you may no longer be able to learn anything new from the past itself – from history.[114] All its diversity and political and ideological contestation has been turned into mere 'transitions' between stages: Demographic, Health, Epidemiologic. For those concerned with Africa's epidemiology and how we can imagine it today, there is so much more to learn from history, including even British history, than this.

Notes

1 Omran, 'The Epidemiologic Transition: A Theory of the Epidemiology of Population Change'. Many subsequent publications by Omran are cited by those discussing the epidemiologic transition theory, but this was the original, full statement. For the most thorough critical intellectual history of Omran's motives in the genesis of the epidemiologic transition theory, see Weisz and Olszynko-Gryn, 'The Theory of Epidemiologic Transition: The Origins of a Citation Classic'. For a critical intellectual history of demographic transition theory and its relation to modernisation theory, see Hodgson, 'Demography as Social Science and Policy Science'; and Szreter, 'The Idea of Demographic Transition'. On the intellectual history of modernisation theory and its persistent afterlife, see Gilman, *Mandarins of the Future*.
2 Omran, 'The Epidemiologic Transition', 511–13.
3 Omran, 'The Epidemiologic Transition', 516–17.
4 Omran, 'The Epidemiologic Transition', 516. This was Omran's formulation despite the fact that diarrhoea is not generally considered primarily an infectious disease, although it is a communicable disease, often acquired from ingestion of contaminated solids and liquids.
5 Omran, 'The Epidemiologic Transition', 518.
6 Omran, 'The Epidemiologic Transition Theory. A Preliminary Update'; Omran, 'The Epidemiologic Transition Theory Revisited Thirty Years Later'; and see, for instance, Olshansky et al., 'Emerging Infectious Diseases'. For an influential alternative reading of Omran's transition as a series of health system responses to changes in diseases, see Frenk et al., 'Elements for a Theory of the Health Transition'.
7 Omran, 'The Epidemiologic Transition', 520.
8 Omran, 'The Epidemiologic Transition', 520.
9 Omran, 'The Epidemiologic Transition', 520.
10 McKeown and Record, 'Reasons for the Decline of Mortality'.
11 Szreter, 'The Importance of Social Intervention', 33–7, discussed this paradox. On the expansive scope of McKeown's wider corpus of work, see Szreter, 'Thomas McKeown', *Dictionary of Medical Biography*.
12 Weisz and Olszynko-Gryn, 'The Theory of Epidemiologic Transition'.
13 By contrast, in Omran's 1998 restatement he did identify public policy as an issue of importance, but that much less-cited reprise of his theme was not the version which attracted so much attention during the 1980s and 90s and it is still the 1971 formulation which is most frequently cited.
14 For a recent historical survey in relation to Britain, see Reid, *United We Stand*. For the international dimension, see Maul, *The International Labour Organization*.
15 McKeown, *The Modern Rise of Population*; Wrigley and Schofield, *The Population History of England*; Hardy, *The Epidemic Streets*; Wrigley et al., *English Population History*; Woods, *The Demography of Victorian England and Wales*; Harrison, *Disease and the Modern World*; Floud et al., *The Changing Body*.
16 Mercer, *Infections, Chronic Disease, and the Epidemiological Transition*.
17 Much of this critical engagement is well summarised in Fleischer and McKeown, 'The Second Epidemiologic Transition'. There is also to be noted a distinct variant developed by Vallin and Meslé, which they see as compatible with – but more general than – Omran's transition theory. They retain the notion of epidemiological history as progress through 'three major stages': Vallin and Meslé, 'Convergences and Divergences in Mortality', 37–8.
18 Zuckerman (ed.), *Modern Environments and Human Health*.
19 Barrett et al., 'Emerging and Re-emerging Infectious Diseases'.
20 Zuckerman, *Modern Environments*, 1; and Ch.18, Armelagos, 'The Second Epidemiological Transition, Adaptation, and the Evolutionary Paradigm'.
21 Zuckerman and Armelagos, 'The Hygiene Hypothesis and the Second Epidemiologic Transition'.
22 Kitson, 'Industrialization and the Changing Morality Environment', 195.
23 Walter and Schofield, 'Famine, Disease and Crisis', 64.
24 Flinn, *The European Demographic System*, Ch.4; Bourdelais, *Epidemics Laid Low*, Chs.1–2.
25 Bourdelais, *Epidemics Laid Low*.
26 Flinn, *The European Demographic System*, Ch.4.
27 Walter and Schofield, 'Famine, Disease and Crisis'.

28 Galloway, 'Basic Patterns in Annual Variations'. Galloway's findings have since been confirmed: Morgan and Ó Gráda, 'The Poor Law of Old England'; Healey, *The First Century of Welfare*, 218–20, 240–54.
29 Sen, *Poverty and Famines*.
30 Walter and Schofield, 'Famine, Disease and Crisis Mortality', 46.
31 For the best short overview of the genesis of the English Poor Laws, see Slack, *The English Poor Law 1531–1782*; see also Brundage, *The English Poor Laws 1700–1930*.
32 Solar, 'Poor Relief and English Economic Development'.
33 Snell, *Annals of the Labouring Poor*; Slack, *Poverty and Policy in Tudor and Stuart England*; Hindle, *On the Parish?*; Williams, *Poverty, Gender and Life-Cycle*; Healey, *The First Century of Welfare*.
34 Walter and Schofield, 'Famine, Disease and Crisis Mortality', 48–56.
35 See Risse, 'Medicine in the Age of Enlightenment'; also Rosen, 'Cameralism and the Concept of Medical Police'; Rosen, 'Mercantilism and Health Policy'.
36 Brezis, 'Mercantilism'. Thomas Mun (1571–1641) was the oldest of the group, which included Sir Josiah Child, Charles Davenant, John Locke, Sir William Petty and, on the continent, Jean Baptiste Colbert, Louis XIV's finance minister, and the German cameralist Johann Joachim Becher.
37 Guyer and Eno Belinga, 'Wealth in People as Wealth in Knowledge'.
38 Hilton, *The Age of Atonement*; Mandler, *Aristocratic Government in the Age of Reform*.
39 Brundage, *England's Prussian Minister*.
40 Hamlin, *Public Health and Social Justice*.
41 Hardy, 'Cholera, Quarantine and the English Preventive System'; Maglen, *The English System*.
42 Szreter, *Health and Wealth*, 122, 127, 222.
43 Wohl, *The Eternal Slum*, Ch.4.
44 Wohl, *Endangered Lives*, Ch.11.
45 Davis, *Planet of Slums*.
46 Dyos and Reeder, 'Slums and Suburbs'.
47 There have been many studies demonstrating the wide range of such provision; for an excellent recent publication offering a particularly wide-ranging geographic coverage, see King, *Sickness, Medical Welfare and the English Poor*.
48 Brundage, *The Making of the New Poor Law*.
49 Szreter and Mooney, 'Urbanisation, Mortality and the Standard of Living Debate'.
50 Szreter and Mooney, 'Urbanisation, Mortality and the Standard of Living Debate'.
51 Hennock, *Fit and Proper Persons*; Szreter, *Health and Wealth*, Chs.4, 7, 9.
52 Garrett et al. (eds.), *Infant Mortality*; Mooney, *Intrusive Interventions*.
53 The interpretation and information cited throughout this section is principally derived from: Ó Gráda, *Ireland: A New Economic History*, Ch.8; and Gray, *Famine, Land and Politics*.
54 The Act of Union occurred in 1800 and the union of the Irish and British economies was completed in 1826 with internal free trade and monetary integration. This lasted until December 1922 when the Irish Free State came into existence (while the northern Ulster counties, where Protestants predominated, remained within the United Kingdom).
55 Total famine-related excess deaths have been estimated at approximately 1 million. Total emigration to N. America 1845–55 was 1.5 million, which was about double the previous normal annual rate of emigration and represented about one-third of the rising generation. Thus, where the 1841 census had shown an Irish population total at 8.2m, the 1851 total was 6.8m. Ó Gráda, *Ireland: A New Economic History*, Ch.8.
56 Gray, *Famine, Land and Politics*, 14.
57 Ó Gráda, *The Great Irish Famine*, 31.
58 Ó Gráda, *The Great Irish Famine*, 45.
59 Ó Gráda, *Ireland: A New Economic History*, 196, 199–204.
60 This move to place the financial burden back on Irish landlords was also in part influenced by concerns over an acute, short-term finance crisis at the Bank of England (because the value of cotton was down by a quarter in 1847 and bad harvests were producing a run on Bank bullion and a rising interest rate). See Read, 'Laissez-faire, the Irish Famine, and British Financial Crisis', 411–34.
61 Gray, *Famine, Land and Politics*, 276.
62 *The Times* 23 April 1847, cited by Gray *Famine, Land and Politics*, 277.
63 Gray, *Famine, Land and Politics*, 278–9.

64 Ó Gráda, *The Great Irish Famine*, 46.
65 Ó Gráda, *The Great Irish Famine*, 70.
66 Ó Gráda, *Ireland*, 197.
67 Ó Gráda, *The Great Irish Famine*, 56.
68 Ó Gráda, *Ireland: A New Economic History*, 253.
69 Gray, *Famine, Land and Politics*, 331.
70 Gray, *Famine, Land and Politics*, 331.
71 Gray, *Famine, Land and Politics*, 331. Gray argues that English government policy, though couched in the language and terms of political economy, was most strongly influenced by the evangelicalism of a coterie of 'Christian economists', notably Thomas Chalmers and J.B. Sumner. Their primary concern was with religious salvation and the moral nature of economic laws: adapting the moral philosophy of Adam Smith to the ominous world of Malthus. Their primary policy goal was *not* to promote economic prosperity, like Adam Smith, but to facilitate a more static, retributive and purgative world: to remove all restrictions on individuals' moral choices in the economic market place in order to reveal the operation of the natural moral law. This was economic competition as means to moral and spiritual education. Their prescriptions frequently mirrored those of classical economy and the utilitarian Benthamites, such as the immensely powerful Edwin Chadwick, as with the making of the New Poor Law for England and Wales in 1834, because they shared a rigorous 'moral individualism'. The Whig-Liberals were responsible for British government policy from March 1846 onwards, encompassing the passing of the Irish Poor Law Extension Act with its Gregory Clause, and they included prominent providentialist evangelicals, such as Charles Trevelyan, Charles Wood and Sir George Grey.
72 Devereux, *The New Famines*.
73 Davis, *Late Victorian Holocausts*.
74 Beckert, *Empire of Cotton*, 337.
75 Cooper, *Africa Since 1940*, Chs.1–5.
76 Evidence and sources: Cooper, *Africa Since 1940*, Ch.5; World Bank, 'Fertility Rate'; 'World Bank, 'World Development Indicators'.
77 Shaxson, *The Finance Curse*, 52–9.
78 Eichengreen and Lindert (eds.), *The International Debt Crisis*.
79 Easterly, 'IMF and World Bank Structural Adjustment Programs and Poverty'.
80 Thomson, Kentikelenis, and Stubbs, 'Structural Adjustment Programmes'; Forster et al., 'Globalization and Health Equity'.
81 Iliffe, *The African AIDS Epidemic*, Ch.2.
82 A process itself surrounded by profound mythification: see McKay, *Patient Zero*.
83 Packard, *A History of Global Health*, Ch.13 and in particular the case study of Zambia, 262–4.
84 Cueto, Brown, and Fee, *The World Health Organization*, 179–80, 240, 245.
85 I wish to acknowledge that the discussion of the evolution of World Bank health policy in this section is indebted to the account in the unpublished Cambridge M.Phil dissertation by Phoebe Heathcote, 'The World Bank's Health Policy Process, 1970–1993'.
86 Packard, *A History of Global Health*, 254–5.
87 Ayres, *Banking on the Poor*, 7.
88 Toye, 'Solow in the Tropics'.
89 *Accelerated Development in Sub-Saharan Africa: An Agenda for Action* (World Bank 1981). The report's co-ordinator was named as Elliot Berg.
90 The counter-evidence of dependency theory, that free trade primarily benefited the developed world at the direct expense of the less developed, had been presented as a compelling statistical analysis of the trends in relative prices of manufactures and primary products by two UN employees, Singer and Prebisch, in 1950 – see Toye and Toye, 'The Origins and Interpretation of the Prebisch-Singer Thesis'. Furthermore, as Chang has more recently emphasised, it was long known to historians, but apparently overlooked by policymakers, that all twentieth-century developed nations in Europe, North America and the Far East had nurtured their early economic development behind protectionist barriers, not through free-trade policies: Chang, *Kicking Away the Ladder*.
91 UNICEF, *Adjustment with a Human Face*; and for an important further critique, see Mosley, Harrigan, and Toye, *Aid and Power*.

92 As pointed out by de Waal and Whiteside, in African communities HIV/AIDs has itself been the cause of food insecurity and lowered resilience to drought and other famine conditions: de Waal and Whiteside, 'New Variant Famine'.
93 Not until a further ten years of deaths had accumulated did a subsequent Republican US President, G.W. Bush, successfully request Congress to circumvent the free market's principles so that antiretroviral treatment be supplied to the African poor for free: The President's Emergency Plan for Aids Relief (PEPFAR).
94 By 2000 the Bank had, since its first loans to Kenya and Turkey in 1980, made 537 adjustment loans to 109 countries totalling nearly $100 billion: Sharma, 'Bureaucratic Imperatives and Policy Outcomes', 669.
95 Amrith, *Decolonising International Health.*
96 Balabanova, McKee, and Mills, *Good Health at Low Cost 25 Years On.*
97 Szreter, 'The History and Development of Public Health'.
98 On internal political disputes at the Alma-Ata meeting, see Birn, 'Back to Alma-Ata'.
99 Szreter, 'Economic Growth, Disruption, Deprivation, Disease and Death'.
100 Frenk et al., 'Elements for a Theory', 34.
101 Although the latest volume of revisionist studies does offer a number of critiques and modifications of epidemiologic transition theory, it does not touch on the main issues addressed here, regarding the role of ideology and politics: Zuckerman and Armelagos, 'The Second Epidemiologic Transition'.
102 Mazzucato, *The Value of Everything.*
103 On the way in which the financial services sector of the British economy has successfully appropriated the concept of national competitiveness, see Shaxson, *The Finance Curse*, 8–14.
104 Alston, 'Statement on Visit to the United Kingdom'.
105 Case and Deaton, 'Rising Morbidity and Mortality'.
106 Wacquant, 'Class, Race & Hyperincarceration in Revanchist America'.
107 Piketty, *Capital in the Twenty-First Century*; Atkinson, *Inequality. What Can be Done?*; Dorling, *Peak Inequality*; Hickel, *The Divide*; Milanovic, *Global Inequality.*
108 See the recent critical survey, Packard, *A History of Global Health*; and on India, for instance, see Amrith, *Decolonising International Health.*
109 Defo, 'Beyond the "Transition" Frameworks'.
110 For critical new thinking, see in particular, Mercer, 'Updating the Epidemiological Transition Model'; and Mercer, *Infections, Chronic Disease, and the Epidemiological Transition*; and for much relevant general wisdom, see Kunitz, *The Health of Populations.*
111 Alkema et al., 'Global, Regional, and National Levels and Trends in Maternal Mortality'.
112 Binagwaho, 'Twenty Years of Improving Access to Healthcare in Rwanda'; Sayngoza and Bijlmakers, 'Drivers of Improved Health Sector Performance in Rwanda'.
113 Brazelton, *Mass Vaccination.*
114 For examples of such 'lessons from history' relevant to development policy and a general introduction, see Bayly et al. (eds.), *History, Historians and Development Policy.*

Bibliography

Alkema, Leontine et al. 'Global, Regional, and National Levels and Trends in Maternal Mortality Between 1990 and 2015, with Scenario-Based Projections to 2030: A Systematic Analysis by the UN Maternal Mortality Estimation Inter-Agency Group', *Lancet*, 387 (2016): 462–74.

Alston, Philip. 'Statement on Visit to the United Kingdom, by Professor Philip Alston, United Nations Special Rapporteur on Extreme Poverty and Human Rights', Office of the United Nations High Commissioner for Human Rights, Geneva: 16 November 2018, https://www.ohchr.org/Documents/Issues/Poverty/EOM_GB_16Nov2018.pdf.

Amrith, Sunil. *Decolonising International Health. India and Southeast Asia, 1930–65.* London: Palgrave Macmillan (Cambridge Imperial and Post-Colonial Studies Series), 2006.

Armelagos, George J., 'The Second Epidemiological Transition, Adaptation, and the Evolutionary Paradigm'. In *Modern Environments and Human Health: Revisiting the Second Epidemiologic Transition*, edited by Molly Zuckerman, 339–52. Hoboken, NJ: John Wiley, 2014.

Atkinson, Anthony B. *Inequality: What Can Be Done?* Cambridge, MA: Harvard University Press, 2015.

Ayres, Robert L. *Banking on the Poor: The World Bank and World Poverty*. Cambridge, MA: MIT Press, 1983.

Balabanova, Dina, M. McKee, and A. Mills. *Good Health at Low Cost 25 Years On: What Makes a Successful Health System?* London: London College of Hygiene and Tropical Medicine, 2011.

Barrett, R. et al. 'Emerging and Re-Emerging Infectious Diseases: The Third Epidemiologic Transition', *Annual Review of Anthropology*, 27 (1998): 247–71.

Bayly, Christopher A. et al. (eds.). *History, Historians and Development Policy*. Manchester: Manchester University Press, 2011.

Binagwaho, Agnes. 'Twenty Years of Improving Access to Healthcare in Rwanda'. In *African Health Leaders*, edited by F. Omaswa and N.Crisp, 235–47. Oxford: Oxford University Press, 2014.

Beckert, Sven. *Empire of Cotton. A New History of Global Capitalism*. London: Allen Lane, 2014.

Birn, Anne-Emmanuelle. 'Back to Alma-Ata, From 1978 to 2018 and Beyond', *American Journal of Public Health*, 108 (2018): 1153–5, doi.org/10.2105/AJPH.2018.304625.

Brazelton, Mary. *Mass Vaccination. Citizens' Bodies and State Power in Modern China*. London: Cornell University Press, 2019.

Brezis, E. S. 'Mercantilism'. In J. Mokyr (ed.), *The Oxford Encyclopedia of Economic History*. Oxford: Oxford University Press, 2003.

Brundage, Anthony. *The Making of the New Poor Law: The Politics of Inquiry, Enactment and Implementation, 1832–39*. New Brunswick, NJ: Rutgers University Press, 1978.

Brundage, Anthony. *England's Prussian Minister: Edwin Chadwick and the Politics of Government Growth, 1832–54*. University Park, PA: Pennsylvania State University Press, 1988.

Brundage, Anthony. *The English Poor Laws 1700–1930*. London: Palgrave, 2001.

Bourdelais, Patrice. *Epidemics Laid Low*. Baltimore, MD: Johns Hopkins University Press, 2006.

Case, Anne and Angus Deaton. 'Rising Morbidity and Mortality in Midlife among White Non-Hispanic Americans in the 21st Century', *Proceedings of the National Academy of Sciences of the United States of America*, 112 (49) (2015): 15078–83.

Chang, Ha-Joon. *Kicking Away the Ladder – Development Strategy in Historical Perspective*. London: Anthem Press, 2002.

Cooper, Fred. *Africa Since 1940: The Past of the Present*. Cambridge: Cambridge University Press, 2002.

Cueto, Marcos, Theodore M. Brown, and Elizabeth Fee. *The World Health Organization: A History*. Cambridge: Cambridge University Press, 2019, doi.org/10.1017/9781108692878.

Davis, Mike. *Late Victorian Holocausts: El Nino Famines and the Making of the Third World*. London: Verso, 2002.

Davis, Mike. *Planet of Slums*. London: Verso, 2006.

Defo, Barthelemy K. 'Beyond the "Transition" Frameworks: The Cross-Continuum of Health, Disease and Mortality Framework', *Global Health Action*, 7 (2014): 24804. Published online: 5 May 2014, http://dx.doi.org/10.3402/gha.v7.24804.

Devereux, Stephen. *The New Famines: Why Famines Persist in an Era of Globalization*. London: Routledge, 2006.

Dorling, Danny. *Peak Inequality: Britain's Ticking Time Bomb*. Bristol: Policy Press, 2018.

Dyos, H. J. and D. A. Reeder. 'Slums and Suburbs'. In *The Victorian City: Images and Realities*, vol. 1, edited by H. J. Dyos and M. Wolff, 359–86. London: Routledge, 1973.

Easterly, William. 'IMF and World Bank Structural Adjustment Programs and Poverty'. In *Managing Currency Crises in Emerging Markets*, edited by Michael P. Dooley and Jeffrey A. Frankel, Ch.11. Chicago, IL: University of Chicago Press, 2003, doi: 10.7208/chicago/9780226155425.001.0001.

Eichengreen, Barry and Peter H. Lindert. *The International Debt Crisis in Historical Perspective*. Cambridge, MA: MIT Press, 1989.

Fleischer, Nancy L. and Robert McKeown. 'The Second Epidemiologic Transition from an Epidemiologist's Perspective'. Ch.19 in *Modern Environments and Human Health. Revisiting the Second Epidemiologic Transition*, edited by Molly Zuckerman, 353–68. Hoboken, NJ: John Wiley, 2014.

Flinn, Michael. *The European Demographic System, 1500–1820*. Baltimore, MD: Johns Hopkins University Press, 1981.

Floud, Robert et al. *The Changing Body. Health, Nutrition and Human Development in the Western World since 1700*. Cambridge: Cambridge University Press, 2011.

Forster, Timon et al. 'Globalization and Health Equity: The Impact of Structural Adjustment Programs on Developing Countries', *Social Science & Medicine*, 2019, doi: 10.1016/j.socscimed.2019.112496.

Frenk, Julio et al. 'Elements for a Theory of the Health Transition', *Health Transition Review*, 1 (1991): 21–38.

Galloway, Patrick R. 'Basic Patterns in Annual Variations in Fertility, Nuptiality, Mortality, and Prices in Pre-Industrial Europe', *Population Studies*, 42 (1988): 275–303.

Garrett, Eilidh et al. *Infant Mortality: A Continuing Problem*. Aldershot: Ashgate, 2006.

Gilman, Nils. *Mandarins of the Future, Modernization Theory in Cold War America*. Baltimore, MD: Johns Hopkins University Press, 2003.

Ó Gráda, Cormac. *Ireland: A New Economic History 1780–1939*. Oxford: Oxford University Press, 1994.

Ó Gráda, Cormac. *The Great Irish Famine*. Basingstoke: Macmillan, 1989.

Gray, Peter. *Famine, Land and Politics: British Government and Irish Society 1843–50*. Dublin: Irish Academic Press, 1999.

Guyer, Jane and Samuel M. Eno Belinga. 'Wealth in People as Wealth in Knowledge: Accumulation and Composition in Equatorial Africa', *Journal of African History*, 36 (1995): 91–120.

Hamlin, Chris. *Public Health and Social Justice in the Age of Chadwick: Britain, 1800–1854*. Cambridge: Cambridge University Press, 2009.

Hardy, Anne. 'Cholera, Quarantine and the English Preventive System, 1850–1895', *Medical History*, 37 (1993): 250–69.

Hardy, Anne. *The Epidemic Streets. Infectious Disease and the Rise of Preventive Medicine 1856–1900*. Oxford: Oxford University Press, 1993.

Harrison, Mark. *Disease and the Modern World*. Cambridge: Cambridge University Press, 2004.

Healey, Jonathan. *The First Century of Welfare. Poverty and Relief in Lancashire 1620–1730*. Woodbridge: Boydell and Brewer, 2014.

Heathcote, Phoebe. 'The World Bank's Health Policy Process, 1970–1993', MPhil. (unpublished), Cambridge University History Faculty, 2019.

Hennock, E. P. *Fit and Proper Persons: Ideal and Reality in Nineteenth Century Urban Government*. London: Edward Arnold, 1973.

Hickel, Jason. *The Divide: A Brief Guide to Global Inequality and its Solutions*. New York and London: Penguin, 2017.

Hilton, Boyd. *The Age of Atonement*. Oxford: Clarendon Press, 1988.

Hindle, Steve. *On the Parish? The Micro-Politics of Poor Relief in Rural England c.1550–1750*. Oxford: Oxford University Press, 2004.

Hodgson, Dennis. 'Demography as Social Science and Policy Science', *Population Development Review*, 9 (1983): 1–34.

Iliffe, John. *The African AIDS Epidemic: A History*. Athens, OH: Ohio University Press, 2006.

King, Steven. *Sickness, Medical Welfare and the English Poor 1750–1834*. Manchester: Manchester University Press, 2018.

Kitson, Peter. 'Industrialization and the Changing Morality Environment in an English Community during the Industrial Revolution'. In *Modern Environments and Human Health. Revisiting the Second Epidemiologic Transition*, edited by Molly Zuckerman, 179–97. Hoboken, NJ: John Wiley, 2014.

Kunitz, Stephen J. *The Health of Populations: General Theories and Particular Realities*. Oxford: Oxford University Press, 2007.

Maglen, Krista. *The English System. Quarantine, Immigration and the Making of a Port Sanitary Zone*. Manchester: Manchester University Press, 2014.

Mandler, Peter. *Aristocratic Government in the Age of Reform: Whigs and Liberals 1830–1852*. Oxford: Oxford University Press, 1990.

Maul, Daniel. *The International Labour Organization: 100 Years of Global Social Policy*. Berlin: Walter de Gruyter, 2019.

Mazzucato, Mariana. *The Value of Everything. Making and Taking in the Global Economy*. London: Penguin, 2018.

McKay, Rich A. *Patient Zero and the Making of the AIDS Epidemic*. Chicago, IL: University of Chicago Press, 2017.

McKeown, Thomas and R. G. Record. 'Reasons for the Decline of Mortality in England and Wales during the Nineteenth Century', *Population Studies*, 16 (1962): 94–122.

McKeown, Thomas. *The Modern Rise of Population*. London: Edward Arnold, 1976.
Mercer, Alex. *Infections, Chronic Disease and the Epidemiological Transition. A New Perspective*. Rochester, NY: Rochester University Press, 2014.
Mercer, A. J. 'Updating the Epidemiological Transition Model', *Epidemiology and Infection* (2018): 1–8, doi.org/10.1017/S0950268818000572.
Milanovic, Branko. *Global Inequality: A New Approach for the Age of Globalization*. Cambridge, MA: Belknap Press, 2018.
Mooney, Graham. *Intrusive Interventions: Public Health, Domestic Space, and Infectious Disease Surveillance in England, 1840–1914*. Rochester, NY: Rochester University Press, 2015.
Morgan, Kelly and Cormac Ó Gráda. 'The Poor Law of Old England: Institutional Innovation and Demographic Regimes', *Journal of Interdisciplinary History*, 41 (2011): 339–66.
Mosley, Paul, Jane Harrigan, and J. F. J. Toye. *Aid and Power: The World Bank and Policy-Based Lending*. London and New York: Routledge, 1991.
Olshansky, S. J. et al. 'Emerging Infectious Diseases: The Fifth Stage of the Epidemiologic Transition?', *World Health Statistics Quarterly*, 51 (1998): 207–17.
Omran, Abdel R. 'The Epidemiologic Transition: A Theory of the Epidemiology of Population Change', *Milbank Memorial Fund Quarterly*, 49 (1971): 509–38.
Omran, Abdel R. 'The Epidemiologic Transition Theory. A Preliminary Update', *Journal of Tropical Paediatrics*, 29 (1983): 305–16.
Omran, Abdel R. 'The Epidemiologic Transition Theory Revisited Thirty Years Later', *World Health Statistics Quarterly*, 51 (1998): 99–119.
Packard, Randall. *A History of Global Health: Interventions into the Lives of Other Peoples*. Baltimore, MD: Johns Hopkins University Press, 2016.
Piketty, Thomas. *Capital in the Twenty-First Century*. Cambridge, MA: Belknap Press, 2014.
Read, Charles. 'Laissez-Faire, The Irish Famine, and British Financial Crisis', *Economic History Review*, 69 (2016): 411–34.
Reid, Alastair J. *United We Stand. A History of Britain's Trade Unions*. London: Allen Lane, 2004.
Risse, Gunther. 'Medicine in the Age of Enlightenment'. In *Medicine in Society*, edited by A. Wear, 149–96. Cambridge: Cambridge University Press, 1992.
Rosen, George. 'Cameralism and the Concept of Medical Police', *Bulletin of the History of Medicine*, 27 (1952): 21–42.
Rosen, George. 'Mercantilism and Health Policy in Eighteenth Century French Thought', *Medical History*, 3 (1959): 259–75.
Sayngoza, Felix and Leon Bijlmakers. 'Drivers of Improved Health Sector Performance in Rwanda: A Qualitative View from Within', *BMC Health Services Research*, 16 (123) (2016).
Sen, Amartya. *Poverty and Famines: An Essay on Entitlement and Deprivation*. Oxford: Oxford University Press, 1981.
Sharma, Patrick. 'Bureaucratic Imperatives and Policy Outcomes: The Origins of World Bank Structural Adjustment Lending', *Review of International Political Economy*, 20 (4) (2013): 667–86, doi.org/10.1080/09692290.2012.689618.
Shaxson, Nicholas. *The Finance Curse: How Global Finance is Making Us All Poorer*. London: Penguin, 2018.
Slack, Paul. *The English Poor Law 1531–1782*. Basingstoke: Macmillan, 1990.
Slack, Paul. *Poverty and Policy in Tudor and Stuart England*. London: Longman, 1998.
Snell, Keith. *Annals of the Labouring Poor: Social Change and Agrarian England 1660–1900*. Cambridge: Cambridge University Press, 1985.
Solar, Peter M. 'Poor Relief and English Economic Development before the Industrial Revolution'. *The Economic History Review*, 48 (1995): 1–22.
Szreter, Simon. 'The Importance of Social Intervention in Britain's Mortality Decline c.1850–1914: A Re-interpretation of the Role of Public Health', *Social History of Medicine*, 1 (1988): 1–37.
Szreter, Simon. 'The Idea of Demographic Transition: A Critical Intellectual History', *Population and Development Review*, 19 (1993): 659–701.
Szreter, Simon. 'Economic Growth, Disruption, Deprivation, Disease And Death: On the Importance of the Politics of Public Health', *Population and Development Review*, 23 (1997): 693–728.
Szreter, Simon. *Health and Wealth. Studies in History and Policy*. Rochester, NY: Rochester University Press, 2005.
Simon Szreter. 'Thomas McKeown', *Dictionary of Medical Biography*, edited by William F. Bynum and Helen Bynum. Westport, CT and London: Greenwood Press, 2007.

Szreter, Simon. 'The History and Development of Public Health in Developed Countries'. In *Oxford Textbook of Global Public Health*, 7th edition, edited by Roger Detels et al., Ch.1.2. Oxford: Oxford University Press, forthcoming 2021.

Szreter, Simon and Graham Mooney. 'Urbanisation, Mortality and the Standard of Living Debate', *The Economic History Review*, 51 (1998): 84–112.

Thomson, Michael, Alexander Kentikelenis, and Thomas Stubbs. 'Structural Adjustment Programmes Adversely Affect Vulnerable Populations: A Systematic-Narrative Review of Their Effect on Child and Maternal Health', *Public Health Reviews*, 38 (13) (2017): 108.

Toye, John. 'Solow in the Tropics', *History of Political Economy*, 41 (1) (2009): 221–40, doi.org/10.1215/00182702-2009-025.

Toye, John and Richard Toye. 'The Origins and Interpretation of the Prebisch-Singer Thesis', *History of Political Economy*, 35 (2003): 437–67.

UNICEF. *Adjustment with a Human Face*, edited by Andrea Cornia and Frances Stewart. Oxford: Oxford University Press, 1987.

Vallin, Jacques and France Meslé. 'Convergences and Divergences in Mortality. A New Approach to Health Transition', *Demographic Research*, Special Collection 2, Article 2 (2004), 11–44.

Wacquant, Lois. 'Class, Race & Hyperincarceration in Revanchist America', *Daedalus*, 139 (3) (2010): 74–90.

de Waal, A. and A. Whiteside. 'New Variant Famine: AIDS and Food Crisis in Southern Africa', *Lancet*, 362 (9391) (2003): 1234–7.

Walter, John and Roger Schofield. 'Famine, Disease and Crisis Mortality in Early Modern Society'. In *Famine, Disease and the Social Order in Early Modern Society*, edited by John Walter and Roger Schofield, 1–73. Cambridge: Cambridge University Press, 1989.

Weisz, George and Jesse Olszynko-Gryn. 'The Theory of Epidemiologic Transition: The Origins of a Citation Classic', *Journal of the History of Medicine and Allied Sciences*, 65 (2010): 287–326.

Williams, Samantha. *Poverty, Gender and Life-Cycle under the English Poor Law 1760–1834*. Woodbridge: RHS Boydell Press, 2011.

Wohl, Anthony S. *The Eternal Slum. Housing and Social Policy in Victorian London*. London: Edward Arnold, 1977.

Wohl, Anthony S. *Endangered Lives. Public Health in Victorian Britain*. London: J. M. Dent, 1983.

Woods, Robert I. *The Demography of Victorian England and Wales*. Cambridge: Cambridge University Press, 2000.

World Bank. *Accelerated Development in Sub-Saharan Africa: An Agenda for Action*. World Bank, 1981.

World Bank. 'Fertility Rate, Total', last modified 2019, http://data.worldbank.org/indicator/SP.DYN.TFRT.IN.

World Bank. 'World Development Indicators: Health Risk Factors', last modified 2017, http://wdi.worldbank.org/table/2.17.

Wrigley, Edward A. and Roger S. Schofield. *The Population History of England, 1541–1871: A Reconstruction*. Cambridge: Cambridge University Press, 1981.

Wrigley, Edward A. et al. *English Population History from Family Reconstitution, 1580–1830*. Cambridge: Cambridge University Press, 1997.

Zuckerman, Molly (ed.). *Modern Environments and Human Health: Revisiting the Second Epidemiologic Transition*. Hoboken, NJ: John Wiley, 2014.

Zuckerman, Molly and George J. Armelagos, 'The Hygiene Hypothesis and the Second Epidemiologic Transition'. In *Modern Environments and Human Health. Revisiting the Second Epidemiologic Transition*, edited by Molly Zuckerman, 301–20. Hoboken, NJ: John Wiley, 2014.

2

Demographic and Disease Shifts

Kavita Sivaramakrishnan

Scholars have been increasingly rethinking the demographic and disease shifts that have been occurring worldwide, such as the global ageing of populations and shifts in incidence and patterns of chronic disease. This has led to a growing interest among social scientists, and particularly historians of health and disease, in probing the deterministic models and assumptions that experts have articulated about these shifts in patterns of disease conditions, the ageing of populations and the social and health challenges that have been associated with these global shifts.

How can we understand the power of experts in deploying contingent and uncertain knowledge, rather than bounded certainties and permanent transition narratives, regarding social changes in other societies and their dynamic historical situations? How did discussions, led by experts at an international and national level, about transitions and social shifts reconcile universal frames with local, contextual factors? These questions form a crucial part of the process of rethinking the teleological models that are inherent in Abdel Omran's thesis of the epidemiological transition, including mulling over its critique by Julio Frenk (1989) and others: Gaylin and Kates (1997), Kahn and Tollman (1999).[1]

This chapter historicises demographic and modernisation theories and projections that emerged through the 1950s–80s in South Asia and South Africa as a broad and intense focus of attention for social scientists, both as end goals and also as processes of social change. It discusses how experts and activists understood, framed and debated the processes and ends of the modernisation of societies worldwide.[2] Indeed, as historians have demonstrated, some ideas and concepts such as projections of stages and models of fertility, as well as data on standards of living and class, were already informing the writings of middle-class experts in Asia. They were engaged in defining a neo-Malthusian agenda in the 1920s and 1930s, even before the articulation of modernisation theories after the Second World War.[3]

By the 1950s and later, these social theories and projections assumed a more global, reductionist form. They focused on characterisations of diseases and health risks in Asia and Africa, and also understandings of disease prevalence, urban migration, fertility transitions and ageing in the South. Experts and professionals from the US and those in Asia and Africa saw this as a progressive agenda consisting of demographic certainties and convincing projections. In the case of both the epidemiological and demographic transitions, scientists tried to 'capture' and manage these processes. However, it is clear that these knowledge-making and evolutionist narratives were characterised by differing and shifting objectives, discontinuities, and anxieties about populations and societies. International experts, who were articulating these theories and models, aimed to predict based on their universalising transition paradigms, but aberrations or shifts in these predictions could be conveniently blamed on local, contextual factors.

In this chapter, I trace demographic debates at several scales and from different perspectives: among international urbanisation experts, demographers in India, and social workers in South Asia and Africa. Through the 1970s–80s it was clear to them that the 'traditional' to 'modern' transition was not happening in the near and immediate future. Not all of them, however, relinquished the idea of a more complete, industrial modernisation in the distant future. Without necessarily wanting to exit or reject this paradigm of transitions, they attempted to control it by shaping it and adding complexity and context to its implications.

Attempts by experts to articulate a progressive teleology of non-western societies were constantly being revised and reorganised based on encounters with local diversity and dissonance in patterns and speed of urbanisation or of demographic ageing. Susan Greenhalgh's work, for instance, has analysed the challenges faced by US demographers and the pervasiveness of modernisation theory in their work which has often been characterised by scholars as reflecting ignorance of the theoretical limits of their discipline, and/or of the flaws in their methodologies. Instead, she argues that their work has to be situated within 'the historical contingency of knowledge creation' that they faced.[4]

What is also significant, and less well brought-out in studies of demographers and epidemiologists in the US at this time, was that the scale and modelling of these studies *needed* to study Asia and Africa comparatively in order to be complete and influential conceptually and scientifically in the West. The need to devise 'transition' models and trajectories and stages of modernisation served a crucial, dual purpose of critical reflectivity for western experts. Most crucially, it served as an effort to shape the postcolonial futures of Asia and Africa by defining them as being in a state of lag or being behind, and 'different' from those of western industrialisation. Through comparative analysis, there was reinforcement of normative trajectories of social and industrial development that had occurred earlier in the US and Europe.

At times, American sociologists and demographers, undertaking world surveys of stages of urbanisation and fertility, were aware that the abstract promise of development for the 'less developed' South was being offered at a historical conjuncture when lasting problems were already associated with industrialised and modern 'futures' in the West. These problems included social, environmental and urbanisation crises, and fears of ageing and dependency among deprived minorities in the US. By the late 1960s and early 1970s there were deep-seated challenges relating to industrialisation in the US. Notions of transition as elaborated, for instance, in the writings of Kingsley Davis (whose private papers form a significant source for this paper) were not envisaging a transformative change and shift in Africa but hinted more towards an inevitable, contingent shift and improvement that could spiral into more complex problems and challenges.

Theories of transition or shifts in patterns of disease, population trends and urbanisation were interrelated and overlapped because they reflected the tensions within the ideas and evidence-building tools that were being used to shape modernisation projects. Together, they help us analyse the contingencies in making and remaking future-centred predictions that were to be repeated across societies, often at dire social costs, and that have often been neglected by scholars.

American demographers and the futures of populations and diseases

In the mid-1940s and later, American demographers Frank Notestein and Kingsley Davis, who were based at the Population Research Bureau at Princeton and Columbia University respectively, began to share their analyses of demographic changes in 'developing' societies across the world in their research. They were trying to understand worldwide interrelations between populations and shifts in fertility, migration and life expectancy.[5] They argued '...that fertility is high in poor, traditional societies because of high mortality, the lack of opportunities for individual advancement and the economic value of children. All these things change with modernisation or urban industrialism, and individuals, once their viewpoints become reoriented to the changes that have taken place, can make use of the new opportunities.'[6] They noted that shifts in population that were brought on by processes of 'modernisation'[7] had been key in the west and were mediated by factors such as the deepening growth of urban, industrial society, technology and the rise of 'rational social movements'.

Notestein and Davis's work was drawn from dominant strands of social science thinking and theorising in the US, which held that there were common, singular routes to social change that could be followed in an accelerated path to industrialisation in newly independent, decolonised states as they transitioned from their 'traditional' societies to 'modern' avatars. Their demographic predictions and modelling were based on these binary assumptions. They were particularly concerned with identifying the chief characteristics of traditional, pre-transition societies: mortality was high, social insecurity was pervasive, the cost of children was low, and they were based on filial piety, and 'primitive' social ties or attitudes, beliefs and traditions that were not rational and kept in place high fertility behaviour.[8]

These generalisations regarding demographic shifts offered models of how modernisation and shifts in patterns of populations and diseases represented a 'continuum of progress' for societies as they industrialised. This involved sequential changes as societies transitioned from being 'pre-modern', or high-fertility and high-mortality focused, to progressing towards low fertility and low mortality. These changes were due to a reduced death rate and longevity; control of epidemics and infections; shifts to lifestyle diseases; and new patterns of urbanisation and of work and labour for both men and women.

The growing interest in demographic projections, in calculating dependent and productive populations in modernising societies, also spurred other experts to trace and anticipate shifts in disease and morbidity patterns, and also to try and map the growth of ageing populations. Abdel Omran's work on shifting patterns of disease or epidemiological transition was initially aimed at addressing international population studies (1971).[9] Later, the work of ageing experts and sociologists such as Donald Cowgill (discussed later in this chapter) extended and tied these predictions to their implications for ageing populations worldwide.[10] These framings were extremely influential among demographic experts and UN organisations who, in turn, influenced population policies in Asia, Africa and Latin America.

Demographic transition models and the ambivalence of experts

Modernisation elicited doubts and ambiguities in the transition models that were offered by experts, including admissions that their knowledge regarding predicted shifts was still incipient and uncertain. However, as we shall see in the course of this chapter, taking the path or passage to transition was not in doubt. Projects and predictions of modernisation were still pursued because international experts were of the view that, if development goals were shifted midway, they would be faced with unintended or unforeseen complications.

Kingsley Davis's sociological expertise made him an international expert whose inputs were in demand both within the US and in Asia and Africa, as his work bridged the links between demographic evolution and industrialisation that were captured in transition theory. In 1968, Davis gave the concluding address to a meeting on cities and world urbanisation models that was held in South Africa. In his speech, he shared an interesting critique of expert-led development planning and compared its impacts with his South African audience.[11] Davis reflected that he could see that South Africa was on an incipient and early path to modernisation and development, on a trajectory that promised what might be regarded as development or despair. He said he envied South Africa's emerging economic stage and lack of complex, industrialised problems because it did not yet reflect the manifold challenges of infrastructural complications, environmental pollution and social tensions that were in evidence at a later, mature and 'developed' stage such as that experienced by the United States.[12]

Davis's ideas, as he elaborated on them in his speech, tended to infantilise South Africa and the 'simplicity' of its current social and economic condition, and they echoed paternalistic notions about colonial subjects and their reform. In his speech, Davis was assuming the role of the disinterested development expert who could mentor and guide this change and modernising transition. He compared stages of development between the two societies (the US and South Africa), and asserted his mixed thoughts about the ends and benefits of development.[13]

Davis's comments also highlight the priorities that influenced the questions posed by social scientists in the US. Our understanding of the work of social science experts, such as Davis, Omran, Cowgill and others, needs to locate them in a postwar university milieu in the US when social science disciplines were under pressure to create overarching disciplinary theories, technical tools and training programmes for a new generation of social science researchers.[14] In the 1950s, Davis was well funded by these philanthropies that were urging an empirical, objective and practical focus to social science questions, especially on long-range problems and predictions to understand societies beyond the US that were undergoing social change.[15] Davis was also vocal in his work in discussing the constraints posed by the demands from development-supporting institutions, such as the Ford Foundation in the US, and the protracted discussions regarding models and generalisations that were the focus of these meetings. Based on these experiences, Davis turned to question the goals of development itself. He wrote, 'I have often observed that economic development in truth, is no goal at all, because it is absolutely neutral as to what the economic gains are to be used for.' The promised end of development and its transition models represented a 'dummy goal', he reflected, with experts speaking vaguely about 'development' and progress as a catch-all phrase but it was not clear who this development was serving, and if it was serving redistributive ends at all.[16]

Studying South Africa and listening to discussions at this conference enabled Davis to make other crossings and linkages that were also somewhat unsettling, such as reflections relating to the US. Models of transition, and mapping the timing and effects of shifts in Africa and Asia, therefore served to complete analytical reflections at home, in the US, on the implications of population and industrial transitions, to reflect on their credibility, and also the fractures and shortcomings associated with these changes.

Demographic models explained stages of modernisation, facilitated discussions relating to differences in stages of development and identified the means to effect these changes; they also brought out the variability and contingency in these models. Davis, for instance, reflected on the pathways that advanced and post-transition societies such as the US had followed. He noted that in the US one observed 'a more crowded, complex, and conflictful condition ... One feels the necessity to point out again that an ever-higher level of living is used in even greater proportion simply to obviate the discomforts and hazards of an ever-higher level of living. At some point, human beings will have to ask how they can control themselves. Not simply how they can control and use their environment.'[17]

It was also clear to Davis after his visit and talks in South Africa that there was a specific deployment of the social sciences and their analytical tools – such as forecasting, modelling and the choice of 'technological fixes' – that was specifically American in orientation and these perspectives were absent in South Africa. The 'solutions' that were proposed, to enable shifts and modernising transitions in populations, health or urbanisation, offered a quick and finite solution when, in fact, they were often only multiplying problems. Davis offered vivid illustrations when he made this critique, saying:

> In South Africa you go far less for what one might call unrestrained technological imagination. In the United States we have people who call themselves experts of the future or futureologists. One of them told me that while other people study the present or the past, he studies the future. When the physicists, engineers, and public health people go to the laboratory they come up with a plastic gimmick that will fix it. If the problem is overpopulation, a small plastic device inserted in the right organ, or a pill taken orally, will solve the problem ... My only complaint about this is that the 'technological fix' often creates two problems when one existed before ... the superhighways stimulate traffic and thus spread congestion while helping to create more smog; the birth control pills become a public hazard. Little attention is paid to the varied social and economic consequences of the proposed technological innovation.[18]

Davis's critique of development planning and of futuristic forecast models was rooted in debates on urban deprivation and environmental disasters that were deepening in the late 1960s in the US. This implied that he realised that this futurology and models of change, interventions to effect modernisation of populations and health, were contingent and uncertain. How does one interpret this rethinking of agency and social change by Davis who was comparing the US and South Africa as well as, in effect, other industrialising societies?

For Davis these inconsistencies and the technocentric, fix-it approach neither fully undermined nor raised questions about the ends of modernisation itself.[19] It demonstrated, I argue, the visualised role of an international expert whose role was not simply to effect change or transition. The expert, as Davis's ideas implied, saw himself as interpreting and shaping change as it evolved. This also meant that complex and modern capitalist societies such as the US had experienced conflicts and compromises between demographic shifts, technology and environmental stress but they were self-rectifying and regenerative. Societies in Africa and Asia needed experts to guide and shape their development through certain paradigms, models and analytical categories to demonstrate that they could not only guide and shape universal models but could also understand and adjust these modernisation plans to local specificities.

The role of experts and expertise ensured that modernised societies could solve their own problems, albeit in complicated ways.[20] Davis was frank in admitting that modernisation and development planning in the US was characterised by competing and often contradictory views advanced by various disciplines. Some disciplines that were involved in 'practice' were interested in propelling change and they assumed that they did not have to build consensus and prove the validity of their claims and practice. Other disciplines were more focused on taking into account differences in context, attitudes and behaviour, as well as the process of effecting development itself. He wrote, 'There is conflict between the scientific (or at least the scientific-in-aim) disciplines such as the social sciences and the clearly applied professional fields such as city-planning, architecture, highway engineering, business analysis, and public health.' The reasons for this cleavage are well worth considering: 'It is not simply lack of communication, (the representatives of different disciplines shout at each other all the time); it is rather that the tasks are different. The aim of the planner or the engineer is to get ahead with the task and consensus is assumed as is human and social "needs". The social scientists act differently, without this assumption and to understand human behaviour, without much practical responsibility.'[21]

What do Davis's ideas serve to explain about the persistent pursuit of transition models and modernisation? Davis understood that numerical shifts in life expectancy, fertility and disease patterns or biology would imply social challenges such as in the organisation of families, work, competitiveness, urbanisation and mobility; but, despite setbacks, modern societies at the end of transition were societies that were more progressive as they were self-reflective, and were able to find and suggest solutions for themselves.

In a later article on the challenges posed by demographic shifts and ageing populations in the US, he expressed these ideas in a more concrete manner, observing that American society would cope with the sociological threats posed by ageing as mature societies had both 'learned to appreciate and initiate social change'.[22] Demographic shifts towards 'advanced' stages of the demographic transition were closely tied to qualities such as enhanced social resilience or coping that came from a mature society that had reduced its mortality and fertility, and such a society with a great proportion of old people in the population, was also '... a society that had science, education, cities, and industrial technology, and was therefore radical in the fundamental sense of the term... .'[23]

Tracing Davis's ideas helps us understand that transition models were envisaged not only as demographic, epidemiological or gerontological projects that pursued and explained modernisation of populations and diseases but were also political and social in nature. Davis's remarks about 'mature' societies and their 'radical' nature were not alluding to the radicalism and counter-culture movements of the 1960s and later in the US but, rather, a postwar technocentric vision of the US offering developmentalism as means of innovative reinvention, and characterised by a self-direction and initiative that newly decolonised nations 'lacked'.

American experts simultaneously voiced generalised transition theories and garnered philanthropic support for their research, but they also articulated their doubts. These two approaches did not overtly contradict one another, and the two threads need to be traced and understood together. Furthermore, Davis's visions also allowed no real space for alternative visions or orientations because this was an America-centric vision, and his efforts to cast South Africa in America's industrialised self-image implied a lack of alternatives and inevitability as decolonised societies contemplated their futures.

Between the 1970s and 80s, Kingsley Davis was succeeded by a new generation of international demographers, who were widely invested in international health programmes and commented on demographic transition theories and their assumptions, often in controversial ways. They argued that transition theories and their projections of temporality and change needed to draw from contextual, culturally informed evidence. John C. Caldwell, an influential demographer and sociologist (a recipient of the United Nations Population Award in 2004), who worked for many decades in Asia and Africa, commented about the criteria advanced by transition theory:

> the criteria employed are highly ethnocentric and are laden with Western values. It is assumed that it is rational for a man or a couple to maximize the expenditure on the individuals in his or their nuclear family; but there are any number of non-Western societies

> in which there is greater pleasure in spending on some relatives outside the nuclear family, and in which children are happier to spend on parents than are parents on children ... What demographic transition theory has always regarded as rational are primarily Western social ends with economically logical steps to maximize satisfactions given those ends.[24]

Caldwell's research brought out the overlaps between demographic and disease transitions, and challenges and barriers to both processes that were drawn from specific examples from South Asia and Africa based on his work and travels there. In a paper on demographic behaviour in Africa, which Caldwell contributed at a conference organised by the Centre of African Studies at the University of Edinburgh (1977), his views on shifts in behaviour were termed by later reviews as bordering on 'guesswork' as they were based on sparse data and evidence, drawn also from his extensive travels in the region. In a restatement of demographic theory (1976), based on broad-based assumptions about behaviour change in 'traditional' societies, he also argued that fertility decline was occurring in these societies due to a reversal of wealth flows that were no longer from children to parents, but in a reverse direction.[25]

Caldwell's work tried to make demographic theory more anchored in local, social and cultural differences but his research also demonstrates how transition theory was often realigned only to be re-inscribed with notions of race and culture relating to fertility and sexuality that demonstrated a limited understanding of local divergences in behaviour, and the uneven nature of data collection that underlay generalisations about change.

Ageing societies and the gerontological transition

Nevertheless, attempts to build, amend and advance transition models still kept proliferating. Emerging disciplines such as gerontology in the 1970s, led by American social gerontologists, were less deterred by the challenges and doubts that were being raised about these generalisations. They were seeking to identify and compare the pace of social and demographic changes and urbanisation worldwide, and these experts were also turning their focus to non-western settings. American gerontologists worried especially about the changing place of older persons in their own society due to increasing concerns about welfare support. They feared the 'obsolescence' of the 'aged', and sought to explain ageing, social adjustment and family support in Asia, noting that ageing populations were 'a by-product of a demographic revolution which is usually called the demographic transition'.[26]

Donald Cowgill, a leading sociologist and social gerontologist, was influenced by Kingsley Davis's work and other models of the demographic transition. His pioneering work, in turn, shaped research on stages in the modernisation and ageing of societies worldwide, premised on the notion that a linear transition to modernisation implied and assumed a decline in the status of older persons due to the effects of urbanisation, migration and industrialisation.[27] He had an interest in urbanisation in Africa, in Rhodesia particularly, and his research on urban social change also overlapped with his efforts to investigate the impacts of ageing populations worldwide on families. Around 1977–8, Cowgill spent sojourns teaching in Thailand and travelling across the world and, on his return, he offered a commentary in the American press and in research journals on rising concerns about older populations.

Cowgill distinguished old age partly by longevity in individuals that was the result of demographic shifts, but he observed that it was also characterised in and across societies by socioeconomic features such as growing intergenerational competition, new technologies and job-related obsolescence, retirement and social segregation due to the mobility promoted by urbanisation.[28] He observed that modernisation at various stages brought in certain contradictions:

> One of the dilemmas of modern societies is that, while sociological processes have fostered a devaluation of old people, demographic processes have led to increasing numbers and proportions of aged in their populations. Thus, such societies have larger proportions of older people than ever before, while at the same time older people have less value and utility to those societies. These countertrends give rise to the further anomaly that societies whose relative affluence permits them to provide the greatest comfort and security to their aged members instead deprive them of useful roles and consign high proportions of them to relative poverty.[29]

Sociologists like Donald Cowgill took easily to the predictive aspects of the demographic transition model, and its determinism regarding modernisation, because it conveniently echoed their perceptions of the wider mission of gerontology and the role of social gerontologists as a new field. They saw their field as being oriented to solving problems and offering 'social remedies' relating to modernisation (as discussed by

Davis earlier in this chapter), with an eye to the present and also to shape the future. In the context of a growing critique of the generalisations and assumptions inherent in modernisation-related predictions – both demographic and social – Cowgill offered what he termed a 'curvilinear rather than a unidirectional trend in the status of the elderly' with cultural values being a key variable in this modification.[30]

The concern and urgency to understand ageing in Africa stemmed from trying to understand the intimate influence of a shared 'common African heritage' among the African-American elderly in the US, and to compare the influence of modernisation-related variables. Donald Cowgill and sociologists such as Marjorie Cantor, Rose Gibson and others were engaged in revising prior interpretations of the social, modernisation processes underlying the demographic transition.[31] They debated whether racial discrimination was a more powerful explanatory variable in the US, in changes associated with ageing, as compared to Africa. This had important implications as it implied a 'reversal' of modernisation theory. Gibson argued that this implied that the black elderly were not in decline in the US, and she and others suggested that the receipt of the first, secure welfare pensions and independence from stressful, 'dead-end' work implied that these groups were better off than younger blacks, and even older white populations. Marjorie Cantor reflected on Cowgill's work and wrote: 'The relatively stronger position of the black elderly when compared to younger blacks suggests that something besides modernization is operating as an explanatory variable...in the case of blacks...it is hard, even impossible to disentangle the impact of political and social discrimination from the effects of technology, change in family structure, and other criteria of modernisation employed by Cowgill.'[32]

These efforts to recast modernisation theory tried to bring in more nuanced analysis of transition and modernisation in the US but often resulted in stating that there were racialised differences in behaviour and dependence of the African-American elderly in the US. These American scholars reached out to noted researchers on demographic ageing and studied African gerontocracies in Ghana and Liberia, but these comparative studies were limited to trying to understand modernisation as being either detrimental to and leading to the obsolescence of older generations, or reiterating that it was the young rather than the old who needed 'remedial assistance'.[33]

Both the African-American elderly and older populations in Africa were not therefore conforming to the transition models envisaged for them, and they represented a deviance from the norm. But the identification of these differences did not focus on the amassing of latent, accumulated disadvantages across the life course in the case of the African-American elderly, and the health and psychological effects. Instead, contemporary writing in the US focused only on labour and occupations, and the relief and redressal offered by welfare pensions for older blacks. Nor did these research collaborations probe and unpack conceptual categories such as 'traditional dependence' and its changes between generations in the context of colonial legacies of capital accumulation and uneven development. They interpreted changes in African societies as a form of decline and marginalisation for the old, or implied that younger and dependent populations in Africa were leading disadvantaged lives.[34]

Even with the flaws mentioned, efforts by these experts to initiate comparative studies and to nuance the factors underlying modernisation in non-western societies, and among minority populations in the US, were rare. More visibly and consistently, social scientists who were building the field of social gerontology and its predictive strengths saw their intellectual mission as using demographic theories as reference points regarding fertility transitions. They offered social remedies and solutions based on the prior and predetermined experiences of ageing in western societies. There were many discussions at their professional meetings that reveal how and when Cowgill's colleagues in social gerontology began to see a wider role for their social science expertise.

At the first international course on gerontology in Lisbon (1970), for instance, a speech made by a leading French gerontologist about the mission of gerontology had an interesting resonance with the comments made by Kingsley Davis some years before. At the conference on urbanisation in South Africa two years earlier, Davis had observed the tendency in the US among experts from the applied social science disciplines to see themselves as offering developmental models and generalisations regarding the future. They intended to solve certain 'problems' in the present through technological and scientific interventions from above. They assumed, he had noted, that there was a consensus regarding the processes or social events that were at work and how 'problems' were defined and approached. In their professional address delivered at Lisbon, gerontologists perceived themselves as deploying a 'science of national interest'. They projected their gerontological approach as being 'clearsighted' and objective and it served the end of 'futurology' or predicting how societies would be transformed.[35]

The main problems of ageing, the French demographer Alfred Sauvy observed, were related to the social passage from a traditional society of underemployment and agrarian economy to migration, urban employment and pensions, which posed social challenges in terms of inactivity and segregation in older years in modern, industrialised societies.[36] Moving a step further, after discussing 'how western societies had become rather heavily involved in...the needs presented by their older populations', the meeting ended with thoughts about international support to disseminate these views about societal ageing and its future.[37] A speaker at this meeting reflected on the UN Declaration on Social Progress and Development (issued in 1969 by 113 member countries of the United Nations) and he noted that the UN declaration had listed 'old age' only once (along with illness and disability), and sought redress of this marginalisation in programmes for the aged, urging the identification of common problems of aged persons across the world.[38]

Statements and papers on ageing that were produced by the WHO during this time reflected these dilemmas regarding ageing and modernisation that had been voiced by gerontological researchers in Europe and the US, and UN experts chose to strategically project them as a wider, international concern relating to ageing and modernisation.[39] The representation of ageing as a universal, human problem that reflected the demographic inevitability of convergent problems relating to modernisation met with resistance from several activists and experts in South Asia and Africa. Some of them accepted the notion of traditional societies with strong solidarities and did not necessarily challenge the assumptions of a modernising transition, but they wanted to reshape its metanarrative and assumptions regarding the individual and social life course.

State bureaucrats and transitions in India

Sripati Chandrasekhar, a well-known Indian demographer and sociologist, was a controversial figure and a relentless advocate of population control who was appointed as Union Health Minister by Indira Gandhi.[40] Chandrasekhar, a demographer who was trained at New York University, worked at the American Office of Strategic Services (the forerunner of the Central Intelligence Agency) as an expert on Indian demography, and returned soon after to India.[41] He gradually assumed senior positions of expertise and was involved in the analysis of demographic and health data, and supervised their collection and reporting at various levels. Chandrasekhar often discussed the systemic flaws in collecting demographic data in India, and the problems that experts faced in accurately predicting death rates and fertility.

Being trained in demography in the US, he understood the importance of intervening, reordering and gaining influence over these predictive models, often by asserting the contingency of knowledge collection in the field in India. It was clear from his writings that there were several scales of transition-related knowledge that it was important to recognise and analyse. Chandrasekhar leveraged conceptual predictions of transitions and their determinants in different ways from experts including Davis, Cowgill and others, such as Omran.

For Chandrasekhar, demographic and disease transitions were changeable and contingent and they were not transformative generalisations. They represented a continuum of forecasting that gave experts the power to weigh in on the development process and goals. His approach was that he highlighted mistakes and technical errors and brought out the problems in training census enumerators to collect statistics, or in public resistance to development programmes. All of this led to efforts to recalibrate the means and priorities that were needed to affect a demographic and medical modernisation.

One of Chandrasekhar's colleagues, in an introduction to a book on demographic *Statistics for Educational Planners* (1965),[42] reassured readers, who were mainly trainees at the Asian Institute for Planning, that 'Statistics are necessary not only for the formulation of schemes and drawing out the plan but also for watching the progress of the plan and for making necessary adjustments from time to time. As a matter of fact, planning to be successful and realistic has to be on a continuing basis and not an ad hoc phenomenon.' A constant flow of basic statistics had, therefore, to be ensured.

At times, beginning to achieve the stated predictions of transition models only served as a leverage for further bureaucratic interventions. Partial failures, or incompleteness or inconsistencies in projections, only built the case for further interventions (and did not negate these projections and developmental plans) and forecasting by national-level experts. Sripati Chandrasekhar and others were interested in looking beyond data that conveyed demographic shifts, such as a rise in life expectancy in India. A report in *The Hindu*, for instance, announced that 'the rise in the average expectation of life at birth during the past ten years has been hailed as one of the striking achievements of the post-Independence era. It is certainly a gratifying index of progress.' However, a rise in life expectancy implied mostly that the high rate of infant mortality (before 1947) had seen a large fall due to better child and maternal welfare and improved living conditions. This report also announced that the health and education ministries were introducing new, nationwide surveys and metrics – in the form of a National Physical Efficiency Drive – for better understanding these transitions in terms of the real health and efficiency of the Indian population, which would be more directly valuable to industrialisation and modernisation.[43] Transition-related achievements and benchmarks were interpreted by government bureaucrats in divergent ways. They were important to demonstrate that political independence at the time of decolonisation was also yielding further on economic visions, and they were keen to assert that scientific data collection guided their agenda. At the same time, even the meeting of certain benchmarks, such as a rise in national life expectancy in the 1960s, was treated simply as a starting point for other industrial, developmental projects rather than planning to sustain the improved health of this longer-lived working class.

Transitions, social development visions and local activists

However, there were alternative critiques and doubts voiced regarding transition models and predictions that were emerging from the locality, emanating from social workers and health activists. These views were not influential in changing the course of dominant models that were advocated and published by international researchers, and they did not challenge the contingent knowledge of transitions articulated by national experts and bureaucrats such as Sripati Chandrasekhar. However, these ideas were influential in shaping a growing critique that was demanding community-based and social-medicine-based approaches to modernisation and development. These perspectives informed and engaged with a more equity-focused approach to modernisation. They also brought out the importance of addressing existing structures of poverty and deprivation among vulnerable populations, rather than advocating changes in behaviour relating to fertility through state-enforced family planning, or criticising old-age dependency and unhealthy lifestyles and habits as most international and national demographers and sociologists were tending to do.

I will examine here the writings of two urban social workers, based in Harare and Delhi respectively, to compare their responses voiced in the late 1970s to early 1980s when belief in developmental projects and experts was increasingly on the wane, and social workers were speaking about 'social development' that was inclusive of the disadvantaged.[44]

Father Joseph Hampson in Zimbabwe had campaigned through a social-work school, supported by a Jesuit order based in Harare, to establish welfare programmes for the elderly (he also conducted several of the earliest studies of 'the experience of ageing' among old populations in Zimbabwe, many of whom had migrated from Zambia, Malawi, Mozambique and South Africa).[45] Hampson countered generalised narratives of modernisation and ageing, which were based on normative, western experiences of population ageing, in his writings by tracing the unstable and partial urbanisation taking place in Zimbabwe. Western experiences of social change, he noted, were characterised by concerns that were centred around retirement, pension rights, housing, changing family relationships, mental health and adjustment.[46] Citing contemporary studies in the US that spoke of ageing as a process of withdrawal and disengagement (especially disengagement from work), Hampson pointed out that society and life for the old in Zimbabwe had been marked by transitions that were complicated shifts and reversals from a pre-industrial society. Social life in a traditional past had been characterised by beliefs in the old as being repositories of knowledge, marked by Shona attitudes to death and mediation by the old, and by vital relationships of responsibility for older persons in the extended family.

Father Hampson's Jesuit and social-work background is significant because church politics were deeply segmented by race, class and ideology as the liberation struggle in Zimbabwe intensified. Catholic priests had been radicalised during the civil war in the 1960s–70s, but their politics were also often ambiguous and divided.[47] Once Mugabe came to power, with new legislative and political powers, oppressive laws were put into place, and 'in the name of "development" land reform focused more on productivity and export markets than poverty alleviation'.[48] Hampson referred to these fast-paced changes in his work: the spread of a cash economy, tremendous land and population pressures and, finally, a brutal liberation struggle that had led to independence and also to violent changes and killings. Regarding the effects on old people, he observed, 'There even grew in Rhodesia a shameful reversal whereby those who had worked the hardest and longest on farms or factories in laboring jobs were the very ones who had least security in old age.'[49]

Demographic statistics meant little, he noted, as birthdays were insignificant for most of the old and deprived population and 'measuring chronological age is not an easy undertaking' but the elderly population was also growing in numbers. Hampson's interviews and research focused especially on migrants, on elderly persons whose status as Malawian migrants was impermanent and precarious and who often could not return from their work places in neighbouring countries. There were also other older persons who could not adjust to town life and missed the customs and life in the Tribal Trust Lands (peasant farming areas), and were deeply affected by the loss of life, disorder and lack of civility and safety (including a pervasive fear of violent party elements). The ageing process that Hampson tracked consisted of a population that lacked resources and a majority that was in 'abject destitution', and were living on the borders of informal, illegal activities (if they were active), and lacked pensions.

Hampson spoke of an individual life course that was in disarray and unstable, and intersected with complex social and political transitions. Ageing and modernisation for the majority did not imply retirement and social ageing as in the west. He wrote, 'In the Zimbabwean context… destitution drives the elderly to seek employment, no matter what kind of employment it is. The search for a job and money is relentless, consuming the energies of the elderly as well as the young, the disabled and frail as well as the able-bodied, the loner as well as the family person. This drive means many other considerations are subservient: health, interest and ability take a backseat.' He added that social disengagement and loneliness was mostly not an option and there was often an increase in involvement, as the grandparents were faced with the care and parenting of grandchildren or young relatives. ('Sometimes the double burden of being old and also caring for these dependents is too great, and the elderly person sees death as a pleasant escape from a future that can only bring more problems and less energy to resolve them.')[50]

Hampson's views were also echoed by activists in South Asia. Walter Fernandes, a sociologist and founding member of the Indian Social Institute who worked on ageing and urban displacement, wrote that, apart from a few elderly in India and Nepal who enjoyed security after retirement and found 'social ageing' traumatic (as in the case of older persons/pensioners in the west), for the rural and urban poor working in the informal sector, 'employment itself may be a game of survival' as the bottom 20 per cent living below the poverty line had to spend 85 per cent of their income on food alone. Of this population, the lowest castes and bonded labourers were an even greater proportion and were doubly disadvantaged; these were the aged who were affected by migration after the loss of rural jobs and seeking informal work in the city and they were ageing in precarity. This category, he noted, were said to euphemistically die of old age, 'and may in reality die of starvation'.[51] They worked for survival and not for comfort like the middle-class pensioners. Poverty was itself the chronic root cause of illness and morbidities, as 'most illnesses affecting people in the informal and rural sectors are what can be called "deficiency illnesses" caused by poor hygienic conditions, lack of drainage in slums, malnutrition, and absence of health services'. The old and aged were further compromised by their lack of resistance, and those who were poor, Fernandes noted, were marginalised from doctors who belonged to the upper classes, and their attitude to diseases was that they would go until their disease symptoms disappeared, not till they were cured, due to expenses, wage loss, and difficulties of movement with old age.

Fernandes conveyed a socially complex picture of ageing in societies in South Asia that had not fully modernised. He also linked an unequal colonial past and its legacies to ongoing struggles, an approach that distinguished him from experts who stressed transitions in the future but rarely acknowledged the continuing effects of the past. In his writings, both individual and social transitions were not homogenous or discrete and, unlike others who referred to a more ethical, socially inclusive traditional past, Fernandes focused on an immediate past (a colonial one) that had been exploitative. He also focused on a present characterised by cumulative inequalities of class, caste, place (rural/urban), poverty and malnutrition that were experienced by the old; and a work life in the informal sector that extended without 'retirement' until death. He also placed ageing within the larger framing of a changing international economic order and the politics of colonisation and partial, inequitable industrialisation:

> In the West, the main problem of the aged is their social marginalization after their retirement and the need for re-integrating them in the political and cultural life of the country, and helping them get over loneliness caused by the loosening of the child-parent bond and the consequent distance between generations. In the South Asian and Third World countries it is a question of the economic survival of the family as a unit.[52]

Hampson and Fernandes also made references to the aged poor in South Asia and Zimbabwe and their ill health, and they pointed out that diseases of poverty, such as malnutrition and infectious diseases, were important causes of death for this population. Though growing rates of chronic diseases and lifestyle risks were associated with industrialised societies, social workers and medical researchers pointed out that infectious diseases continued to have high rates of incidence in societies that were also seeing a rise in life expectancy.

Conclusion

Transition-focused tropes about ageing populations and disease patterns were persistent and served a range of political and scientific projects. They were recast and interpreted at several scales by international demographers and experts, whose work was often supported by US philanthropic funding for the social sciences, and by demographer-experts and bureaucrats at the national level. Unexpectedly, they drew reactions from social workers and activists in the global south who saw theories and generalisations about modernisation and development as a means to introduce more local initiative and social, developmental goals.

In global health today, a growing focus on the challenges of chronic disease and on the growing numbers of an ageing population implies that the focus is on measuring, forecasting and anticipating the costs of morbidities, risk estimations and long-term care and dependency.[53] A renewed focus on middle age has also emerged in the biology of ageing-related research over the past few years. Early interventions to slow ageing are viewed as being critical because they allow researchers to study 'the pace of ageing' in individuals and populations who are in the first half of the life course, when people are beginning to diverge in their life trajectories.

The growing focus in global health, and among demographic and disease experts, is to highlight new temporalities that have emerged due to a changing, extended lifespan globally, a new life course of work and dependency that is now pervasive across a globalising world. Risky lifestyles and chronic diseases are no longer associated with specific spaces and populations, or differentiated by differences between industrialised, affluent nations and poorer, emerging societies as depicted in transition models. Specific, centralised disease control and demographic interventions, which were planned by state agencies and assisted by international philanthropy for a transition from traditional to modern societies in past decades, are now absent or retrenched due to the privatisation of health services.

This has implied the growing replacement of universalised, transition-focused conceptual frameworks by an approach that focuses on *continuums rather than transitions*. The approach is to plan on extending functionality and working lives, on linking generational support ('generativity') to ensure care for morbidities and frailty, and on guided behavioural change across the life course to control disease risks (both embodied and lifestyle-related) turning into disease.[54]

This implies that the contingent visions of experts, as they guided state-centred modernisation projects that addressed population and disease transitions, have now waned. But the deployment of new and revised technical models, which link disease and ageing populations with labour and productivity, persists as experts redeploy their scientific framings and institutional affiliations in global health through newer initiatives and alignments, and these perspectives continue to ignore the realm of the political and of collective responsibility.

Notes

1 Bell and Chen, 'Responding to Health Transitions'. I also refer to a chapter in the same book by Frenk et al. See Frenk et al., 'Elements for a Theory of the Health Transition', 21–38 and a previous article authored by Frenk et al., 'Health Transition in Middle-Income Countries'. On HIV-related complications and challenges, see, Gaylin and Kates, 'Refocusing the Lens'. I also draw from the complex findings of the Agincourt Study in South Africa: Kahn et al., 'Mortality Trends in a new South Africa'; Tollman et al., 'Reversal in Mortality Trends'.

2 For the latter, I will draw on examples mostly from cancer and heart disease in South Asia based on my research into both.

3 See the work of Ramsam, founder of the Madras Neo-Malthusian League and the 'globalization of middle class fertility' discussed in the following works: Hodges, *Contraception, Colonialism and Commerce*; Dejung, Motadel, and Osterhammel, *The Global Bourgeoisie*, 84–96.

4 Greenhalgh, 'The Social Construction of Population Science'.

5 Their work was preceded by that of Landry in France in the 1930s, and others such as Cowgill (1963) modified and expanded it. The term 'demographic transition' refers to the secular shift in fertility and mortality from high and sharply fluctuating levels to low and relatively stable ones. 'This historical process ranks as one of the most important changes affecting human society in the past half millennium, on a par with the spread of democratic government, the industrial revolution, the increase in urbanization, and the progressive increases in educational levels of human populations. During the transition, mortality typically begins to decline first, followed some decades later by fertility decline, leading to a series of changes in population growth rates, size, and age distribution that continues for many decades. This pivotal process started in many European countries and parts of the Americas well over a century ago and is currently underway in most of the world. The presumption is that it will eventually affect all countries. The transition transforms the demography of societies from many children and few elderly to few children and many elderly.' Extract from Lee and Reher, 'Introduction: The Landscape of Demographic Transition'. See attempted reformulations of transition theory, in Cochran and O'Kane, 'Urbanization-Industrialization'.

6 A summary of these references to demographic shifts in the writings of Notestein (1945) and Landry (1934) referred to a transition in world population that would occur sequentially in pre-modern and modern societies, and is discussed in Kirk, 'Demographic Transition Theory'. Notestein, 'Population: The Long View', 39 refers to the demographic transition. Also, see Davis, *Human Society*. Notestein offered a twofold explanation for why fertility had begun to decline. Fertility in pre-modern countries had been kept, if not artificially high, then high only by the maintenance of a whole series of props: 'religious doctrines, moral codes, laws, education, community customs, marriage habits and family organizations ... all focused towards maintaining high fertility'. For an excellent summary and critique of Notestein's work, see Caldwell, 'Toward a Restatement of Demographic Transition Theory'. These lines are quoted from Caldwell who cites Notestein. See also Davis, 'The World Demographic Transition', 1–11.

7 Even though they did not always use the term.

8 Caldwell, 'Toward a Restatement of Demographic Transition Theory' and Caldwell, 'Population Health in Transition'.

9 Omran cited Notestein's work through a secondary source: David Reisman's somewhat dated work, *The Lonely Crowd: A Study of Changing American Character* (1950), which deployed social evolution theories. See Weisz and Olszynko-Gryn, 'The Theory of Epidemiologic Transition', 312.

10 As Weisz points out, Omran's paper was contributing to the emerging field of population epidemiology, and he was primarily addressing the WHO's international family planning agenda and its predictions regarding the links between populations and shifts from infectious to chronic diseases in the context of economic development. Weisz and Olszynko-Gryn, 'The Theory of Epidemiologic Transition'.

11 Davis, 'Closing Speech'.

12 Davis, 'Closing Speech'.

13 Arturo Escobar's work analyses the representational strategies of developmental discourse in producing ideas of 'underdevelopment' and the making of the 'Third World' as a historically specific space and population characterised by deficiency and lack. Escobar, *Encountering Development*. See also Breckenridge and van der Veer, *Orientalism and the Postcolonial Predicament*; Nandy, *The Intimate Enemy*; James, 'Review of "Orientalism"'.

14 Geiger, 'American Foundations'.

15 Geiger, 'American Foundations', 320–8.

16 However, Davis's ideas regarding redistribution were not racially inclusive. In this case, he was talking about addressing the challenges of persistent poverty and poorer classes who were not beneficiaries of development. He also made comparisons about social change and mobility, desegregation and race relations in South Africa and the US that make it clear that he overlooked the lasting historical legacies of colonial rule and continuing racialised exploitation in South Africa. Instead he saw certain contradictions: America was more developed than South Africa in terms of racial relations and representation but its assimilative doctrines had also made it more like South Africa due to representation and rights based on 'community' and groups rather than as individuals based on their 'talent' and merit – see Davis, 'Closing Speech', 495. For an insightful historical background, and comparative analysis more generally, see Frederickson's influential work, *White Supremacy*. I am grateful to Fred Harris for taking the time to discuss these comparative perspectives and drawing from his own work.

17 Davis, 'Closing Speech'.

18 Davis, 'Closing Speech'.

19 Modernisation would still alleviate and improve economic circumstances, especially poverty, and in the long run relative poverty would be more significant than absolute poverty. He added, 'Economic development simply means the multiplication of the means available to a society', Davis, 'Closing Speech'.

20 I draw on Cooper's work in my analysis. Cooper, 'Development, Modernization, and the Social Sciences'.

21 Cooper, 'Development, Modernization, and the Social Sciences'. He added, 'In addition to the usual switch blade slashing that occurs whenever anthropologists, sociologists and economists get together for teamwork, there is in the case of the cities a somewhat deeper interdisciplinary cleavage – a sort of fundamental war in which poison gas and automatic weapons are used instead of switch blades.'

22 Davis and Combs (eds.), *The Social and Biological Challenge*.

23 Davis and Combs (eds.), *The Social and Biological Challenge*.

24 Caldwell, 'Towards a Restatement'.

25 Caldwell, Caldwell and Quiggin, 'The Social Context of AIDS in Sub-Saharan Africa'; Doyle, *Before HIV*; Parker and Reid (eds.), *The Oxford Handbook of Modern African History*; Caldwell, 'Major Questions in African Demographic History'.

26 The following discussion of Cowgill's international work on ageing, changes in family structure, and discussions and mapping of the spread of ageing research and methodologies worldwide are mostly drawn from his private papers (Accession CA4791) consulted at the library at the University of Missouri Library Collections, St Louis. Cowgill spent long stretches of time in Northern Rhodesia trying to understand demographic changes, urbanisation and social structure; and, later, in Thailand. His most often cited research on transition models is 'The Aging of Populations and Societies', quote from page 5.

27 His work on ageing and social impacts across societies as they modernised was widely quoted and later elaborated in UN reports. See Cowgill and Holmes (eds.), *Aging and Modernization*; Cowgill, 'Aging in Cross-Cultural Perspective'.

28 Interestingly, demographers are late comers to writing about ageing, especially in a global context: Haaga writes, 'The 1987 program of the Population Association of America had no sessions primarily devoted to aging. In 2007, by contrast, *Demography* published nine articles dealing primarily with aging, the elderly, or adult mortality and disability, about a fifth of the journal's total.' Haaga, 'What's Next for the Demography of Aging'; International Center for Social Gerontology, *First International Course in Social Gerontology*, J.A. Huet, President of CIGS, Foreword – Opening Address; Adamchak, 'Aging in Sub-Saharan Africa'; Cowgill quoted in Adamchak, 'Aging in Sub-Saharan Africa'; for a discussion of Cowgill and gerontological visions of ageing across the non-western world, see also Sivaramakrishnan, *As the World Ages*; Adamchak and Friedmann, 'Societal Aging and Generational Dependency Relationships'; Treas and Logue, 'Economic Development and the Older Population'; United Nations Department of International Economic and Social Affairs, *World Population Trends and Policies*.

29 Cowgill, 'Black Aging in Cross-cultural Perspective'.

30 Cowgill, 'Black Aging in Cross-cultural Perspective'.

31 They (including Cowgill) were reviewing older work, including Cowgill's writings in the 1970s on modernisation theory.

32 Cowgill, 'Black Aging in Cross-cultural Perspective'.

33 In a conference held in 1987, these US sociologists were joined by Apt, an African sociologist from Ghana and Teitelbaum, an anthropologist, known for her work among the Kpelle in Liberia. See *conference proceedings* in Cowgill, *Aging in Cross-cultural Perspective* with contributions by Teitelbaum, 'Singing for Their Supper and Other Productive Work of African Elderly', and Apt, 'Aging in Africa'.

34 Ferguson, *Expectations of Modernity*.

35 International Center for Social Gerontology, *First International Course in Social Gerontology*.

36 Sauvy, 'The Passage from Activity to Inactivity'.

37 Sauvy, 'The Passage from Activity to Inactivity'.

38 International Center for Social Gerontology, *First International Course in Social Gerontology*, 9–10; UN-related comments by Van Zonneveld, 'Programs for the Aged', 119–21.

39 Roth, 'Mental Health Problems of the Aging and the Aged'. Loneliness, social segregation and stress were important themes that were raised as being associated with ageing in modern societies: 'Mental illness among the aged presents one of the clear examples of social stress, a new and significant theme in medicine. In particular "social isolation", which often recurs in the field of psychiatry in other contexts, offers a challenge for more precise definition and practical action. Here the aged pose the problem of loneliness, a major cause of unhappiness and ill health in modern society.'

40 For a reference to Sripati and a broader context to his career as founder of the Family Planning Association in India, see Matthew Connelly's discussion of population control and its multiple, complex political projects in 'Population Control Is History', 147.

41 Martin, 'Sripati Chandrasekar Dies at 83', *New York Times*, June 23, 2001, 11.

42 *Sripati Chandrasekhar Papers*, University of Toledo, *Statistics for Educational Planners*.

43 Chandrasekhar, 'Physical Efficiency'; Chandrasekhar, 'Convocation Address: Death Control', Poona, October 20, 1968, B27, F1, Sripati Chandrasekhar Papers.

44 These perspectives were influential in producing a wide range of social-work and development-focused writing based in Zimbabwe and South Africa. Dr Edwell Kaseke, Father Joseph Hampson's student, and the first non-Jesuit Principal of the School of Social Work in Harare (he was appointed in 1988, and he moved later to the University of Witwatersrand), was influenced by Hampson and worked on social security for vulnerable populations in South Africa. See Kaseke, 'Repositioning Social Workers in South Africa'; Lombard and Wairire, 'Developmental Social Work in South Africa and Kenya'; Patel, *Social Welfare & Social Development in South Africa*.

45 Hampson, *Old Age*. I have interviewed Father Joe Hampson several times and am deeply grateful for his inputs.

46 Hampson, *Old Age*, 10–11.

47 Dorman, *Understanding Zimbabwe*; Mamdani, 'State and Civil Society in Contemporary Africa', 49; Raftopoulos, 'Beyond the House of Hunger'; Charumbira, *Imagining a Nation*; Barnes, 'History Has to Play Its Role'; Ranger, 'Nationalist Historiography, Patriotic History and the History of the Nation'; Scarnecchia, *The Urban Roots of Democracy*; Thompson, *A History of South Africa*.

48 Dorman, *Understanding Zimbabwe*, 35–8.
49 Dorman, *Understanding Zimbabwe*, 35–8. In the current post-HIV context in Sub-Saharan Africa, ageing is affected not only by fertility but also by mortality and counter-transition effects (where epidemiological and demographic changes have been protracted and concurrent), and is further disguised by the impact of HIV/AIDS deaths on the age structure of the population as there are age pyramids that have been affected dramatically by the death of young adults and changed kin relations and living arrangements due to orphans.
50 Dorman, *Understanding Zimbabwe*, 68.
51 Fernandes is quoting Djurfeldt and Linberg's study, *Pills Against Poverty*. See De Souza and Fernandes, *Aging in South Asia*, 17.
52 De Souza and Fernandes, *Aging in South Asia*, 1–23; Fernandes, 'Aging in South Asia as Marginalization', 1–13.
53 Alwan et al., 'Monitoring and Surveillance of Chronic Non-communicable Diseases', 1853. ('the ageing of the populations of these countries will lead to a substantially increased overall number of deaths'); World Health Organization, *Preventing Chronic Diseases*; Mbanya et al., 'Mobilising the World for Chronic NCDs' ('The 9 million deaths such diseases cause in people younger than 60 years of age each year ... represent nothing less than a development emergency in slow motion').
54 Whitmarsh terms this 'regimes of compliance'. Whitmarsh, 'The Ascetic Subject of Compliance', 302–24.

Bibliography

Adamchak, Donald J. 'Aging in Sub-Saharan Africa: The Effects of Development on the Elderly', *Population and Environment*, 10 (3) (1989): 62–176.

Adamchak, Donald J. and Eugene A. Friedmann. 'Societal Aging and Generational Dependency Relationships: Problems of Measurement and Conceptualization', *Research on Aging*, 5 (1983): 319–38.

Alwan, Ala et al. 'Monitoring and Surveillance of Chronic Non-Communicable Diseases: Progress and Capacity in High-Burden Countries', *Lancet*, 376 (9755) (2010): 1861–8.

Apt, Nana A. 'Aging in Africa', *South African Journal of Gerontology*, 8 (1) (1999): 23–4.

Barnes, Teresa. 'History Has to Play Its Role: Constructions of Race and Reconciliation in Secondary School Historiography in Zimbabwe, 1980–2002', *Journal of Southern African Studies*, 33 (2007): 633–5

Bell, D. E. and L. C. Chen, 'Responding to Health Transitions: From Research to Action'. In *Health and Social Change in International Perspective*, edited by L. C. Chen, A. Kleinman, and N. C. Ware, 491–510. Cambridge, MA: Harvard University Press, 1994.

Breckenbridge, C. and P. Van Der Veer (eds.). *Orientalism and the Postcolonial Predicament: Perspectives on South Asia*. Philadelphia, PA: University of Pennsylvania Press, 1993.

Caldwell, John C. 'Toward a Restatement of Demographic Transition Theory', *Population and Development Review*, 2 (3/4) (1976): 321–66.

Caldwell, John C. 'Population Health in Transition', *Bulletin of the World Health Organization*, 79 (2001): 159–60.

Caldwell, John C. 'Major Questions in African Demographic History', *Population and Development Review*, 42 (2016): 343–58.

Caldwell, John, Pat Caldwell, and Pat Quiggin. 'The Social Context of AIDS in Sub-Saharan Africa', *Population and Development Review*, 15 (1989): 185–234

Chandrasekhar, Sripati. 'Physical Efficiency', *The Hindu*, 21 October 1963. In S. Chandrasekhar Private Papers, 1879–2001, MSS-189, University of Toledo.

Charumbira, Ruramisai. Imagining a Nation: History and Memory in Making Zimbabwe. Charlottesville and London: University of Virginia Press, 2015.

Cochran, Lillian T. and James M. O'Kane. 'Urbanization-Industrialization and the Theory of Demographic Transition', *The Pacific Sociological Review*, 20 (1977): 113–34.

Connelly, Matthew. 'Population Control Is History: New Perspectives on the International Campaign to Limit Population Growth', *Comparative Studies in Society and History*, 45 (1) (2003): 122–47.

Cooper, Frederick. 'Development, Modernization, and the Social Sciences in the Era of Decolonization: The Examples of British and French Africa', *Revue D'Histoires Des Sciences Humaines*, 1 (2004): 9–38.

Cowgill, Donald. 'The Aging of Populations and Societies', *Annals of the American Academy of Political and Social Science*, 415 (1974): 1–18.

Cowgill, D. 'Aging in Cross-Cultural Perspective: Africa and the Americas'. In *Aging in Cross-Cultural Perspective: Africa and the Americas*, edited by E. Gort, 110–32. New York: The Phelps Stokes Fund, 1988.

Cowgill, D. 'Black Aging in Cross-cultural Perspective', *Ageing International*, 15 (2) (1988): 39–41.

Cowgill, Donald O. and Holmes Lowell (eds.). *Aging and Modernization*. New York: Appleton-Century-Crofts, 1972.

Davis, Kingsley. 'The World Demographic Transition', *Annals of the American Academy of Political and Social Science*, 237 (1945).

Davis, Kingsley. 'Closing Speech: Focus on Cities Conference, 1968', 1968. 83035, Box 2, 495–6. Kingsley Davis Papers, Hoover Institution, Stanford, CA.

Davis, Kingsley. *Human Society*. New York: Macmillan, 1973.

Davis, Kingsley and J. W. Combs (eds.). *The Social and Biological Challenge of an Aging Population*. Proceedings of the Eastern States Health Conference, 31 March–1 April 1949. New York: Columbia University Press, 1950.

De Souza, Alfred and Walter Fernandes. *Aging in South Asia: Theoretical Issues and Policy Implications*. New Delhi, Indian Social Institute, 1982.

Dejung, Christof, David Motadel, and Jürgen Osterhammel. *The Global Bourgeoisie: The Rise of the Middle Classes in the Age of Empire*. Princeton, NJ: Princeton University Press, 2019.

Djurfeldt, Göran and Staffan Lindberg. *Pills Against Poverty: A Study of the Introduction of Western Medicine in a Tamil Village*. Scandinavian Institute of Asian Studies Monograph: Curzon Press, 1975.

Dorman, Sara R. *Understanding Zimbabwe: From Liberation to Authoritarianism*. Oxford and New York: Oxford University Press and Hurst, 2016.

Doyle, Shane. *Before HIV: Sexuality, Fertility and Mortality in East Africa, 1900–1980*. Oxford: Oxford University Press, 2013.

Escobar, Arturo. *Encountering Development: The Making and Unmaking of the Third World*. Princeton, NJ: Princeton University Press, 2012.

Ferguson, James. *Expectations of Modernity: Myths and Meanings of Urban Life on the Zambian Copperbelt*. Berkeley, CA: University of California Press, 1999.

Fernandes, Walter. 'Aging in South Asia as Marginalization'. In *Aging in South Asia: Theoretical Issues and Policy Implications*, edited by Alfred De Souza and Walter Fernandes, 1–24, New Delhi: Indian Social Institute, 1982.

Frederickson, George. *White Supremacy: A Comparative Study in American and South African History*. New York: Oxford University Press, 1981.

Frenk, Julio et al. 'Health Transition in Middle-income Countries: New Challenges for Health Care'. *Health Policy and Planning*, 4 (1) (1989): 29–39.

Frenk, Julio et al. 'Elements for a Theory of the Health Transition', *Health Transition Review*, 1 (1991): 21–8.

Gaylin, D. S. and J. Kates. 'Refocusing the Lens: Epidemiologic Transition Theory, Mortality Differentials, and the AIDS Pandemic', *Social Science and Medicine*, 44 (5) (1997): 609–21.

Geiger, Roger L. 'American Foundations and Academic Social Science, 1945–1960,' *Minerva* 26 (1988): 315–41.

Greenhalgh, Susan. 'The Social Construction of Population Science: An Intellectual, Institutional, and Political History of Twentieth-Century Demography', *Comparative Studies in Society and History*, 38 (1996): 26–66.

Haaga, John. 'What's Next for the Demography of Aging: A Symposium', *Population and Development Review*, 35 (2009): 323–30

Hampson, Joe. *Old Age: A Study of Aging in Zimbabwe*. Harare: Mambo Press, 1982.

Hodges, Sarah. *Contraception, Colonialism and Commerce: Birth Control in South India, 1920–40*. London: Routledge, 2008.

International Center for Social Gerontology, *First International Course in Social Gerontology*. Paris: International Center of Social Gerontology, 1970.

James, Clifford. 'Review of "Orientalism": History and Theory', *Studies in the Philosophy of History*, 19 (1980): 204–23.

Kaseke, E. 'Repositioning Social Workers in South Africa for a Developmental State', *International Social Work*, 60 (2) (2017): 470–8.
Kahn, K. et al. 'Mortality Trends in a New South Africa: Hard to Make a Fresh Start', *Scandinavian Journal of Public Health*, 69 (2007): 26–34.
Kirk, Dudley. 'Demographic Transition Theory', *Population Studies*, 50 (1996): 361–87.
Landry, Adolphe. *La Révolution Démographique*. Paris: Sirey, 1934.
Lee, Ronald D. and David S. Reher. 'Introduction: The Landscape of Demographic Transition and Its Aftermath', *Population and Development Review*, 7 (2011): 1–7.
Lombard, A. and G. Wairire. 'Developmental Social Work in South Africa and Kenya: Some Lessons from Africa', *The Social Work Practitioner Special Issue* (2010): 98–111.
Mamdani, Mahmood. 'State and Civil Society in Contemporary Africa: Reconceptualizing the Birth of State Nationalism and the Defeat of Popular Movements', *Africa Development*, 15 (1990): 47–70.
Martin, Douglas. 'Sripati Chandrasekar Dies at 83', *New York Times*, 23 June 2001.
Mbanya, Jean Claude et al. 'Mobilising the World for Chronic NCDs', *Lancet*, 377 (2011): 536–7.
Nandy, Ashis. *The Intimate Enemy: Loss and Recovery of Self under Colonialism*. Delhi: Oxford University Press, 1988.
Notestein, Frank W. 'Population: The Long View'. In *Food for the World*, edited by Theodore W. Schultz. Chicago, IL: University of Chicago Press, 1945.
Omran, Abdel. 'The Epidemiologic Transition: A Theory of the Epidemiology of Population Change, 1971', *Bulletin of the World Health Organization*, 2001 (republished), 79(2): 161–70.
Parker, John and Richard Reid (eds.). *The Oxford Handbook of Modern African History*. New York: Oxford University Press, 2013.
Patel, L. *Social Welfare & Social Development in South Africa*. Cape Town: Oxford University Press, 2005.
Raftopoulos, Brian. 'Beyond the House of Hunger: Democratic Struggle in Zimbabwe', *Review of African Political Economy*, 54 (1992): 64.
Ranger, Terence. 'Nationalist Historiography, Patriotic History and the History of the Nation: The Struggle over the Past in Zimbabwe', *Journal of Southern African Studies*, 30 (2) (2004): 215–34.
Riesman, David in collaboration with Reuel Denney and Nathan Glazer. *The Lonely Crowd: A Study of Changing American Character*. New Haven, CT: Yale University Press, 1950.
Roth, Martin. 'Mental Health Problems of the Aging and the Aged', *Bulletin of the World Health Organization*, 21 (1959): 527–61.
Sauvy, 'The Passage from Activity to Inactivity as it was in the Past and as it is Today'. In International Center for Social Gerontology, *First International Course in Social Gerontology*. NP, 1970: 48–9.
Scarnecchia, Timothy. *The Urban Roots of Democracy and Political Violence in Zimbabwe, Harare and Highfield, 1940–1964*. Rochester, NY: University of Rochester Press, 2008.
Sivaramakrishnan, Kavita. *As the World Ages: Rethinking a Demographic Crisis*. Cambridge, MA: Harvard University Press, 2018.
Sripati Chandrasekar Papers, 1879–2001, MSS-189, Ward N. Canaday Center, Toledo, OH.
Sripati Chandrasekhar Papers, Ward M. Canaday Center, University of Toledo, MSS-189, Series 8, Box 72, *Statistics for Educational Planners* (1965), 2.
Thompson, Leonard. *A History of South Africa*, 3rd edition. New Haven, CT: Yale University Press, 2001.
Tollman, S. M. et al. 'Reversal in Mortality Trends: Evidence from the Agincourt Field Site, South Africa, 1992–1995', *AIDS*, 13 (1999): 1091–7.
Treas, Judith and Barbara Logue. 'Economic Development and the Older Population', *Population and Development Review*, 12 (1986): 645–73.
United Nations Department of International Economic and Social Affairs. *World Population Trends and Policies: 1981 Monitoring Report, 2*. New York: United Nations, 1983.
Van Zonneveld, R. J. 'Programs for the Aged'. In *International Center for Social Gerontology, First International Course in Social Gerontology* (NP, 1970).
Weisz, George and Jesse Olszynko-Gryn. 'The Theory of Epidemiologic Transition: The Origins of a Citation Classic', *Journal of the History of Medicine & Allied Sciences*, 65 (3) (2010): 287–326.
Whitmarsh, Ian. 'The Ascetic Subject of Compliance: The Turn to Chronic Diseases in Global Health'. In *When People Come First: Critical Studies in Global Health*, edited by Joao Biehl and Adriana Petryna, 302–24, Princeton, NJ: Princeton University Press, 2013.
World Health Organization: *Preventing Chronic Diseases: A Vital Investment*. Geneva: WHO, 2005: 51.

3

Transition Theory, Health of the Mother and Epidemiology: An African Perspective

Shane Doyle

Introduction

Maternal health fits awkwardly within medical history, contemporary medical provision and epidemiological transition theory. Maternity is not a disease, yet it is one of the primary causes of death for women of reproductive age in much of the developing world; the lifetime risk of dying in pregnancy or childbirth for a woman from sub-Saharan Africa is one in thirty-six.[1] How maternal deaths have been defined has varied significantly over time, as the category expanded beyond deaths immediately connected to childbirth to include all deaths related to pregnancy and post-delivery complications within 42 days of a birth. Although the medical subfield is entitled maternal health, in Africa attention focuses heavily on maternal mortality, not morbidity. In addition, whereas maternity care was a medical priority for mission and secular medicine for much of the twentieth century, in recent decades maternal health across sub-Saharan Africa has been a secondary concern. Approximately a quarter of all international development aid in 1990 was designated for maternal healthcare; by 2017 this had fallen to around a twelfth, a decline unmatched among other health focus areas.

Since 2000 international aid has focused heavily on HIV/AIDS, malaria, tuberculosis, and newborn and child health. National governments and international agencies have recognised the relative neglect of maternal health so that, for example, the UN made reducing Maternal Mortality Ratios (MMRs) per 100,000 live births to 70 one of its Millennium Development Goals (MDGs). Kenya, like several other countries, has identified high maternal mortality as one of its national health priorities. But national interventions have frequently been underfunded and public facilities have suffered intense shortages of staff and supplies. Only two African countries (Cape Verde and Rwanda) achieved their MDG maternal mortality target; 18 experienced very slow or no change between 1990 and 2015, with, for example, Kenya's MMR falling from 687 to 510 during this period. Across sub-Saharan Africa as a whole, MMRs had fallen by 45 per cent by 2015, but were still 34 times higher than that recorded in Europe. Africans' experience of maternity appears to fit uncomfortably with narratives of progress.[2] Even within Abdel Omran's initial development of epidemiological transition theory, his discussion was less concerned with maternal morbidity and mortality per se than with the impact of women's illness or death during their reproductive years on overall levels of fertility.[3]

This chapter will suggest that the incongruity that characterises maternal health may also reveal particular flaws within theories of epidemiological transition. First, there exists the possibility that the recent identification of African divergence from a global maternal mortality norm of improvement is a statistical artifice, generated by the mass institutionalisation of delivery, rather than changing prevalence of morbidity and mortality per se. This hypothesis will be tested by examining the enormous decline in institutional maternal mortality in the 1950s and 1960s within East Africa. While this transformation seemingly fits the model of transition, it is possible that apparent improvements were a product of the rapid change in the frequency of institutional delivery which occurred over this period. It is necessary to consider whether there existed consistency over time related to whether patients felt particular conditions merited institutional care, and how such institutions recognised and recorded medical problems. If variation in the availability, accessibility and understanding of (potentially successful) treatment did exist, and if trends within individual institutions were affected by fluctuations in levels of referral, then it seems unlikely that such inconsistency will have been confined to the maternal field. The narratives of evolution which underlie epidemiological transition theory may then be based upon statistical trends that are partially misleading. Second, maternal mortality has been categorised by epidemiological transition theorists as one of the Group 1 (ancient) causes of death, alongside perinatal, communicable and nutritional mortality.[4] In recent years, however, medical researchers have focused on the growing incidence of maternal mortality attributed to non-communicable (Group 2) diseases.[5] Yet, while there exists a broad narrative of transition from maternal death due to infection or undermanaged risk, towards a pattern dominated by problems associated with chronic conditions such as diabetes or obesity, there is, within East Africa, extreme variation by region (and within region) in the causes of maternal mortality. The national trend is an aggregate of extremely diverse local trends, and generates a false impression of consistent, teleological change. Third, transition theory, in its later iterations, has tended to exaggerate the centrality of the present, the individual and the cohort. Yet, for some women, maternal health-seeking behaviours are influenced by corporate or discordant advice from senior kin, that is, in part by experiences and knowledge which date from one or two generations earlier.

Since the early twentieth century, maternal mortality has featured prominently, but never centrally, in Africa's 'epidemiological imagination'. As early colonial regimes emerged from their initial, existential struggles with outbreaks of sleeping sickness, smallpox and other contagions, maternal health symbolised European empires' self-proclaimed mission to move African societies towards a future defined by morality and rationality. Maternal deaths within communities were held up as the inevitable outcomes of indigenous ignorance, squalor or superstition. Preventing such 'waste' reflected a culture of governance shaped by the logics of national efficiency. Africa's colonial governments were typically pro-natalist, anxiously combating the perceived causes of supposed population decline, and dependent on social stability. Maternal deaths threatened these core goals, and helped to justify policies characterised by radical interventionism. In reality, however, the relative rarity of maternal mortality, and the limited efficacy of biomedical obstetrics before the 1950s, ensured that it was only one part of a package of medical problems that justified sweeping reform. Women were encouraged to attend ante-natal and post-natal clinics, mothercraft clubs and delivery suites out of risk-averting self-interest. But secular and mission medicine regarded maternal healthcare primarily as a vehicle to achieve other ends. These larger goals evolved over time, reflecting the changing ambitions of church and state before and after decolonisation. Between the wars, the reduction of infant mortality, the improvement of sexual morality and an increase in levels of fertility typically took priority. After 1945, attention shifted towards utilising maternal health provision as a means of stabilising marriage and addressing endemic childhood health problems such as malnutrition. After independence, new goals, including meeting international targets for childhood immunisation, monitoring and controlling HIV infection, and, in some cases, developing a new model of postcolonial citizenry, increasingly took precedence. Over this century of shifting goals, the moral politics of maternal mortality has evolved. Narratives of individual and communal failing have not disappeared, but they have been supplanted in recent decades by a rights-based discourse of governmental and medical neglect, within which maternal deaths have been portrayed as avoidable and emblematic of gendered and generational health inequalities.[6]

This chapter will illustrate how these broad themes played out in local contexts through an examination of two case studies. It will compare the recent history of Kisumu County, formerly part of Nyanza Province, in western Kenya, with the experiences of mid-twentieth-century Buganda, the region around Kampala in Central Uganda. These two societies, lying on the eastern and western shores of Lake Victoria/ Nyanza, were intimately linked in the mid-twentieth century by rail and steamer, migration and trade. At that time, both regarded themselves as educationally advanced, economically significant and politically crucial to their respective countries' futures. Both societies have experienced fluctuating fortunes since independence but, since the late 1960s, Kisumu has consistently defined itself as structurally marginalised, whereas Buganda has driven Uganda's economic resurgence since the late 1980s. The first part of the chapter focuses on Buganda during the middle decades of the twentieth century. This was a time when the rapid development of missionary and secular maternity units, in combination with the emergence of a cohort of research-oriented physicians linked to East Africa's first university at Makerere, created a body of archival material of exceptional richness. The chapter's later sections focus on Kisumu's more recent past, and draw on a series of interviews and focus groups to supplement a documentary record which has not yet been fully disciplined by the archivist's structuring of knowledge. In both cases, attention focuses on women's changing views and practices in relation to pregnancy and birthing. While epidemiological transition theory places emphasis on the role of lifestyle choices in shaping patterns of morbidity and mortality in the recent past, this chapter suggests that neither choice nor trends are straightforward phenomena. The past is not abandoned in the process of cultural shift, but is actively reimagined in the creation of new opportunities and constraints. Indigenous foodstuffs, for example, are redefined in relation to diabetes and hypertension; traditional birth attendants repackage themselves as nurturing companions in contrast to the technical impersonality of biomedical midwifery. Above all, the meaning of care is endlessly debated within societies experiencing the marketisation of health provision, the repurposing of families and peer groups, and the recategorisation of who and what is deserving and undeserving. Shifts in the values attached to care, and in its accessibility, underlie both what is recorded and how trends are shaped.

Measuring a transition

Since 1990 the UN has sought to standardise how maternal mortality is categorised and recorded around the world. That its major report on this project was subtitled 'Estimates by WHO, UNICEF, UNFPA, the World Bank and the United Nations Population Division' is suggestive of the multiple techniques used to measure MMRs, and their limitations. Most of the report focused on the difficulties in estimating MMRs rather than on discussing their causation. Indeed, only 18 per cent of African countries recorded data on maternal causes of death. Nonetheless, the report was able to state with some precision on page 1 that sub-Saharan Africa accounted for 62 per cent of global maternal mortality. On page 39 it stated that Kenya had made 'insufficient progress' since 1990, given that its recorded MMR had declined by only 17 per cent by 2013.[7] However, given that maternal health has been made a national priority over this period, with a series of high-profile policy innovations including the decision to make delivery in public units free, it is necessary to consider whether the changes in national MMRs should be taken at face value. To what extent might the popularisation of institutionalised childbirth have skewed the data on institutional maternal mortality?

To address this question, this chapter will begin by evaluating a body of historical data from East Africa, analysing the rapid decline in institutional maternal mortality seen in central Uganda from the late 1940s into the 1960s. Maternal mortality was reported to be extremely common in the kingdom of Buganda in the early twentieth century. European doctors, such as the great medical missionary Albert Cook, frequently bemoaned the huge loss of life associated with pregnancy and childbirth. Medical experts, typically employing rather dubious statistical evidence, associated reproductive failure with immorality and ignorance. It was often claimed that almost all Ganda were syphilitic, and that traditional birthing practices were unhygienic and dangerous to both mother and baby.[8] Arguing that the Ganda faced extinction unless their reproductive health improved, medical professionals enlisted the support of the missions and both colonial state and local chiefs in a campaign to press Ganda women to seek ante-natal guidance and to give birth in the clinic. By the early 1920s an impressive network of maternity centres had been created, but they were far from overwhelmed with eager new mothers. Rather, early reports indicate that initially the women who did seek their help were probably not very representative of the female population as a whole. One constituency consisted of the great and good of Ganda society, wives of chiefs and mission workers, for whom medicalised childbirth formed part of a package of demonstrated modernity and devotional Christianity. The majority of attendees though could be characterised as the desperate. It was common for doctors to comment on women's tragic reproductive histories. In 1919 at Mengo hospital one woman reported that she had had seven successive miscarriages. Another woman had had seven live births, but all her babies had died in infancy. Overall women attending the hospital in that year reported that 65 per cent of the children they had previously given birth to had already died.[9]

Between the wars, giving birth in the clinic grew only gradually in popularity. Maternity cases at Mengo in the 1930s were about 40 per cent higher than in the previous decade, a rate of increase far inferior to that of non-maternity medical attendances. This relative lack of enthusiasm among expectant mothers reflected in part the limited efficacy of biomedical maternity provision in Africa in this period. In Mengo between the wars the proportion of women who died during childbirth remained more or less constant at around 5,000 per 100,000. Neo-natal mortality among newborns fluctuated between 4 and 10 per cent. The proportion of babies which were stillborn meanwhile rose steadily from 9 per cent in 1919 to 14 per cent in 1939. All in all, these were grim statistics given that this was the leading maternity hospital in East Africa. Hospital maternity centres were regarded by many women with a degree of antagonism in this period. Women believed that being required to give birth while lying on your back was more painful than the traditional method, resting on all fours. Some resented the moral criticism they received when they were tested positive for syphilis – with good reason given that the consensus in the 1950s was that interwar STD testing was systematically inaccurate. And they associated the clinic with death.[10]

After the Second World War, however, the popularity of medicalised childbirth soared. The proportion of all births which took place in a medical facility in Buganda rose from approximately 20 per cent in 1947 to 30 per cent in 1958 and 40 per cent in 1967. No doubt the exceptional availability and visibility of maternity services facilitated the growth in attendances. As early as 1926 there were 19 maternity centres, state and mission, in rural Buganda. By 1959 Buganda had 969 maternity beds in 45 centres. Throughout Uganda an enormous expansion in ante-natal and mother and child services had begun in the early 1950s, successfully portraying institutionalised childbirth as a normal part of modern life, not something reserved for the elite or the despairing. Nsambya mission hospital in Kampala accordingly saw the number of deliveries increase by 600 per cent between 1954 and 1969.[11]

This expansion in both the demand for, and the provision of, medicalised childbirth coincided with a remarkable reduction in pregnancy-associated mortality, contrasting sharply with what has happened in Kenya since public maternity care was made free in 2013. Comparing outcomes from Kampala's mission hospitals in the decades before and after 1950, the proportion of babies that were stillborn fell from 13 to 3 per cent, neo-natal deaths fell from 8 per cent of all live births to 3 per cent, while the maternal mortality rate per 100,000 fell from c.4,500 to 500. Doctors at the time believed that the key innovations that facilitated this huge improvement in survivorship were the use of penicillin to reduce post-partum infection, the introduction of blood transfusions to respond to haemorrhage, and the adoption of the lower segment caesarean section and, subsequently, vacuum extraction to deal with cases of obstructed delivery and foetal distress. It is likely though that a steady increase in birthweights over this period would also have played a role in increasing babies' robustness, while Buganda's educational advantages meant that adult female literacy had reached 36 per cent by the 1950s, greatly enhancing the likelihood that women would be able to look after their health during pregnancy.[12] This would seem then to reinforce the argument developed in Simon Szreter's chapter, that focused medical interventions, supported by the state or religious institutions, can have very rapid effects on morbidity and mortality, particularly where technological change broadly aligns with social change.

Yet there remains the very real possibility that this apparent improvement in outcomes in Buganda was simply a function of changes in the population at risk. It is conceivable that a lower proportion of women and babies died during and immediately after assisted childbirth because hospitals were suddenly swamped with normal women, rather than those with tragic reproductive histories or chronic poor health. This factor must have had some impact on the outcomes, but there are several approaches which indicate that survivorship probably did improve significantly during the later colonial period.

The first is that Mengo and Nsambya from the 1920s through to the 1960s served as referral hospitals for a network of rural maternity centres scattered across Buganda. Frequent references to referrals within the maternity registers indicate that this referral system was still fully functional – if anything it is likely that it operated more effectively given the huge expansion in ante-natal care that began in the 1940s. Women who were identified as high risk because of their history or stature were despatched to Kampala for expert assistance. That this system worked well is indicated by data from the 1930s which showed the rural mission centres achieving rates of stillbirth and neo-natal and maternal mortality that matched those of England and Wales – an exceptional performance, but one achieved in large part by the rapid despatch of any abnormal cases. Yet survival rates at the rural centres declined three times more slowly through the 1950s and 60s than in the Kampala referral hospitals, suggesting that it was technical improvements in care at the higher level units which lowered mortality rates.[13]

The second method which can be employed to evaluate to what degree the decline in recorded institutional mortality rates reflected actual trends is to examine cause-specific mortality. If patients with the same condition experienced declining mortality rates over time, then that could suggest that specific medical interventions were reducing maternal deaths overall. The best example to use is the treatment of obstructed delivery. Buganda was famous in obstetric circles during the colonial period for having the highest recorded rates of obstructed delivery, and of mortality relating to it, in the world. In the 1930s it was found that an unusually large proportion, 18 per cent, of Ganda women had compressed pelvises, probably due to childhood malnutrition. Overall the average Ganda pelvic outlet was 14 per cent smaller than that of women in England and Wales, yet the average foetal skull was only 5 per cent smaller. It seems that the improved diet and health of small-framed women had resulted in a sharp increase in birthweights, and therefore in the size of babies' skulls, provoking a situation where disproportion was endemic. Maternal exhaustion and uterine rupture, followed by shock, haemorrhage and infection, meant that disproportion was the most important cause of maternal death and stillbirth in Uganda's hospitals before the 1950s. Surgical interventions between the wars were notable for their lack of success. Babies stillborn due to cranial injury following the use of forceps appeared in the registers with depressing regularity. By the 1950s the crisis had eased. The average Ganda pelvis was now 14 per cent bigger than it had been in the early twentieth century. Better nutrition in utero had been sustained through to adulthood. As babies' birthweights had only increased by 4 per cent, the frequency of disproportion reduced but, just as importantly, the medical response to the problem improved radically. Women of small stature were automatically identified during ante-natal checks as requiring assisted delivery, while the introduction of the lower segment caesarean section in the 1950s, and vacuum extraction in the 1960s, resulted in the proportion of ruptured uterus cases in Kampala ending in maternal death falling from 90 per cent in 1951 to 29 per cent in 1959. Much of the improvement in survival rates in this period then was due to enhanced treatment for this one condition, which was only indirectly affected by the general expansion of maternity care.[14]

How does this historical perspective shape our understanding of Kenya's MMR situation of recent decades? It is of course risky to compare institutional MMRs from different countries and periods. Intense pressure on bedspace in Kisumu's referral hospitals since delivery was made free to the user has led to patients being discharged a few hours after being delivered, fostering the impression that the current system prioritises quantity over quality. By contrast, in the 1960s, patients were typically retained for a day. Therefore, the likelihood that a maternal death would occur in hospital today is lowered simply because the period of risk has been reduced. Moreover, cultures of data recording may also have fluctuated over time. It is possible that the recent shift towards performance-related funding would encourage the false recording of (successful) admissions into the medical system. Whether such motivations would affect maternity cases, given the exceptional detail required for maternity admissions, including cross-referencing to carefully monitored data such as HIV status, is uncertain. What seems more likely, as suggested in various conversations with Kisumu senior medical staff, is that the attempt to reduce maternal mortality by implementing intensive reviews of each institutional death, as well as growing community anger at the frequency of maternal death, had encouraged staff at lower-level institutions to pass patients with complications up the referral chain, even where a transfer was not in the patient's best interests. The desire to avoid responsibility for maternal mortality, in other words, acted to increase MMRs overall, but particularly in the referral hospitals. Referral, moreover, is also more likely to occur where complications relating to a non-communicable disease (NCD) are present. The increasing perception among high-level specialists that NCDs are on the rise may reflect a referral system of increasing efficiency rather than radically changing prevalence.[15] There are therefore forces at work skewing institutional rates in different directions, making assumptions about epidemiological transition over time problematic.

Nonetheless, it does seem striking that institutional MMRs in Kenya's major referral hospitals during this decade are similar to, or higher than, those recorded in Uganda's referral hospitals in the 1960s. Kenyatta National Hospital's MMR in 2017–18 was 700 per 100,000. National rates, too, may have fluctuated to some degree since 1990 in East Africa, but they are not substantially lower than the figures from the 1960s. If these figures are comparable, then their congruity is unusual. Indeed, since 2000 in Kenya, MMRs and the intimately related Neonatal Mortality Rate have declined much more slowly than other major health indicators. Strikingly, for example, Kenya's Crude Death Rate is now lower than Europe's.[16] While maternal mortality may be revealing, it is important to note that it may not be representative of wider statistical trends. But the relative exceptionalism of maternal health trends is suggestive of gendered disadvantage, a phenomenon characteristic of more extreme 'counter transitions'.[17]

NCDs and maternal mortality

Epidemiological transition theorists tend to assume that their model of change is universally applicable. Societies, it is argued, tend to move in the same direction, both in comparative terms and with regard to internal consistency. It is more the pace of change on which scholars have focused, since Omran first identified three models of transition: the classical western, the accelerated, and the delayed.[18] It is natural that the measurement of progress or regress in health indicators is organised by the nation-state. The nation-state legitimises itself in part by its capacity to assemble data, which can be used to evaluate its position in regard to its peers. Yet the internal representativeness of data compiled at the level of the nation-state is not the same everywhere. While the nation-state emerged in Europe several centuries ago as part of a project aimed at the achievement of domestic cohesion, rarely have pressures towards cultural homogenisation been sustained for long in sub-Saharan Africa. Given Africa's exceptional ethnic diversity, and the extreme regional inequality of socioeconomic development which is part of its colonial legacy, there exists a fundamental flaw in the national statistics used by governments and international agencies to measure changes in health trends. In Uganda, for example, 43 indigenous languages are spoken, and regional variation from the national mean is extreme. Thus, in 2017, the per capita share of GDP in that country's wealthiest region, South Central Uganda, was 10.9 times higher than in the region of Karamoja, where 61 per cent of the population lived in absolute poverty. In 2016 female literacy across Uganda also varied sharply, again from highs of 92 per cent in Kampala and 82 per cent in South Central to a low of 18 per cent in Karamoja.[19] In most African countries a national average is an amalgam of wildly fluctuating local rates and trends. Relatively few regions are located near the mean, so that there exists little real sense of a norm in relation to a range of indicators. This is as true of measurements of health and demography as it is of social and economic development. Thus in Kenya, for example, the 2014 DHS report indicated that the national Total Fertility Rate was 3.9, but local rates ranged widely from Kirinyaga's 2.3 births per woman to Wajir's 7.8. HIV prevalence averaged 6 per cent but ranged from 0.4 per cent in Wajir to 26 per cent in Homa Bay. Childhood diarrhoea averaged 15 per cent but ranged from 3 per cent to 28 per cent.[20] And in terms of maternal mortality ratios in 2010 Kenya's national average was 495 deaths per 100,000 births, but the range varied from Mandera's enormous 3,795 to Nairobi's 160. If the timing of maternal mortality is considered, again major differences can be seen, with post-partum mortality accounting for 43 per cent of all maternal deaths in Nyanza Region, but only 15 per cent in Northeastern Kenya. Even if these internal differences were ignored, it would be difficult to derive any sense of transition from reported national MMRs, which fell from 590 per 100,000 in 1990 down to 414 in 2003, but then rose to 495 in 2010.[21]

Policymakers in Kenya are well aware of these extremes, and the impossibility of developing national plans which can encompass the range of situations found across the country. 'Mandera and Kirinyaga are like two different countries' was how one demographic advisor to the Kenyan government put it.[22] Yet national plans are required, and within Kenya's policy on maternal health, growing emphasis has been placed on the risks associated with NCDs, particularly diabetes, hypertension and obesity.[23]

The increasing significance of NCDs in Africa should not be ignored, and they remain under-researched and underfunded in a continent where the structural primacy of infectious disease continues.[24] With specific reference to maternal mortality, NCDs such as anaemia, cardio-vascular conditions and diabetes are implicated in increasing numbers of pregnancy-related deaths across the global south, with obesity identified as an underlying factor of growing significance. Moreover, women of African descent suffer disproportionately from pre-eclampsia compared to those from other parts of the world.[25] It should be noted though that, where NCDs do affect maternal health, their manifestation is often indicated as an episode of crisis, rather than chronic illness, further complicating visions of transition. It is also necessary to consider whether the perception that changes in diet and lifestyle have fundamentally altered patterns of morbidity and mortality has, to some degree, deflected attention away from pre-existing, perhaps more mundane, causes of maternal illness and death. It is not unusual in western Kenya for people to initially emphasise that the local diet used to be extremely healthy when asked why maternal deaths occur. Contamination of foodstuffs and rising consumption of processed staples are significant health risks in Kenya but, in this region, the incidence of obesity and diabetes among women is relatively low (6.8 per cent and 0.7 per cent, far below the national rates), and hypertensive disorders are important but not the primary causes of maternal mortality. Nyanza region had the second-lowest level of hypertension among women of reproductive age in Kenya in 2014. Moreover, eclampsia and pre-eclampsia are the result of a range of factors, including genetic predisposition and stress.[26] To consider stress as a fundamentally modern phenomenon is problematic in itself; to assume that causes of stress during pregnancy are universal is even more dubious. Pregnancy in western Kenya is often the factor which leads to women discovering they are HIV positive; it is commonly expected that women continue with their normal work until childbirth; verbal and physical abuse of maternity patients is far from unusual; and most women know that emergency medical care is of uneven quality and availability. To go into labour at night when it is raining, a far from unusual situation, in many cases makes transportation impossible. In recent research Jane Plastow asked dozens of women near Kisumu what their emotional response was to their most recent pregnancy; almost all reported fear and anxiety.[27]

This tendency to highlight NCDs is not confined to popular discourse. Opportunities for specialism, advancement and research funding shape policy and practice. So, too, do the patterns of morbidity observed in research-oriented referral hospitals. The finding that hypertensive disorders were the primary cause of death at Kenyatta National Hospital has been interpreted by Kenya's leading obstetricians as an indication of a major shift from haemorrhage to eclampsia/pre-eclampsia reflecting underlying change in morbidity patterns and improvements in the treatment of severe bleeding. Country-wide statistics which show that this transition is confined to the institution at the apex of the national referral system are acknowledged, but not with the enthusiasm reserved for the new.[28]

This intellectual interest in the emerging problem of NCDs among maternal health experts contrasts with the assumption among the broader elite of Nairobi that high maternal mortality among the Luo was simply a product of HIV, poverty and what is perceived as a stubborn traditionalism, reinforced by low educational standards.[29] Such assumptions broadly tally with what are categorised as indirect causes of maternal death, which undoubtedly do play a role in the former Nyanza region's high MMRs. In 2013, for example, HIV was implicated in a third of all maternal deaths in one study in rural Nyanza. Arguably, it was the catastrophic scale of the HIV epidemic which turned Luo culture inwards, and certainly in the past the Luo were among Kenya's best-educated ethnic groups. Despite decades of impoverishment in terms of income and public school provision, the former Nyanza region falls in the middle rather than at the bottom of Kenya's education scale. This false sense of unchanging 'backwardness' distracts attention from a core issue within the current crisis of high maternal mortality ratios: why has substantial investment in maternal health since 2010 seemingly not reduced mortality rates more significantly? How should the similarity in institutional maternal mortality rates in the recent past to those recorded in East Africa 40 to 60 years ago be understood? Are such medical data comparable over time, and if so, how should this apparent consistency be interpreted?[30]

Epidemiological transition theory, the present and the individual

Epidemiological transition theorists have often made assumptions about disease risk, patterns and interventions which exaggerate the centrality of the current period, the autonomy of the individual or the capacity of a cohort to act in social isolation. Such suppositions were not expressed overtly in Omran's original 1971 statement, although they were implicit in his theory's deterministic logic, and his reference to the impact of modernisation on 'national and individual aspirations'. In Omran's later writings, however, his analysis of epidemiological change moved beyond the societal level, noting variation by large social categories, such as class, age group, gender or ethnicity, and associating the introduction of female schooling with enhanced childcare.[31] Still, it is in the writings of other scholars that what was implicit in Omran's work has been more fully drawn out. Assessments of the factors which put individuals at risk of developing specific NCDs have placed heavy emphasis on individual life choices such as smoking, unhealthy diets and lack of exercise. Mental illness, suicide, substance abuse, cirrhosis of the liver and other conditions have been labelled as socio-pathological and lifestyle-related by scholars such as Rogers and Hackenberg. This stress on individual action (or inaction) has been accompanied by a recognition that individual risk is shaped by socioeconomic context, with, for example, the sharp declines in heart disease and stroke observed in various Northern societies in recent decades being much more evident among groups of higher social status. Scholars such as Salomon and Murray have modelled how variation in income levels shapes mortality levels by cohort over the life course.[32]

This is not to deny that factors such as income, education or employment significantly influence an individual's health status. However, for some women in East Africa maternal health-seeking behaviours are influenced by mothers, aunts or mothers-in-law, or their own or their partner's grandmothers or great-aunts. Receiving information about maternal health from traditional birth attendants (TBAs), who are often elderly women, also remains extremely common. This engagement with the elderly seems to occur less often among women who are well-educated and relatively financially stable, where peer groups seem to carry more influence, but even among such relatively autonomous women the role of elders is frequently significant.[33] In other words, the response to medical problems in the present is in some cases shaped partly by experiences and knowledge which date from one or two generations ago.

The durability of beliefs and attitudes around maternity is perhaps unsurprising, given how emotionally and physically extreme experiences of childbirth typically are. During interviews, very elderly women could relate the story of their first births, which occurred sometimes six or seven decades previously, in great detail.[34] For women who had very negative experiences, lessons learned were to be shared, not retained. One woman recounted how one evening, at the age of 16, she went to the regional referral hospital as soon as her labour pains started. On admission she was told she was not yet ready to deliver and should wait. No-one attended her through the night – the informant believed the nurses were sleeping – even when she called for help as her contractions strengthened. Only when she was in the final stages of childbirth did her screams attract attention, and her baby was delivered by a nurse-midwife. As the terror of the night subsided, the morning brought intense resentment. She resolved that she would never deliver again in a hospital, and shared her experiences with her own daughters, warning them of the dangers of putting themselves in the care of those viewed as uncaring.[35]

Even more common than the sharing of narratives of neglect is the recounting of stories of abuse. Elderly grandmothers contrasted their experiences of childbirth supervised by a TBA with those where they had been institutionalised. In these morality tales, TBAs comforted and reassured women, whereas nurse-midwives humiliated those who failed to fit their model of the ideal mother. Recurring themes included accounts of nurse-midwives slapping and pinching women who made too much noise during contractions, complaining that village women smelt 'bushy', and questioning the sexual self-control of both very young and very old mothers. Many women reported that when they asked for attention during labour, nurse-midwives asked if they had needed their help on the night they had conceived.[36] Of course, not all women had negative experiences of medicalised childbirth in the past. But even some of these women used their positive memories to counsel their daughters and granddaughters about the risks of attending the clinic. Within this cohort it was generally agreed that nursing staff in the past had typically been conscientious and that 'only a few bad ones' abused patients. Today, by contrast, elders held that rudeness and carelessness had become the norm. Nursing, it was agreed, was no longer a calling, but a job for those who had nothing else to do.[37]

Such intergenerational transfer of wisdom is not always welcomed, and even where its relevance is acknowledged, pregnant women in western Kenya do not necessarily follow the advice given. Since the Kenyan government made delivery in public hospitals (technically) free in 2013, the proportion of women who give birth in a medical unit has risen by 20 per cent, and more than 90 per cent of women attend an ante-natal clinic at least once. But these statistics convey a false sense of compliance, or indeed transition. Many younger women who engage with maternity services do so reluctantly. They attend ante-natal only once, to be registered in the system, because they know they might otherwise be refused admission to the delivery ward should their homebirth develop complications. Some fail to attend the recommended post-natal checkups, deterred by their own negative experiences of the maternal healthcare system.[38] Elderly TBAs reported that, while they were no longer called upon so frequently to assist during childbirth, their services during pregnancy were as popular as ever. That most of these services were nurturing (reassurance, counselling, massage) is indicative of the perceived failings of the biomedical system, which help explain why patient engagement with it is often limited.[39]

The repurposing of the TBA is suggestive of some of the complexities at play in the evolution of narratives and support mechanisms around reproduction in western Kenya. Elderly informants tend to highlight the tenderness of the TBA for the purpose of condemning the coldness of the biomedical professional. When elderly women were asked to tell their own birth stories, it was not unusual for TBAs to be presented in a different light. Luo women might have been relatively cosseted during their pregnancies, but delivery itself was defined as an opportunity to demonstrate both physical and emotional endurance. TBAs' role in part was to train Luo women to adopt the self-control of motherhood, by teaching them to avoid displaying fear or discomfort: 'the first birth is always painful; it just needs courage'. One informant remembered her treatment in the 1960s and 1970s, 'Well mine wasn't that bad since I was very strong. Some could abuse you, slap you and all sort of things.'[40] Since TBAs were forbidden from delivering women as part of Kenya's push for universal institutionalised delivery, they have redefined their roles, shifting away from discipline towards the provision of emotional and physical comfort. This has been accompanied by a monetisation of their services. In the past, the TBA was rewarded for her services with gifts of food or small stock. In recent years, theirs has been a cash-based service. Not all TBAs have managed these transitions effectively but, for those who have, their removal from the act of childbirth itself seemingly has not significantly affected their income levels. Some younger informants sought massage and counselling from TBAs every fortnight through their pregnancies, such that the most successful providers of these services struggled to manage demand.[41] The traditional birth attendant today is not so traditional. Narratives of change within the biomedical world should be considered in relation to the separate, but intersecting, evolution of 'traditional medicine'.[42]

While this chapter has so far argued that intergenerational influence challenges the linear assumptions which underpin transition theory, it is important to note that relationships between the generations are also subject to change. The sub-group which is most vulnerable to risk of maternal mortality today consists of adolescent girls. Teenage mothers are at risk not only because of their physiological immaturity, but also because of the lack of support they receive from medical staff *and* their senior kin. Kisumu County has one of the highest rates of teenage pregnancy in Kenya, which seems to have sharpened rather than reduced social condemnation. Very young mothers repeatedly report being mocked when they attended ante-natal clinics, by older mothers in the waiting area, and then by medical staff: 'Come and see this! A baby having a baby!' Teenage girls state that it is the norm for their fathers to beat and verbally abuse them, and often to drive them away. This is not because the age of sexual debut has changed significantly over the decades – in one focus group of six Luo grandmothers all had conceived by the age of seventeen – nor even that sex before marriage is a new phenomenon. But in the past only non-penetrative pre-marital sex was legitimate, and early marriage for girls was the norm. The age at marriage has risen, and *codo* (adolescent thigh sex) has been forgotten, but pre-marital conception remains much more of a taboo among the Luo than is the case in many other East African societies.[43]

In the past the role of guiding adolescent Luo girls towards womanhood typically fell to grandmothers, particularly where, as was often the case, girls moved from their parental home to live with their grandparents on reaching puberty. Grandmothers today feel sharply their failure to sustain this practice. From their perspective, young women have chosen to isolate themselves from familial support. A recurring theme of the elders' focus groups was that 'the world has turned sour because people have lost their morals.'[44] In grandmothers' narratives, that 'the world is nowadays rotten' was linked to their assertion that their granddaughters 'are digital so they don't ask [for guidance] … I haven't seen them coming'. In fact, further discussion revealed that conversations did occur, but seemed unproductive. 'These modern women can't be taught. [I just] tell them to go to the hospital because if I try to explain anything traditional to them then they get furious and can start war with you.' 'Sometimes you'd wonder what is up with the woman, she came when she's okay, later on you realize it is the chemicals they insert in their bodies.'[45] This reference to chemical imbalance relates to a larger sense of the inauthenticity of the young Luo woman related within elders' accounts. Several focus groups referred to the young as being digitized. The common use of contraceptive implants across Kenya was associated with a loss of personhood. 'What is more dangerous to our daughters-in-law, granddaughters and even you is the digitalisation of the world. These metals [implants] inserted in the body … And this metal also kills babies nowadays … The metal has a chemical that I don't understand how it works. It has been a cause of death amongst young women.' From elders' perspective, these women were lessened rather than enhanced by their bionic status. 'Nowadays, you see, your daughter-in-law is brought and she gives birth to only how many kids? One. Then she swears not to give birth again.'

This weak maternal instinct was, in grandmothers' eyes, often compounded by moral and physical inadequacy: 'you can find a woman with the metal [implant] in her arm and the husband is not even aware.' Then, if she does become pregnant, 'she is unable to give birth [naturally] and she is operated', because young women are too weak to push.[46] The insufficiency of the young was blamed, in part, on their bodily contamination by medicine and diet that was synthetic, convenient and therefore corrupting. 'Maybe it is what the young eat, and the medicine they take, but those days there weren't as many maternal deaths as today.' The healthfulness of the traditional lifestyle was contrasted repeatedly in interviews with that experienced by the young – farmwork rather than urbanity, herbal medicines rather than chemotherapeutics, boiled rather than fried food, millet not maize, porridge not tea, ghee instead of oil of doubtful provenance. Young women 'take light foods that can't strengthen them during birth. Sometimes you find the baby is heavier, therefore they lack the strength to push the baby.'[47]

It is not unique to Luoland, nor to the recent past, to find the elderly complaining of the corruption of the young in East Africa.[48] In this case, what elders observe is not a complete disengagement between the young and their seniors, nor the absolute individualisation of health-related decision-making. Rather, it seems to be more a shift from young women relying primarily on guidance from grandmothers, towards a greater engagement between adjoining generations. Until the mid-twentieth century, Luo women's lives were shaped by normative rules that sought to impose a degree of separation between post-pubescent girls and mothers. As one elderly informant remembered, 'When a girl was old enough to start her menstrual cycle then you were not allowed to sit on your mother's bed, not even in her bedroom for if the blood spilled on your mother's bed then it was believed that this may prevent the girl from being able to give birth. A girl was only allowed to sleep in her grandmother's hut who taught her everything.'[49] In recent years, according to female elders, they tend only to hear of their granddaughters' reproductive lives indirectly. 'Most of them, they only believe their mothers are the ones to help them.' 'Their mother is the one who can tell you.' Yet for all the agency that female elders believe young women to have, young mothers often presented a sharply different perspective during interviews. Rather than achieving autonomy over their bodies and the making of decisions about their health, marriage had placed them under the authority of their mothers-in-law. Recently pregnant Luo women asked by Jane Plastow to identify key themes for a community theatre production about maternal health stated that the change they desired most was a reduction in the extent to which their husbands' mothers controlled their reproductive lives. Not all young women feel able to express their resentment. Nurse-midwives frequently complained that young women of limited education felt unable to authorise medical interventions. One interview in a hospital was interrupted when the senior nurse was called to persuade a first-time mother that she did not need her mother-in-law's permission to have a caesarean section. As the nurse recounted afterwards, 'I explained that she had rights as an adult to make the decision. She said "Do I?" Still, I had to phone the mother-in-law and husband so she could hear them say it was OK.'[50] Reliance on elders' experience of maternal health has not disappeared, then, but nor is it an unchanging obstacle to the smooth transition towards some form of epidemiological modernity.

That individuals make health-related decisions following discussions with their relatives should not in itself be a cause for concern. A person's medical treatment often has implications for other family members, while navigating through Kenya's healthcare system without the benefit of lay experience is a difficult task. Maternal health is an especially complex sector within the medical system, as a series of policy changes have left many women unsure of their currently valid entitlements and choices. Rutenberg and Cotts Watkins have observed that women's desire for non-expert guidance in their reproductive health planning is above all a reflection on the often opaque, disengaged and generic nature of the medical information provided by health professionals.[51] But women do not always seek or desire guidance, and unsolicited familial instruction is less welcome than the requested sharing of peer experience. It is argued here that the cross-generational nature of familial advice-giving works against the logic of epidemiological transition theory. Focusing on shifts in medical technology or coverage is of more relevance for some health categories than others – for fields such as maternal health, societal attitudes and mechanisms of knowledge transmission are also key. Large-scale changes in 'development' indicators, such as the proportion of births attended by a medical professional, do not automatically translate into substantially different health patterns. Maternal mortality remains so high in western Kenya largely because of late diagnoses of, or responses to, emergencies. Some of these crises result from underlying diseases commonly associated with modernisation, such as diabetes, hypertension, and of course AIDS. Others can be linked to understaffing and under-resourcing. But an underappreciated factor seems to be the conflictual relationships, tying present to past, which shape childbirth for so many women.

Care has been contested throughout the past century, in terms of its meaning, provision and gatekeeping. Maternity presents health challenges which are measured out in a series of fixed, relatively short-term, consecutive phases – three trimesters of pregnancy, three stages of childbirth, and the six weeks of the post-partum period. But the monitoring of progress and management of risk is shaped not only by the immediacy of gestation and recovery, but also by longer-term narratives, shaped locally by perceptions of cultural change, and nationally by policy development influenced by notions of epidemiological transition.

Conclusion

Epidemiological transition theory, which emerged out of modernisation and demographic transition theories, argues that all societies will replicate the western transition from epidemics of infectious disease to a health pattern dominated by chronic, lifestyle conditions.[52] A series of important works have critiqued the epidemiological transition model, arguing that African experience does not fit a linear pattern of change. Notkola, Timaeus and Siiskonen, for example, offer an unusually detailed case study of falling mortality within one society. They note that the African 'transition' varied from the standard model both in the unusually high mortality among adults in the past, and in the resurgence of infectious disease since the 1980s, in the form of HIV/AIDS.[53] Whether the distinctive character of chronic disease in Africa, meanwhile, is best explained by ancient genetic adaptations to infectious disease, local socioeconomic adaptation to changes in food preparation and availability, or contemporary global inequalities remains as yet uncertain. But the theme of inequity applies beyond the realm of income and property, with Prince and Marsland, and Livingston illustrating how chronic conditions are neglected within a medical system which remains heavily focused on contagion. Livingston further challenges Omran's model by noting that chronic conditions in Africa often result from infection and criticising universalist epidemiological theories which underplay the significance of local contexts of disease causation and response.[54]

An analysis of maternal mortality reinforces many of these critiques, but it reminds us that adult mortality patterns are heavily gendered, and that NCDs are rapidly increasing in significance within high-level policy discussions. It also permits an engagement with epidemiological transition theory's emphasis on the role of cultural shift in the rise of NCDs, in the form of individual or cohort choices around lifestyle and consumption. Maternal healthcare is perhaps unusually shaped by local cultural assumptions, by intergenerational relations and knowledge transfer, and by group decision making.[55] But such factors are certainly not limited to pregnancy and childbirth.

A focus on maternal health also reinforces criticisms of depictions of epidemiological transition as a homogeneous global phenomenon.

But it further highlights the sharp divergence which can be observed in patterns of morbidity and mortality between different regions within many African countries. In the field of maternal health, extreme sub-national variation exists firstly in the timing of maternal death: whether this occurs most frequently during pregnancy, childbirth or the post-partum period. Secondly, while sub-Saharan Africa suffers the largest number of maternal deaths due to indirect causes in the world, within African countries different indirect causes dominate in different regions. In Kenya, for example, most indirect causes around Kisumu relate to infectious diseases such as HIV and malaria, whereas NCDs such as diabetes are dominant in the central region.[56]

An examination of maternal mortality over time, and as it is discussed between the generations, highlights other problematic aspects of epidemiological transition theory, such as its assumptions of a linear relationship between, for example, education and health attitudes, and that health-related decision making is best understood in terms of logic and rational choice.[57] In rural Kenya health options are often poorly explained, and what may appear as a choice may prove in practice to be unavailable. Patients, unsurprisingly, frequently seek, or receive, advice and reassurance elsewhere, often from senior kin. Sometimes such lay guidance aligns with current medical recommendations. Not uncommonly, however, lay advice reflects the experiences or moral codes of previous generations, challenging the idea of clear chronological progression which lies at the heart of epidemiological transition theory. Achieving good healthcare, therefore, requires negotiation in domestic but especially institutional settings. Personal networks as well as educational attainment influence how effectively individuals navigate through a highly complex system of healthcare provision, constantly remade through decentralisation, experiments with vouchers, 'free' care, and the incorporation, exclusion and repurposing of TBAs. Meanwhile the trust which underlies logic-based choice is, often, tentative. Reproductive health in Kenya is a subject of intense scepticism in many communities, where rumours of malintent and malpractice are recurrently, but ephemerally, challenged by public health interventions, from radio advertising campaigns to the provision of free goods to patients.[58] In contrast to the neatness of transitions, rumours disrupt the periodisation and localisation central to historical reconstruction. Moral narratives, like rumours, spread and survive shaping behaviours far from the time and place where lessons to be learned applied directly. Attitudes and behaviours are governed by moral debates as well as 'hard' data. Elders see changes differently from statisticians – they may recognise, for example, that AIDS mortality has fallen significantly, but HIV remains high and narratives of crisis and moral decline remain relevant. Equally, MMRs are unlikely to be higher today than half a century ago, yet they are highly publicised in the media now, they occur in public spaces rather than private homes, and again they are discussed within a moral framework of decadence. Clinical advances in societal health can be complicated by perceptions of societal decline.

Notes

1 This research was funded by the AHRC-MRC award 'Maternal Mortality in East Africa' (MC_PC_MR/R024502/1). Filippi et al., 'Levels and Causes of Maternal Mortality'.

2 Dieleman et al., 'Spending on Health and HIV/AIDS'; WHO, UNICEF, UNFPA, World Bank and United Nations Population Division, 'Trends in Maternal Mortality'; Alkema et al., 'Global, Regional, and National Levels and Trends in Maternal Mortality'.

3 Omran, 'The Epidemiologic Transition: A Theory'. See Weisz and Olszynko-Gryn, 'The Theory of Epidemiologic Transition', for discussion of Omran's use of epidemiological transition to promote population control. Omran did note that maternal mortality affected the relative risk of female survival over a woman's life course.

4 Murray and Lopez, *The Global Burden of Disease*.

5 See for example McCaw-Binns, 'Epidemiologic Transition in Maternal Mortality and Morbidity'.

6 Hunt, *A Colonial Lexicon of Birth Ritual*; Doyle, *Before HIV*; Prince, 'Introduction: Situating Health and the Public in Africa', 3.

7 WHO, UNICEF, UNFPA, World Bank and United Nations Population Division, 'Trends in Maternal Mortality'; UN, 'The Millennium Development Goals Report 2015'. In many African countries the quality of the data collection was so poor that little confidence should be placed in the precision of the reported change between 1990 and 2015. In Nigeria, for example, the point estimate for the relative reduction in MMR 'suggests a decrease of 39.6 per cent', according to one study. But the estimates generated with 80 per cent uncertainty intervals indicate that Nigeria's MMRs might have fallen by more than 80 per cent, or risen by 5 per cent; Alkema, 'Global, Regional, and National Levels'.

8 Cook, 'An Urgent Need in Uganda'; Lambkin, 'Mission to the Uganda Protectorate'; Cook, 'Obstetric Medicine in Uganda'; Cook, 'Recent History'; Uganda, 'Annual Medical Report, 1932'. For broader discussion see Tuck, 'Venereal Disease, Sexuality, and Society in Uganda'; Vaughan, *Curing their Ills*.

9 Cook, 'A Social Purity Campaign in Uganda'; Mengo Maternity Register for 1919; Musisi, 'Transformations of Baganda Women'. See also Summers, 'Intimate Colonialism'.

10 Mengo Maternity Registers 1919–39, Mengo Hospital Archive, Albert Cook Library, Mulago, Kampala; Interview (Int.) HW, Female (F), retired doctor, UK, 31 July 2008 (all interviewees were promised anonymity, so names have been changed and abbreviated); Billington, 'Neurosyphilis in Natives of East Africa', 32; Davies, 'Pathology of Central African Natives'; Davies, 'Causes of Death in African Children', 228; Doyle, *Before HIV*, 260–78.

11 Uganda Protectorate, *Annual Report of the Medical Department, 1947*; Uganda Protectorate, *Annual Report of the Medical Department, 1958*; Grech et al., 'Maternal Mortality in Uganda'; Buganda Annual Report 1926; Franciscan Missionary Sisters of Africa, 'The History of our Mission Work'.

12 Doyle, *Before HIV*, 273–5, 294, 302–4; Rendle Short, 'Causes of Maternal Death'; Everett, 'Causes of Stillbirth'; Grech, 'Review of the Treatment of Ruptured Uterus'.

13 Annual Medical Report Mengo District 1958; Grech et al., 'Maternal'; Nsambya Maternity Registers 1945–69; Nkokonjeru Maternity Registers 1954–69; Doyle, *Before HIV*, 262.

14 Rendle Short, 'Rupture of the Gravid Uterus'; Mengo Hospital Maternity Records, 'Report of the Lady Coryndon Maternity Training School'; Allbrook, 'Some Problems'; Billington, *A Tune*,

13, 92–7; Int. HW, F, retired doctor, UK, 31 July 2008; Rendle Short, 'Causes'; Everett, 'Causes'; Marasha, 'Causation and Prevention of Stillbirths and Postnatal Deaths', 20, 32; Akerele, 'Review of Present MCH Services', 23; Grech, 'Review', 508–15.

15 Workshop on Maternal Mortality in East Africa, Kisumu, 7 Aug. 2018. See also Adams' work on the sometimes deliberate miscategorisation of deaths. Adams, 'Saving Tibet?'

16 Workshop on Maternal Mortality; 'Statistics Kenya'.

17 Salomon and Murray, 'The Epidemiologic Transition Revisited', 207.

18 For an early statement, see Preston, *Mortality Patterns in National Populations*; Omran, 'The Epidemiologic Transition: A Theory of', 732. The possibility of divergence is emphasised by McMichael et al., 'Mortality Trends and Setbacks'.

19 Rafa et al., *Estimating District GDP in Uganda*, 13; Uganda Bureau of Statistics, 'Uganda Demographic and Health Survey 2016', 55. Kampala, Uganda's capital city, was excluded from these calculations. It contained the best-educated but not the wealthiest population.

20 Kenya National Bureau of Statistics, 'Kenya Demographic and Health Survey 2014'; National AIDS Control Council, Kenya HIV County Profiles 2016. See also Okiro, 'Estimates of Subnational Health Trends in Kenya'.

21 UNFPA, 'Burden of Maternal Mortality'; Muchemi et al., 'Trends in Health Facility Based Maternal Mortality', 259; Akhasakhala et al., 'Estimating Maternal Mortality in Kenya'.

22 Int. JA, M, Kisumu, 7 Aug. 2018.

23 Kenya National Bureau of Statistics, 'Women and Men in Kenya'.

24 Livingston, *Improvising Medicine*.

25 Say et al., 'Global Causes of Maternal Death'; Nakimuli et al., 'Pregnancy, Parturition and Preeclampsia'.

26 Focus Group Discussion Tura 1151, F, 19 Oct. 2018; Kenya National Bureau of Statistics, 'Kenya Demographic and Health Survey 2014', 178, 259; Anorlu et al., 'Risk Factors for Pre-eclampsia in Lagos'. In 2018 concerns around refined foods and contamination in the Kenyan diet converged with the revelation that the nation's sugar supply had been contaminated with mercury. *Daily Nation*, 'Contraband Sugar Contains Mercury'.

27 Personal communication, Jane Plastow.

28 Workshop on Maternal Mortality in East Africa.

29 Personal communication, CM and JA.

30 Desai et al., 'An Analysis of Pregnancy-Related Mortality'; Kenya National Bureau of Statistics, 'Kenya Demographic and Health Survey 2014', 26; Salomon and Murray, 'The Epidemiologic Transition Revisited'.

31 Omran, 'The Epidemiological Transition: A Theory of', 754; Omran, 'Epidemiological Transition: Theory'.

32 Rogers and Hackenberg, 'Extending Epidemiologic Transition Theory'; Murphy and Di Cesare, 'Use of an Age-Period-Cohort Model'; Salomon and Murray, 'The Epidemiologic Transition Revisited'.

33 Int. CMN, F, Nyeri, 11 Dec. 2017.

34 Focus Group Discussion, Konywera 1327, 12 Sept. 2019.

35 Focus Group Discussion 2, 9 Aug. 2018.

36 Focus Group Discussion, 29 July 2018; Focus Group Discussion 3, 9 Aug. 2018.

37 E.g. Focus Group Discussion 1, 9 Aug. 2018.

38 E.g. Focus Group Discussion, 2 Aug. 2018.

39 Focus Group Discussions 1 and 2, 7 Aug. 2018.

40 Focus Group Discussion, Central Bwanda Kabonyo Kanyagwal, 17 Sept. 2018.

41 Int. MAO 1328, F, Bondo, 16 Jan. 2019; Focus Group Discussion, Ahero, 4 July 2018. For discussion of the ebb and flow of institutionalised childbirth globally, see Adams et al., 'Alternative Accounting in Maternal and Infant Global Health', 280.

42 See Janzen, 'Ideologies and Institutions', 320.

43 Personal communication, Saudah Namyalo; Evans-Pritchard, 'Marriage Customs of the Luo of Kenya'; Doyle, *Before HIV*.

44 Focus Group Discussion Tura 1316, 27 Oct. 2018.

45 Focus Group Discussion Tura 1119, 27 Oct. 2018; Focus Group Discussion Kogony 1144, F, 29 Oct. 2018; Focus Group Discussion Central Bwanda Kabonyo Kanyagwal, F, 17 Sept. 2018.

46 Focus Group Discussion Central Bwanda Kabonyo Kanyagwal, 17 Sept. 2018.

47 Focus Group Discussion Tura 1119, 27 Oct. 2018; Focus Group Discussion Kogony 1144, 29 Oct. 2018; Focus Group Discussion Central Bwanda Kabonyo Kanyagwal, 17 Sept. 2018.

48 See for example Berman and Lonsdale, 'The Labors of "Muigwithania"'.
49 Focus Group Discussion Konywera 1327, F, 12 Sept. 2018; Focus Group Discussion Central Bwanda Kabonyo Kanyagwal, 17 Sept. 2018; Focus Group Discussion Tura 1119, 27 Oct. 2018. Even where informants agreed that grandmothers were designated as the primary source of information on womanhood in the past, they observed that following this norm was not always possible due to migration or mortality. Moreover, grandmothers were not granted exclusive rights of communication on reproductive and sexual morality, with various elderly informants reporting conversations in their adolescence with other senior relatives, including paternal uncles. Nor is the marginalisation of elders universal: one young woman whose mother had died and who had no aunts received advice on pregnancy from her grandmother. Int. SA, F, Tura, 27 Oct. 2018.
50 Focus Group Discussion Central Bwanda Kabonyo Kanyagwal, 17 Sept. 2018; Focus Group Discussion Tura 1119, 27 Oct. 2018; personal communication, Jane Plastow; Int. CO, F, Bondo, 23 May 2019.
51 Rutenberg and Cotts Watkins, 'The Buzz outside the Clinics'.
52 For a classic introduction see Omran, 'Epidemiologic Transition: Theory'.
53 Notkola et al., 'Impact on Mortality of the AIDS Epidemic'.
54 Cruickshank et al., 'Sick Genes'; Prince and Marsland, *Making and Unmaking Public Health*; Livingston, *Improvising*.
55 See Bledsoe, *Contingent Lives*; Boddy, *Wombs and Alien Spirits*; Hunt, *A Colonial Lexicon*; Johnson-Hanks, *Uncertain Honor.*
56 Say, 'Global Causes', e328.
57 Barrett et al., 'Emerging and Re-emerging Infectious Diseases'; Omran, 'The Epidemiological Transition: A Theory', 749.
58 Int. PO, F, Kisumu, 15 May 2019. On rumours and healthcare see White, 'They Could Make Their Victims Dull'.

Bibliography

Adams, Vincanne. 'Saving Tibet? An Inquiry into Modernity, Lies, Truths, and Beliefs', *Medical Anthropology*, 24 (1) (2005): 71–110.

Adams, Vincanne et al. 'Alternative Accounting in Maternal and Infant Global Health', *Global Public Health*, 11 (3) (2016): 276–94.

Akerele, C. Olayiwola. 'Review of Present MCH Services in West Mengo'. DPH dissertation, Makerere University, 1971.

Akhasakhala, Anne et al. 'Estimating Maternal Mortality in Kenya from Reported Households Deaths', last modified 29 July 2019, https://uaps2015.princeton.edu/papers/150239.

Alkema, Leontine et al. 'Global, Regional, and National Levels and Trends in Maternal Mortality between 1990 and 2015, with Scenario-based Projections to 2030: A Systematic Analysis by the UN Maternal Mortality Estimation Inter-Agency Group', *Lancet*, 387 (10017) (2016): 462–74.

Allbrook, David. 'Some Problems Associated with Pelvic Form and Size in the Ganda of East Africa', *The Journal of the Royal Anthropological Institute of Great Britain and Ireland*, 92 (1) (1962): 103–13.

Anorlu, Rose et al. 'Risk Factors for Pre-eclampsia in Lagos, Nigeria', *Australian and New Zealand Journal of Obstetrics and Gynaecology*, 45 (4) (2005): 278–82.

Annual Medical Report Mengo District 1958 (Albert Cook Archive, Kampala).

Barrett, Ronald, et al. 'Emerging and Re-emerging Infectious Diseases: The Third Epidemiologic Transition', *Annual Review of Anthropology*, 27 (1) (1998): 247–71.

Berman, Bruce and John Lonsdale. 'The Labors of "Muigwithania": Jomo Kenyatta as Author, 1928–45', *Research in African Literatures*, 29 (1) (1998): 16–42.

Billington, Roy. 'Neurosyphilis in Natives of East Africa'. MD dissertation, University of Cambridge, 1945.

Billington, Roy. *A Tune on Black and White Keys. Partnership in Healing: the Story of Mengo Hospital*. London: Janus, 1993.

Bledsoe, Caroline. *Contingent Lives: Fertility, Time, and Aging in West Africa*. Chicago, IL: University of Chicago Press, 2002.

Boddy, Janice. *Wombs and Alien Spirits: Women, Men and the Zar Cult in Northern Sudan*. Madison, WI: University of Wisconsin Press, 1989.

Buganda Annual Report 1926, Uganda National Archives, A46/428.

Cook, Albert. 'An Urgent Need in Uganda', *Mercy and Truth*, 12 (1908): 44–50.

Cook, Albert. 'Obstetric Medicine in Uganda', *British Medical Journal* 1 (2789) (1914): 1281–3.

Cook, Albert. 'A Social Purity Campaign in Uganda', *Mercy and Truth* 25 (1921): 271–98.

Cook, 'Recent History', Cook Archives, Mulago, Kampala, c.1933.

Cruickshank, John et al. 'Sick Genes, Sick Individuals or Sick Populations with Chronic Disease? The Emergence of Diabetes and High Blood Pressure in African-Origin Populations', *International Journal of Epidemiology* 30 (1) (2001): 111–17.

Daily Nation. 'Contraband Sugar Contains Mercury, Says Fred Matiang'i', 13 June 2018.

Davies, Jack. 'Pathology of Central African Natives: Mulago Hospital Post Mortem Studies', *East African Medical Journal*, 24 (8) (1947): 289–303.

Davies, Jack. 'Causes of Death in African Children', *East African Medical Journal*, 25 (1948): 228–35.

Desai, Meghna et al. 'An Analysis of Pregnancy-Related Mortality in the KEMRI/CDC Health and Demographic Surveillance System in Western Kenya', *PLoS ONE*, 8 (7) (2013): e68733.

Dieleman, Joseph et al. 'Spending on Health and HIV/AIDS: Domestic Health Spending and Development Assistance in 188 Countries, 1995–2015', *Lancet*, 391 (10132) (2018): 1799–1829.

Doyle, Shane. *Before HIV: Sexuality, Fertility and Mortality in East Africa, 1900–1980*. Oxford: Oxford University Press, 2013.

Evans-Pritchard, Edward. 'Marriage Customs of the Luo of Kenya', *Africa*, 20 (2) (1946): 132–42.

Everett, V. 'Causes of Stillbirth in Mulago Hospital, Kampala, and their Prevention', *Uganda Medical Journal*, 1 (1972): 45–7.

Filippi, Véronique et al. 'Levels and Causes of Maternal Mortality and Morbidity'. In *Reproductive, Maternal, Newborn, and Child Health: Disease Control Priorities*, 3rd edition, vol. 2, edited by Robert Black et al. Washington DC: The International Bank for Reconstruction and Development/The World Bank, 2016, https://www.ncbi.nlm.nih.gov/books/NBK361917/ doi: 10.1596/978-1-4648-0348-2_ch3.

Franciscan Missionary Sisters of Africa, 'The History of our Mission Work', Franciscan Missionary Sisters of Africa Archive, Dundalk, Box 6.

Grech, Edwin. 'Review of the Treatment of Ruptured Uterus at Mulago Hospital, Kampala', *East African Medical Journal*, 45 (7) (1968): 508–15.

Grech, Edwin et al. 'Maternal Mortality in Uganda', *International Journal of Gynaecology and Obstetrics*, 7 (6) (1969): 263–78.

Hunt, Nancy Rose. *A Colonial Lexicon of Birth Ritual, Medicalization and Mobility in the Congo*. Durham, NC: Duke University Press, 1999.

Janzen, John. 'Ideologies and Institutions in the Precolonial History of Equatorial African Therapeutic Systems', *Social Science & Medicine. Part B: Medical Anthropology*, 13 (4) (1979): 317–26.

Johnson-Hanks, Jennifer. *Uncertain Honor: Modern Motherhood in an African Crisis*. Chicago, IL: University of Chicago Press, 2006.

Kenya National Bureau of Statistics. 'Women and Men in Kenya: Facts and Figures 2017', last modified 1 September 2018, https://www.knbs.or.ke/download/women-men-kenya-facts-figures-2017/.

Kenya National Bureau of Statistics. 'Kenya Demographic and Health Survey 2014', last modified 31 July 2019, https://dhsprogram.com/pubs/pdf/fr308/fr308.pdf.

Lambkin, Francis. 'Mission to the Uganda Protectorate on the Prevalence of Venereal Diseases. Summary of Evidence', Dec. 1907, UK National Archives, CO/536/15.

Livingston, Julie. *Improvising Medicine: An African Oncology Ward in an Emerging Cancer Epidemic*. Durham, NC: Duke University Press, 2012.

Marasha, B. 'Causation and Prevention of Stillbirths and Postnatal Deaths at Mulago Hospital, 1970–71'. DPH dissertation, Makerere University, 1972–3.

McCaw-Binns, Alexander. 'Epidemiologic Transition in Maternal Mortality and Morbidity: New Challenges for Jamaica', *International Journal of Gynecology & Obstetrics*, 96 (3) (2007): 226–32.

McMichael, Anthony et al. 'Mortality Trends and Setbacks: Global Convergence or Divergence?', *Lancet*, 363 (9415) (2004): 1155–9.

Mengo Maternity Registers 1919–39, Mengo Hospital Archive, Albert Cook Library, Mulago, Kampala.

Mengo Hospital Maternity Records, 'Report of the Lady Coryndon Maternity Training School, Namirembe, 1932' (Albert Cook Archive).

Ministry of Health, 'Medical Services Statistical Records, 1959' (unpublished TS, Ministry of Health library, Kampala).

Muchemi, Onesmus et al. 'Trends in Health Facility Based Maternal Mortality in Central Region, Kenya: 2008–2012', *Pan African Medical Journal*, 23 (1) (2016).

Murphy, Michael and Mariachiara Di Cesare. 'Use of an Age-Period-Cohort Model to Reveal the Impact of Cigarette Smoking on Trends in Twentieth-Century Adult Cohort Mortality in England and Wales', *Population Studies*, 66 (3) (2012): 259–77.

Murray, Christopher and Alan Lopez. *The Global Burden of Disease*. Cambridge, MA: Harvard University Press, 1996.

Musisi, Nakanyike. 'Transformations of Baganda Women: From the Earliest Times to the Demise of the Kingdom in 1966'. PhD dissertation, University of Toronto, 1991.

Nakimuli, Annettee et al. 'Pregnancy, Parturition and Preeclampsia in Women of African Ancestry', *American Journal of Obstetrics and Gynecology*, 210 (6) (2014): 510–20.

National AIDS Control Council. Kenya HIV County Profiles 2016, last modified 26 July 2019, https://nacc.or.ke/wp-content/uploads/2016/12/Kenya-HIV-County-Profiles-2016.pdf.

Nkokonjeru Maternity Registers 1954–69, Nkokonjeru Hospital.

Notkola, Veijo et al. 'Impact on Mortality of the AIDS Epidemic in Northern Namibia Assessed Using Parish Registers', *AIDS*, 18 (7) (2004): 1061–5.

Nsambya Maternity Registers 1945–69, Nsambya Hospital, Kampala.

Okiro, Emelda. 'Estimates of Subnational Health Trends in Kenya.' *Lancet Global Health*, 7 (1) (2019): e8–9.

Omran, Abdel. 'Epidemiological Transition: Theory'. In *International Encyclopedia of Population*, vol. 1, edited by John Ross, 172–83. New York: The Free Press, 1982.

Omran, Abdel, 'The Epidemiologic Transition: A Theory of the Epidemiology of Population Change', *The Milbank Memorial Fund Quarterly*, 83 (4) (2005): 731–57 [first published in 49, no. 4 (1971): 509–38].

Preston, Samuel. *Mortality Patterns in National Populations: With Special Reference to Recorded Causes of Death*. New York: Academic Press, 1976.

Prince, Ruth. 'Introduction. Situating Health and the Public in Africa: Historical and Anthropological Perspectives'. In *Making and Unmaking Public Health in Africa*, edited by Ruth Prince and Rebecca Marsland, 1–54. Athens, OH: Ohio University Press, 2014.

Prince, Ruth and Rebecca Marsland (eds.). *Making and Unmaking Public Health in Africa*. Athens, OH: Ohio University Press, 2014.

Rafa, Mickey et al. *Estimating District GDP in Uganda*. Denver, CO: USAID, 2017.

Rendle Short, Coralie. 'Rupture of the Gravid Uterus in Uganda', *Obstetrics and Gynecology*, 79 (6) (1960): 1114–20.

Rendle Short, Coralie. 'Causes of Maternal Death among Africans in Kampala, Uganda', *British Journal of Obstetrics and Gynaecology*, 68 (1) (1961): 44–51.

Rogers, Richard and Robert Hackenberg. 'Extending Epidemiologic Transition Theory: A New Stage', *Social Biology*, 34 (3–4) (1987): 234–43.

Rutenberg, Naomi and Susan Cotts Watkins. 'The Buzz outside the Clinics: Conversations and Contraception in Nyanza Province, Kenya', *Studies in Family Planning*, 28 (4) (1997): 290–307.

Salomon, Joshua and Christopher Murray. 'The Epidemiologic Transition Revisited: Compositional Models for Causes of Death by Age and Sex', *Population and Development Review*, 28 (2) (2002): 205–28.

Say, Lale et al. 'Global Causes of Maternal Death: A WHO Systematic Analysis', *Lancet Global Health*, 2 (6) (2014): e323–33.

'Statistics Kenya', last modified 6 Aug. 2019, https://www.unicef.org/infobycountry/kenya_statistics.html.

Summers, Carol. 'Intimate Colonialism: The Imperial Production of Reproduction in Uganda, 1907–1925', *Signs*, 16 (4) (1991): 787–807.

Tuck, Michael, 'Venereal Disease, Sexuality, and Society in Uganda'. In *Sex, Sin and Suffering: Venereal Disease and European Society since 1870*, edited by Roger Davidson and Lesley Hall, 191–204. London: Routledge, 2001.

Uganda, 'Annual Medical Report, 1932', British Library, B.L.SPR.MicB, Group 5, Reel 28.
Uganda Bureau of Statistics. 'Uganda Demographic and Health Survey 2016', last modified 27 July 2019, https://dhsprogram.com/pubs/pdf/FR333/FR333.pdf.
Uganda Protectorate. *Annual Report of the Medical Department, 1947*. Entebbe: Government Printer, 1948.
Uganda Protectorate. *Annual Report of the Medical Department, 1958*. Entebbe: Government Printer, 1959.
UN. 'The Millennium Development Goals Report 2015': 43, last modified 23 September 2019, https://www.un.org/millenniumgoals/2015_MDG_Report/pdf/MDG%202015%20rev%20(July%201).pdf.
UNFPA. 'Burden of Maternal Mortality', last modified 30 April 2017, http://kenya.unfpa.org/news/counties-highest-burden-maternal-mortality.
Vaughan, Megan. *Curing their Ills: Colonial Power and African Illness*. Cambridge: Polity Press, 1991.
Weisz, George and Jesse Olszynko-Gryn. 'The Theory of Epidemiologic Transition: The Origins of a Citation Classic', *Journal of the History of Medicine and Allied Sciences*, 65 (3) (2009): 287–326.
White, Luise. '"They Could Make Their Victims Dull": Genders and Genres, Fantasies and Cures in Colonial Southern Uganda', *The American Historical Review*, 100 (5) (1995): 1379–402.
WHO, UNICEF, UNFPA, The World Bank and the United Nations Population Division. 'Trends in Maternal Mortality: 1990 to 2013', last modified 5 August 2019, https://www.who.int/reproductivehealth/publications/monitoring/maternal-mortality-2013/en/.

4

African Smoking Epidemic and Modernization Theory

David Reubi

Introduction

The critical role that epidemiologists and epidemiology play in global health today has been the focus of a growing body of work in the social sciences and humanities.[1] A lot of this work has been concerned with how epidemiologists have transformed the government of international health efforts over the last 30 years, from innovative techniques to calculate life to new forms of accountability.[2] In contrast to this work, the present chapter examines how political and social theories have shaped epidemiological imaginaries. A few scholars have started to explore this question.[3] The present chapter builds on this burgeoning body of work and examines how modernisation theory, which dominated the field of international development during decolonisation, informs the way epidemiologists and public health experts have imagined the African smoking epidemic.

The hold of modernisation theory on epidemiological and public health imaginaries dates back to the period between the early 1970s and the mid-1990s, when epidemiologists first mapped the incidence of, and attitudes to, smoking in Africa. I begin by charting the expert networks and quantification techniques that underpinned these early mapping efforts and outline how these efforts drew attention to the smoking epidemic spreading across the continent and brought to light a new social category: the African smoker. I then show how these experts drew on tropes associated with modernisation theory to analyse and narrate the epidemic, linking the rise of smoking in Africa with economic development and industrialisation as well as new urban lifestyles and female emancipation. Drawing on modernisation theory to make sense of the smoking epidemic, I also suggest, was not without consequences. First, it led epidemiologists to believe that tobacco use in Africa would necessarily increase as the continent modernised, mirroring the patterns previously recorded in the West. Second and somewhat ironically, it undermined modernisation theory by linking modernity and economic development with new forms of disease and death. Third, it distracted from the examination of the political economy and, especially, the role of the tobacco industry in the making of the smoking epidemic in Africa. To finish, I show how, despite contradictory data, modernisation theory continues today to inform how epidemiologists and global health experts imagine not just the smoking epidemic but also the wider transition from infectious to non-communicable diseases (NCDs) on the African continent.

Mapping the African smoking epidemic

Between the early 1970s and the mid-1990s, there was a growing number of efforts by physicians and epidemiologists to map the incidence of and the attitudes to smoking in sub-Saharan Africa. Many of these researchers worked in hospitals and medical faculties in large African cities like Abidjan, Cape Town, Lagos and Nairobi. For the most part, their interest in smoking stemmed from their own and others' research on the aetiology of cancer in Africa. This was a burgeoning area of medical research during the decolonisation period in Africa, with cancer registries established in many of the region's newly independent nation-states, studies published in leading cancer journals and international conferences organised across the continent. Informed by the tradition of geographical pathology championed by Oxford epidemiologist Richard Doll, this body of research sought to 'contribute to the knowledge of the causes of cancer' by comparing the incidence and types of the disease among populations living in 'different geographical circumstances and exposed to widely varying nutritional, social, economic and other environment factors'.[4] For those working within this tradition, the effect that seemingly rising smoking rates could have on the prevalence of lung cancer, which had hitherto been relatively uncommon across the region, was something worth studying.[5]

Besides these African-based researchers, and often collaborating with them, was a smaller group of physicians and epidemiologists working for the World Health Organization (WHO), international medical associations like the International Union against Tuberculosis and Lung Disease (UITLD) and the International Union against Cancer (UICC) or other research institutions in North America and Europe. Their contribution to the mapping of the African smoking epidemic was shaped by their work in the field of international tobacco control. At first, this field was fundamentally a North American and European affair, with smoking and smoking-related diseases deemed to be a problem that was exclusive to the rich, industrialised societies of the West. This changed from the late 1970s onwards, when public health experts realised that, with the tobacco industry working aggressively to establish new markets for its products outside North America and Europe, the smoking epidemic was quickly spreading to the Third World. This led to a reconfiguration of international tobacco control, with international efforts like the UICC Smoking and Lung Cancer Programme and the WHO Tobacco or Health Programme becoming all about educating doctors and political leaders in the developing world. The importance of knowing the prevalence of and attitudes to smoking, together with the epidemiological expertise to generate this knowledge, were critical to these efforts.[6]

Efforts to map the incidence of and attitudes to smoking in Africa were articulated around two major quantification techniques. The first of these techniques was the social survey. Most of the surveys conducted between the early 1970s and mid-1990s were small-scale and isolated efforts carried out by African-based physicians with some occasional help from international tobacco control experts and organisations. A good illustration is the surveys on smoking carried out by Professor Deji Femi-Pearse and his team at the Department of Medicine, University of Lagos, with the technical support of an eminent figure in the international tobacco control movement, Dr Charles Fletcher from the Royal College of Physicians.[7] Another example is the surveys conducted by Dr W. Lore from the Faculty of Medicine, University of Nairobi, for which he received financial support from the UICC and used one of the WHO's standard smoking questionnaires.[8] In addition to these small-scale, isolated surveys, larger, multi-country surveys began to be conducted in Africa from the late 1980s onwards. An early example was the smoking survey which Professor John Crofton in Edinburgh and his colleague Paul Fréour in Bordeaux coordinated for the UITLD in 42 countries, including five in sub-Saharan Africa.[9] The aim of these different surveys was to measure tobacco use and attitudes towards tobacco among Africans using questionnaires. For example, in their study of smoking habits in Abidjan, Dr D. Schmidt and his team at the Centre Hospitalier Universitaire de Treichville used a questionnaire to record participants' socioeconomic status, tobacco consumption, motivation to smoke and knowledge about the dangers of tobacco.[10] Sometimes, surveys also included physical examinations and histopathological tests in addition to questionnaires, as in Schonland and Bradshaw's work on smoking and lung cancer in Durban.[11] For the most part, surveys conducted during this period focused on social groups that were easily accessible and inexpensive to study – students in the medical faculty, children and teachers in local schools, patients at the city's main public hospital – but not representative of the whole population.[12]

The second major quantification method used in early efforts to map smoking in Africa was estimation techniques, which combined epidemiological modelling with the utilisation of existing data. The main example here is the WHO Tobacco or Health Programme. One of the aims of the Programme was to collect and publish reliable epidemiological information about the smoking epidemic in Africa and elsewhere. Efforts in this area began in the early 1980s but it was only after the arrival of Alan Lopez in the late 1980s, and as part of his work with Oxford epidemiologist Richard Peto on global estimates of smoking-attributable mortality, that they really picked up and became more systematic and sophisticated.[13] A key part of these efforts was to collect and assess the quality of existing data on smoking in Africa. This included: using diplomatic channels to request WHO member states to send their official data on smoking; examining the data on tobacco production, trade and consumption collated by the United Nations' Food and Agriculture Organisation (FAO), the World Bank and the US Department of Agriculture; and searching the scientific literature for any studies on smoking in Africa. Another key part of these efforts was to build epidemiological models of the smoking epidemic in order to compute reliable estimates about smoking prevalence where there was no data or where the existing data was inconsistent. It is as part of these efforts that Lopez and his colleagues articulated their influential model of the cigarette epidemic and produced the WHO's first *Tobacco or Health Global Status Report*.[14]

The picture of smoking in Africa that physicians and epidemiologists painted through their surveys and estimates seemed alarming. It showed that, as some had feared, the continent was in the grip of a serious and mounting epidemic. As Paul Fréour cautioned: 'today's Africa is faced with a smoking pandemic that is developing right in front of our eyes, just as in the Western world'.[15] To start with, drawing on the data collected by organisations like the FAO and the US Department of Agriculture, Fréour and others pointed out how cigarette consumption in sub-Saharan Africa was rapidly growing. Crofton, for example, warned that tobacco use in Africa was 'increasing at an alarming rate'.[16] Specifically, he noted that while 'global consumption had risen by 7 per cent between 1970 and 1985', African countries like Kenya and others had experienced 'formidable rises' of over 30 per cent.[17] In the same way, Professor Monteiro, a physician from Benin who had worked as a consultant for the WHO Tobacco or Health Programme and participated in the UITLD multi-country smoking survey, alerted his readers to 'the worrying rise in tobacco use' in Africa that would lead to 'so much human suffering, deaths and health expenses'.[18]

These physicians and epidemiologists also drew attention to the already disturbingly high smoking prevalence rates among men across the continent. In a report to the WHO Tobacco or Health Programme, a British public health expert stressed that, in Africa, it was 'rare to find less than 40 per cent of males regularly smoking'.[19] Similarly, Crofton pointed out in an article published in the *International Journal of Epidemiology* that, in most African countries, 'some 50 per cent of men are dependent on some form of tobacco use'.[20] The prevalence figures used by these experts came from the small-scale smoking surveys that were being carried out in cities across the region at the time. For example, Femi-Pearse and his colleagues' highly cited study of smoking in Lagos showed that about 40 per cent of adult men in the Nigerian city smoked on a regular basis.[21] These findings echoed those of Henri Baylet and his team in Dakar who reported that 50 per cent of the male population consumed cigarettes.[22] Similarly, a study of black factory workers in Johannesburg documented that over 60 per cent smoked, while a survey at Nairobi's Kenyatta National Hospital showed that 50 per cent of the male staff were regular tobacco users.[23]

It is important to point out that many health experts had doubts about the reliability of the epidemiological data on smoking in Africa, although this did not usually lead them to question the claim that the continent was in the grip of an epidemic. These doubts were fuelled by a variety of factors. First, many experts pointed to 'broad divergences' in recorded smoking prevalence rates that were 'difficult to explain'.[24] So, for example, in Nigeria, recorded prevalence for adult urban males ranged from as low as 7 per cent all the way up to 53 per cent for the same time period.[25] Similarly, in Senegal, recorded prevalence rates for adult urban males ranged from 43 per cent to an incredible 87 per cent.[26] Second, many experts felt that some of the prevalence rates recorded were excessively high compared to what they saw on the ground when travelling across Africa. One consultant who had worked for the UICC Smoking and Lung Cancer Program in Africa in the 1980s remembered in an interview with me that he and his colleagues 'always questioned smoking statistics in those days' as they showed 'much higher smoking rates than we would see in the field'. The usually lower prevalence rates of no more than 30 per cent among adult males that were recorded from the late 1980s onwards seem to corroborate these impressions. The UITLD multi-country smoking survey led by Crofton and Fréour, for example, counted about 20 per cent of smokers among male medical students in Benin, Kenya, Madagascar, Nigeria and Senegal.[27] Likewise, Lopez and his team estimated that, apart from richer countries like South Africa and Mauritius where rates were close to 50 per cent, smoking prevalence among males in sub-Saharan Africa was 'possibly as low as 25 per cent'.[28] Third, experts were acutely aware of the unreliability and tentativeness of much of the data on mortality and health coming out of Africa. Crofton, for example, was always keen to remind his readers that, when 'accessing the prevalence of smoking' in Africa, one 'should always appreciate the difficulty of having reliable and accurate statistics'.[29] Fourth and lastly, experts also stressed the absence of any epidemiological data on smoking for much of the African population. As Alan Lopez and his colleagues at the WHO explained, there is 'very little survey information available' on Africa, with 'reliable data on smoking prevalence' obtainable for no more than '33 per cent' of the continent's adult population.[30]

The African smoker

Besides drawing attention to and measuring the size of the tobacco epidemic spreading across Africa, physicians and epidemiologists also helped trace the contours of a new figure that had emerged with the epidemic – the African smoker. As Joe Pobee, an epidemiologist at the University of Ghana who had studied smoking patterns among civil servants in Accra, explained:

> The African smoker … is an urban male cigarette user who starts in adolescence … He is likely to belong to a lower socio-economic or to a high-income group, but he is likely to smoke more heavily

> if he belongs to the latter group … The female is not much of a smoker.[31]

As Pobee's quote makes clear, gender was a defining trait of this emerging figure of the African smoker. This was repeatedly commented upon by physicians and epidemiologists working in the field. For example, Derek Yach, a South African health expert who would later be critical of the adoption of the WHO's *Framework Convention on Tobacco Control*, and his colleagues at the Centre for Epidemiological Research in Cape Town explained: 'the strongest determinant of smoking [in Africa] is gender', with 'young girls and women smoking at very low level'.[32] Similarly, when discussing the results of their multi-country smoking survey, Fréour, Crofton and their team noted that 'the amount of smoking by women was very different in Europe and Africa', with the proportion of female smokers 'much lower' in the latter.[33] For researchers, the 'very low smoking rate among females' in Africa stemmed from 'socio-cultural factors'.[34] Specifically, they pointed out that most communities across the continent deemed smoking to be 'a very bad behavior for women', which was 'not ladylike' and 'linked with lax morals' and 'professionally promiscuous women'.[35] So, for example, researchers working on smoking among women in Kenya reported that:

> There was nearly universal agreement that it was not acceptable for women to smoke … [It was thought that] women who smoked were prostitutes or might become prostitutes to obtain the money needed to purchase cigarettes … [There was a belief that] women's cigarette smoking [was linked] with sexual promiscuity.[36]

Another, important characteristic of the African smoker besides gender was youth and urbanicity. As Crofton explained, the 'increase in smoking prevalence' in Africa happened 'especially in the young and especially in towns'.[37] In the minds of doctors and epidemiologists working on the issue, cities in Africa – characterised by rapid, chaotic growth; a young, often unemployed population fuelled by migration from the countryside; and new Western forms of living – represented an environment that was propitious to the smoking epidemic. Monteiro, for example, speaking about Cotonou in Benin, lamented that:

> With the introduction of Western customs, and all the attendant false values, young people in the cities imitating film heroes or advertising posters have begun to smoke on a large scale … [It is

> among] this rootless youth of the towns [that smoking has been on the rise in Africa].[38]

This was echoed by Paul Fréour, who believed that 'the new Western forms of smoking' (*le nouveau tabagisme à l'occidentale*) spreading across Africa were an 'urban form of smoking practised by young people' (*un tabagisme citadin, un tabagisme des jeunes*) who lived in the poor, sprawling 'shantytowns' (*bidonvilles*) found in most of the continent's cities.[39]

As the work of physicians and epidemiologists showed, these young, urban smokers started to use tobacco from a very young age. For example, surveys in townships in Cape Town conducted by Yach and his colleagues showed that 'schoolboys take up the smoking habit in their early teens' and that, 'by adulthood, over half of all men are smokers'.[40] For these young urban smokers, the preferred mode of tobacco use was smoking cigarettes rather than smoking pipes or chewing tobacco. As Baylet and his team noted in relation to their work on smoking habits among students at the University of Dakar: 'young people prefer to smoke cigarettes. To be cool in nightclubs or at the movies, you cannot chew tobacco or smoke the pipe.'[41] Similarly, speaking about black male workers in a factory near Johannesburg, Baker, Johnston and Turner reported that 'the younger generation is smoking more and more cigarettes, as opposed to pipes'.[42] Last but not least, the number of cigarettes consumed by these young, male smokers living in cities across the continent tended to be remarkably low. Alan Lopez and his team, for example, noted that 'the number of cigarettes smoked by daily smokers is a low of 10 per day in the African region'.[43] Likewise, Crofton pointed out that, 'because of poverty', smokers in Africa 'can only afford a few cigarettes per day'.[44]

Smoking and modernity

Modernisation theory came to dominate the field of international development and the government of political, economic and social life in Africa during the decolonisation period.[45] Modernisation theory was certainly not the preserve solely of development specialists in Western aid agencies and universities; it was also enthusiastically embraced by political leaders and intellectuals in Africa. As Frederick Cooper has argued, this enthusiasm stemmed from the possibility of change that modernisation theory seemed to encompass.[46] Indeed, while colonial administrators had imagined Africans as immutably fixed in race, customary laws and tribal structures, modernisation theorists believed that Africans could, through the process of development, free themselves from tradition and become, in the words of Swedish economist Gunnar Myrdal, 'new', 'modern men'.[47]

For modernisation theorists and their followers, tradition and modernity referred to societal forms that stood at opposite ends on the scale of human progress and were characterised by contrasting political, economic, social, technological and demographic traits.[48] Specifically, tradition was associated with the simple, rural societies believed to be typical of Africa and distinguished by: extended family and tribal structures where women had few rights and responsibilities outside the home; subsistence, agrarian economies with archaic production methods; residence in villages with poor, unsanitary living standards; fatalism, superstition and religion; as well as young populations with high fertility and low life expectancy. In contrast, modernity was coupled with the imagined advanced societies of North America and Europe characterised by: strong, centralised nation-states where women were educated and emancipated; market-based, industrialised economies centered around technological innovation and mass consumption; residence in cities with high living standards and consumer goods like automobiles and televisions; rationality, science and entrepreneurship; as well as older populations with low fertility and high life expectancy. In the dichotomous world of modernisation theory, the task of development experts and political leaders was to lead Africa's newly independent nations from poverty and tradition to economic growth and modernity by investing in large physical infrastructure and industrialisation projects.[49]

Modernisation theory had a clear influence on the epidemiologists and physicians who sought to map the incidence of and attitudes to smoking in Africa between the early 1970s and the mid-1990s. This influence can be seen in the way these epidemiologists and physicians drew on ideas and models of modernisation to analyse and explain the spread of the African smoking epidemic. To start with, many of them saw a strong causal relationship between industrialisation and economic growth on the one hand and smoking prevalence on the other hand. Femi-Pearse and his collaborators, for example, noted that because of the 'improved cash economy consequent upon industrialisation', 'smoking is on the increase' in many 'African towns'.[50] A case in point, they argued, was 'metropolitan Lagos' where 'the nation's foremost seaport' and over '70 per cent of the nation's industries were located'.[51] Hassam Gareebo at the Ministry of Health in Mauritius made a similar point in relation to their island-state, arguing that increases in smoking prevalence were 'due largely to the rapidly improved economic situation', with the 'economy having shifted from purely agricultural to mainly industrial'.[52] In a similar spirit, Bradshaw and Schonland noted that 'the phenomenal growth of industry in South Africa since the second world war' has 'created economic opportunities', with a 'huge number of African males' becoming 'wage earners' and adopting 'tobacco smoking'.[53] This was echoed by David Nostbakken, the lead of the UICC tobacco control efforts in Africa in the 1980s, who stated that 'economic prosperity and growth [are] important predictors of cigarette consumption' in the region, with 'evidence suggesting that per capita consumption increases as per capita income increases'.[54]

Epidemiologists and physicians working on tobacco in Africa also often associated rising smoking rates with urbanisation and the uptake of Western lifestyles on the continent. For example, drawing on his research on smoking in Senegal, d'Hondt suggested that there is a 'close relationship' between 'tobacco smoking and the growing adoption of Western values and ways of life concomitant with urbanisation'.[55] Similarly, Derek Yach thought that 'urbanisation [and] westernisation' have 'led to an increase in smoking in many African countries'.[56] Specifically, these epidemiologists and physicians believed that rural areas were associated with 'more primitive', 'traditional patterns of life' governed by 'local custom'.[57] People in these areas consumed tobacco but prevalence was low and forms of use were 'traditional' like pipe smoking and tobacco chewing.[58] By contrast, they associated cities with the loss of tradition and the adoption of a more 'advanced', 'Western manner of life'.[59] There, smoking prevalence was higher and took the form of the 'modern', 'industrial cigarette'.[60] So, after surveying and comparing smoking behaviours between 'urban subjects' (*les sujets urbanisés*) in Dakar and 'rural subjects living in customary villages' (*les ruraux des centres coutumiers*) in the Niakhar region of Senegal, Baylet and his team concluded that:

> Urbanisation has led to changes both in the forms of smoking, with people abandoning traditional forms and preferring cigarettes, and in smoking incidence, which is higher in the urban milieu. The urban subject who can afford cigarettes is often in a stronger economic position and has, therefore, taken up a more evolved way of life. With urbanisation, the Western mode of smoking has replaced the traditional form of smoking like the pipe and chewing.[61]

Similarly, McGlashan and Harington remarked that, in South Africa, as 'blacks' migrate from rural towns to 'major cities' for work, their 'exposure to Western customs' and 'urban lifestyles' like 'that of cigarette smoking' increases greatly.[62] Paul Fréour made a similar point for Africa in general:

> Besides traditional forms of smoking (*tabagisme traditionnel*), there are now Western forms of smoking (*tabagisme à l'occidentale*) which spread so rapidly that they represent a real epidemic. The drivers of these Western forms of smoking are industrially manufactured cigarettes (*la cigarette industrielle*) and the large number of young people who do not integrate well in the traditional economy and migrate to cities where they hope to find work and live a Western lifestyle (*vivre à l'occidentale*).[63]

Finally, epidemiologists and physicians also associated smoking patterns among African women with the shift from tradition to modernity in the region. They held that existing low smoking prevalence rates among African women were due to traditional sex roles, which imposed a range of restrictions on female behaviour, including the prohibition of tobacco use. As Waldron argued: 'traditional sex roles, including men's greater social power and generally greater restrictions on women's behavior, has contributed to widespread social pressures against women smoking'.[64] The few women who did smoke on the continent were deemed to be modern, educated and urban. For example, Simon Chapman, who worked for the UICC Smoking and Lung Cancer Programme in Africa, remarked that smoking among African women is generally 'confined to the small proportion who are culturally or economically elite'.[65] Similarly, Baylet and his collaborators noted that the few women who smoked in Senegal were 'very urbanised, young women' (*jeunes femmes très urbanisées*) and 'intellectuals' (*intellectuelles*) who 'contested what they saw as a limit to their liberty'.[66] Given these beliefs, it is no wonder that epidemiologists and physicians predicted that female smoking in Africa would pick up as the region modernised and women liberated themselves. So, Kaplan and her colleagues assumed that 'modernisation [would] lead to increasing sexual equity in the future' and that this would 'result in increased cigarette smoking among women' in Africa.[67] This was echoed by Collishaw and Lopez at the WHO, who believed that the low prevalence rates among women in Africa would 'increasingly be challenged by modernisation and industrialisation'.[68]

The most influential attempt at narrating the African tobacco epidemic within the framework of modernisation was Lopez and his colleagues' model of the smoking epidemic published in the journal *Tobacco Control* in 1994. As I have examined elsewhere,[69] this model was a product of international efforts at WHO and beyond to develop more reliable numbers for global smoking use and mortality. Based on the historical, statistical data available for Western countries, the model outlines how the smoking epidemic develops in any national population in the world over a 100-year period. As with many models of modernisation, such as Rostow's *Stages of Economic Growth*, the Lopez model identifies four successive, 25-year phases – which Lopez and his colleagues call Stage I, Stage II, Stage III and Stage IV – through which the epidemic unfolds. For all four stages, the epidemic is characterised through three explicit variables – smoking prevalence, smoking-attributable deaths, and public attitudes to smoking and the state of tobacco control policies, with the first two of these variables further broken down by gender. Stage I represents the start of the epidemic, when smoking becomes widely acceptable, with male prevalence rising to 15 per cent, while female prevalence remains low and tobacco control measures are non-existent. Stage II sees the epidemic develop further, with male prevalence peaking at 60 per cent, female prevalence jumping to 30 per cent and male smoking-attributable mortality starting to rise, mirroring prevalence with a 20-year time-lag due to the late onset of lung cancer. Stage III is a turning point in the epidemic: male prevalence begins to decline to about 40 per cent; female smoking plateaus; smoking-related mortality continues to climb; there is growing public awareness about the dangers of tobacco; and tobacco control measures are finally put in place. Stage IV represents the tail end of the epidemic as tobacco control measures harden and smoking prevalence for both sexes continues to decline. Crucially for us, the Lopez model further characterises the epidemic along a fourth, implicit variable: the level of economic development of a country, which seems to rise in tandem with smoking prevalence and mortality. So, Lopez and his colleagues thought that 'developing countries … in sub-Saharan Africa are currently in Stage I', while countries that are further in their economic development 'such as China … and other countries of Asia [and] Latin America' are in Stage II and most of the rich, industrialised 'countries of Western Europe along with Australia, Canada and the US are nearing the end of Stage III or [have passed] into Stage IV'.[70]

Analysing and explaining the African smoking epidemic through the lens of modernisation had important consequences. In relation to the smoking epidemic on the continent, it meant that its future development was, in the minds of epidemiologists and physicians working on the issue, already known and established. Specifically, they believed that, as Africa modernised, smoking rates and smoking-attributable mortality on the continent would rise accordingly. For example, a Nigerian colleague of Femi-Pearse claimed that:

> Already young Africans are smoking more than their forebears ... An improved cash economy, industrialisation and aggressive advertising by international tobacco companies are likely to further increase acceptance of the cigarette smoking habit in African countries and the incidence of bronchial carcinoma is likely to increase.[71]

This was echoed by Diop and his colleagues working up the coast in Senegal, who asserted that:

> In the current context, the health consequences of tobacco use are still invisible. But, with the rise of smoking prevalence due to urbanisation, it is to be feared that diseases associated with tobacco use will emerge as countries in Africa develop socially and economically.[72]

Epidemiologists' belief that the African smoking epidemic would spread in the foreseeable future was compounded by their conviction that future smoking patterns on the continent would follow the patterns that had been previously observed in the West. Paul Fréour, for example, believed that the African smoking epidemic was driven by 'Western forms of smoking' (*un tabagisme à l'occidentale*) that were spreading across the continent and contributing to 'tobacco-attributed pathologies' *(une pathologie tabagique*) that 'were very similar to the Western model'.[73] Similarly, American economist and tobacco control specialist Kenneth Warner mused that African countries 'give a sense of déjà vu' because the countries' 'experiences are often quite comparable to our own three decades ago'.[74] But perhaps the best example was the Lopez model itself, which assumed that African countries, now in Stage I, would, if no action was taken, necessarily move to the next stages of the epidemic, which were modelled on how the epidemic had unfolded in North America and Europe in the past.[75] As two epidemiologists working for the US Centers for Disease Control and Prevention (CDC) and specialising in tobacco control explained:

> Africa falls into Stage I [of the Lopez model] where the health consequences are not yet apparent on a large scale and fewer

> women than men have taken up [smoking] ... If the epidemic continues [into the next stages], more women will smoke in the future, and the incidence of smoking related diseases in men and women will increase substantially.[76]

In turn, the belief that smoking prevalence and smoking-attributable diseases would soon be increasing markedly in the region led many epidemiologists and physicians to think that Africa presented them with the opportunity to prevent the tobacco epidemic from happening altogether for the first time in history. Put differently, 'tobacco control in Africa' offered unique 'opportunities for prevention'.[77] So, for example, in an editorial for the WHO Tobacco or Health Initiative's newsletter, the Nigerian Minister of Health, Professor Ransome-Kuti, argued that:

> Tobacco use worldwide is currently killing three million people each year and the African contribution to this figure ... is rising rapidly. [We need to] recognis[e] the need for preventive action to avoid the looming epidemic ... The challenge facing ... African countries is to prevent smoking from reaching the scale found in developed countries.[78]

Lopez and his colleagues made a similar point, suggesting that African countries had the opportunity to 'prevent history from repeating itself' by taking 'strong public health measures to arrest the growth of tobacco consumption'.[79] Indeed, they 'have the advantage of knowing the serious health consequences of smoking' and of having at their disposal an array of already existing 'effective prevention interventions' to address the problem.[80]

The way of reading and narrating smoking in Africa through the lens of modernisation theory also had an important consequence for the latter. Until the 1970s, modernisation and modernity had been viewed as something that nations in Africa aspired to and actively pursued. But this changed thereafter, with modernisation and modernity increasingly questioned and critiqued.[81] This critique came from a variety of sources: neoliberal thinkers opposed to the central role of the state in modernisation efforts; environmentalists concerned about the ecological destruction associated with large physical infrastructure projects and industrialisation; development experts who believed that modernisation efforts should be about social progress, not just economic growth; and Marxists and dependency theorists who held that modernisation efforts simply perpetuated the underdevelopment of the periphery and its exploitation through the metropole. Epidemiologists' and physicians' early efforts to map and understand smoking in Africa further fuelled this critique of modernisation. Indeed, their work suggested that modernisation and modernity was not just something desirable, which brought about prosperity and progress, but also something darker, which led to increased disease and death. Their use of the term 'pathologies of development' (*pathologies du développement*) to refer to smoking-related diseases like cancer made this association between disease and modernity particularly clear.[82] Schmidt and his team in Abidjan, for example, spoke about 'a pulmonary pathology linked to development' when they sought to warn against lung cancer among Africans due to higher cigarette consumption.[83] In the same way, another epidemiologist working in West Africa argued that the advent of smoking-attributable lung cancer in Africa was a typical case of a 'pathology of development', where 'the evolution in the population's mode of life' had transformed 'cancerogenic risk factors' and led to the 'emergence of a new pathology'.[84] Others spoke about a modernisation that was taking place too rapidly or imperfectly to convey this unfortunate relationship between modernity and disease. Warner, for example, suggested that, in their 'rapid adoption of smoking', countries in Africa are 'modernising all too quickly'.[85] Similarly, anthropologist Kenyon Rainer Stebbins argued that 'the rise in chronic diseases' associated with smoking in Africa and elsewhere was best viewed as the product of a 'defective modernisation' that 'prioritises economic growth ahead of human welfare'.[86]

This talk of smoking and smoking-related diseases as pathologies of development echoed but differed in important ways from the belief held by doctors in late-colonial British Africa that 'civilisation was sending Africans mad'.[87] These doctors felt that, in the late-colonial period, the incidence of insanity was rising among 'educated, urbanised' Africans, while it remained very low among 'traditional' Africans. Drawing on theories of acculturation, they thought that the reason for these trends was that Africans were emotionally unstable and could easily become insane when trading their cultural traditions for a Western education and an urban lifestyle. As Megan Vaughan has shown, these ideas were part of wider fears that the upheavals of colonialism – industrialisation, education, urbanisation – were leading to the destruction of traditional African structures and a loss of social control.[88] More importantly, she also showed that these ideas were articulated around a notion of racial difference whereby Africans, unlike Europeans, had an 'innate psychological inferiority' that made them unable 'to cope with civilisation'.[89] In contrast, talk of smoking and smoking-related diseases as pathologies of development was based on a concept of sameness, with modernisation theorists suggesting Africans could be modern on a par with Europeans.[90] There is, in the West, a long history of associating smoking and smoking-related diseases with modernity. Many physicians in Nazi Germany, for example, viewed cancer as a 'disease of civilisation' that could be traced to 'excessive smoking' and was 'rare among the primitive races of the world'.[91] In the postwar period, health experts believed that the rise in chronic disease was exclusive to the West and the result of the 'affluent, self-indulgent American lifestyle' characterised by 'city living', 'driving', 'habits of indolence [and] the abuse of alcohol, tobacco and drugs'.[92] The identification of smoking and smoking-related diseases as pathologies of development made it possible for Africans to now share these health risks and diseases with Europeans.

To finish, it is important to note that, while the modernisation framework made it possible for epidemiologists and physicians to link smoking to economic growth, industrialisation, urbanisation and female emancipation, it did not really encourage them to examine the political economy of the African tobacco epidemic and, especially, the role of the cigarette industry in the making of the epidemic. As a matter of fact, only a few of them made more than a cursory allusion to the impact that transnational tobacco corporations might have on smoking prevalence rates on the continent. This, of course, is not to say that no one recognised and examined the role of the tobacco industry in the making of the African smoking epidemic. Indeed, at about the same time that epidemiologists started mapping smoking in Africa, another network of experts began analysing how transnational tobacco corporations both incited African governments to increase tobacco cultivation and worked hard to establish new markets for their products on the continent.[93] Drawing on ideas from neo-Marxist thought, dependency theory and the environmental movement, the economists, anthropologists and development experts that made up this network were highly critical of the tobacco industry and its impact on African development. They depicted how multinational cigarette companies bankrupted small farmers and pushed them into debt by controlling production and prices thanks to their oligopolistic position in the market. They also outlined how tobacco cultivation led to severe environmental damage, from pesticides poisoning water supplies to soil erosion and deforestation. Furthermore, they described how the tobacco industry lured Africans to smoke through aggressive marketing strategies, vast distribution networks and corruption practices to thwart tobacco control efforts.

These concerns were progressively picked up by international tobacco control activists during the 1980s and 1990s and, by the turn of the century, they had become part of standard public health thinking, where they shared the stage, sometimes uneasily, with modernisation tropes.

The enduring spell of modernisation

Sustained and comprehensive efforts to reduce tobacco use in Africa only really picked up in the new millennium, after the adoption of the WHO's *Framework Convention on Tobacco Control* in 2003 and in tandem with the increasing focus on non-communicable diseases in global health.[94] To begin with, there has been a multiplication of international tobacco control initiatives in the region, from the Africa Tobacco Control Regional Initiative set up by the American Cancer Society together with Cancer Research UK to the Bloomberg Initiative to Reduce Tobacco Use financed by the Gates and Bloomberg foundations. Aimed at strengthening the tobacco control movement in Africa, these initiatives have trained activists across the continent, organised anti-smoking campaigns in countries, coordinated large epidemiological surveys and funded research on regional tobacco taxation policies. Regional organisations like the African Union, the WHO's Regional Office for Africa and the Economic Community of West African States have also expressed a growing concern about tobacco use on the continent, publishing reports and holding high-level meetings on the subject. Similarly, an increasing number of civil society groups across the continent have taken up the issue, drawing the public's attention to the dangers of smoking and lobbying for better tobacco control policies in their countries, often with the support of the African Tobacco Control Alliance. Finally, a growing number of governments in the region, from South Africa, Mauritius and Kenya to Ghana, Senegal and Uganda, have set up national tobacco control commissions and adopted comprehensive tobacco control laws and policies.

The understanding of the African smoking epidemic at the heart of these tobacco control efforts is indistinguishable from the one articulated by epidemiologists and physicians between the early 1970s and mid-1990s and influenced by modernisation theory. Indeed, experts involved in these recent efforts usually assume, drawing explicitly on Lopez' 1994 model, that Africa is in the early stages of the epidemic and that, if nothing is done to prevent it, the region will experience a dramatic rise in smoking, as was the case in the West. For example, at the opening of the Centre for Tobacco Control in Africa (CTCA) in Kampala in 2011, the head of the WHO Tobacco Free Initiative, Douglas Bettcher, argued that the tobacco epidemic in Africa is 'at an early stage of development' and that 'the CTCA can help prevent this relentless epidemic unfolding the way it has done in other parts of the world'.[95] Similarly, Nkosazana Dlamini-Zuma, the African Union's Chairperson and former Health Minister for South Africa, outlined in an editorial in the *South African Medical Journal* that 'Africa is still in the early stages of the tobacco epidemic' and that African governments 'must intervene now to prevent [future] tobacco-related death [and] disease'.[96] This was echoed in a report by the African Union on the impact of tobacco use in Africa which stated that:

> Lopez ... outlined a four-stage model describing tobacco use and its effects ... [While] high-income countries have moved into stage 4 ... [and] middle-income countries such as China ... are in stages 2 and 3, ... the African continent is largely in stage 1 ... [This presents] valuable opportunities for prevention ... Without any systematic intervention to prevent smoking ... [the] trajectory [of the epidemic in Africa will] most likely ... [mirror] the experience of high-income countries.[97]

The Gates Foundation, which is one of the biggest donors in tobacco control in Africa, made the same point in its 'Tobacco Control Strategy Overview', claiming that the 'tobacco epidemic in Africa is at a relatively early stage' and that, 'if strong tobacco control measures are not implemented' now, 'tobacco use could double in the coming years'.[98]

For experts involved in contemporary tobacco control efforts on the continent, the reason why smoking prevalence would soon rise was because the region was modernising and developing at pace. First, they believed that economic growth and rising incomes among some segments of the population meant that a growing number of Africans could now afford to purchase and smoke cigarettes. As the Uganda Tobacco Control Alliance suggested, 'sustained economic growth' will 'drive tobacco consumption in Africa to double within the next ten years'.[99] Likewise, in a report for the Gates Foundation, two economists at the University of Cape Town explained that, in the twenty-first century, 'Africa has experienced some of the strongest economic growth in decades' and that, 'as the economy grows and incomes rise', there is a 'growth in the number of smokers and cigarettes smoked in Africa'.[100] Furthermore, many of these experts also thought that smoking prevalence increased with the continent's rapid urbanisation and adoption of modern sedentary lifestyles. Yussef Saloojee, a South African tobacco control veteran, argued that 'urbanisation' is one of the 'factors facilitating the adoption of cigarette smoking' and other unhealthy, 'Western lifestyles'.[101] In the same vein, development specialists working for the International Development and Research Council in Canada believed that, 'as countries urbanise and modernise', a 'greater numbers of Africans are adopting [unhealthy Western] lifestyles' like cigarette smoking.[102] Finally, many of these experts also associated increased smoking with the emancipation of women in Africa. As two American epidemiologists working on tobacco use in Uganda argued: 'women's empowerment is associated with greater tobacco use'.[103] The same point was made by two Nigerian researchers about smoking among young women in their country:

> [With modernisation,] Western ideas are set as models, traditional culture and ties are weakened and women's emancipation is championed. The effect of these is [women's] adoption of lifestyles simulating that of the West [like] tobacco smoking.[104]

My purpose here is to outline the enduring influence of modernisation theory on epidemiological imaginaries of smoking in Africa, not to assess whether these imaginaries are consistent with the reality on the ground. However, it is still worth noting that the outline of the African tobacco epidemic privileged by modernisation theory – where smoking prevalence rises quickly from a low base and which is best exemplified by the Lopez model – does not seem to fit with the epidemiological data on tobacco use collected in the region. Indeed, if we follow the Lopez model, Africa was in the first stage of the epidemic in the early 1990s with male smoking prevalence at 15 per cent and would now be, about 30 years later, in the second stage with male smoking prevalence at 60 per cent.[105] However, if anything, the epidemiological data available for Africa seems to show a decrease in smoking prevalence over this period. So, for example, the WHO's estimates for the late 1970s indicated 40 per cent for male smoking prevalence while its estimates for the late 1990s showed 25 per cent and its estimates for the late 2010s gave 17 per cent.[106] The data from surveys seem to suggest a similar trend. As mentioned earlier, surveys in the 1970s and 1980s measured male smoking prevalence between 40 and 50 per cent, while surveys in the 1990s counted around 20 to 30 per cent of men who smoked.[107] And more recent surveys, like the Demographic and Health Surveys funded by USAID and the Global Adult Tobacco Surveys run by the CDC, have measured male smoking prevalence rates from about 10 per cent in Ghana, Nigeria and Senegal to about 19 per cent in Kenya, Namibia and Malawi.[108] This downward trend is further confirmed by researchers at the Institute for Health Metrics and Evaluation, who have shown that male smoking prevalence had decreased in most African countries between 1990 and 2015.[109]

These discrepancies between the existing epidemiological data and forecasts based on the Lopez model do not necessarily invalidate the former or other modernisation theory-influenced readings of the African smoking epidemic. Indeed, there are possible reasons that can account for these discrepancies. One, which I mentioned earlier, is the serious doubts that many public health experts have about the reliability of much of the epidemiological data on smoking and health that came out of Africa in the twentieth century. Another is the fact that, because of the global economic recession of the 1970s and the structural adjustment programmes imposed by international lenders, most African countries experienced economic decline throughout the 1980s and 1990s.[110] This meant that Africans, instead of seeing their incomes rise as the Lopez model assumes, became poorer and, in consequence, reduced their cigarette consumption or stopped smoking altogether. This is not the place to ascertain whether these reasons can justify the discrepancies outlined above. But one might want to point out that, while these reasons could account for differences between epidemiological data and projections based on Lopez' model prior to 2000, they do not seem to be able to explain the decline in smoking prevalence across the continent recorded thereafter.

Modernisation everywhere

So far, this chapter has focused exclusively on how modernisation narratives have shaped epidemiological understandings of the smoking epidemic in Africa. Here, I want to move beyond smoking and show how these same narratives also influence the way epidemiologists imagine other health issues in the region. Specifically, I want to show how modernisation theory also shapes the way epidemiologists and global health experts construe the NCD epidemic and the transition away from infectious diseases in Africa. Sustained efforts to address the rising chronic disease burden on the continent began in the early twenty-first century, with the publication of reports, the establishment of new NGOs and the launch of public education campaigns and health programmes.[111] As I outline below, the understanding of the NCD epidemic in Africa on which these efforts are based is very similar, in terms of the arguments, language and concerns, to how epidemiologists and global health specialists have imagined the smoking epidemic in the region.

First, most official reports and scientific articles about the NCD epidemic in Africa start with numbers about the chronic disease burden in the region. For example, *Uniting Against NCDs*, a report published in 2011 by the WHO's Regional Office for Africa, states that, 'in 2008, NCDs were responsible for the death of 2.8 million people' or about '25 per cent' of all deaths 'in the African region'.[112] As with the smoking epidemic, these numbers come from modelling efforts like the Global Burden of Disease (GBD) project or social surveys like the WHO's STEPwise surveys. And, as with the smoking epidemic too, these deaths are imagined to be the beginning of an upcoming epidemic that will grow like it did in the West if nothing is done about it. To quote the WHO's Regional Office for Africa: 'the region is still at an early stage of the [NCD] epidemic', with chronic diseases 'projected to exceed communicable ... diseases as the most common cause of death by 2030'.[113] In the same spirit, epidemiologists working for the GBD project argued that the 'increasing burden of NCDs in Africa shows a growing health iceberg hidden under epidemics of infectious diseases'.[114]

Second, reports and articles on the African NCD epidemic see the rise in chronic diseases in the region as a (harmful) consequence of economic growth, urbanisation and Western lifestyles, in the same way that smoking has been linked to modernisation. The notion of 'health transition' used by the epidemiologists leading the GBD project – some of whom, like Alan Lopez, worked on smoking in Africa – is a good example given the influence that their research has had in drawing awareness to the NCD epidemic in Africa and beyond. Building on Abdel Omran's concept of epidemiological transition, these epidemiologists use the term 'health transition' to refer to the 'displacement of infections by accidents and chronic diseases' taking place in developing countries in Africa and elsewhere in the global south and which, they believe, is a consequence of the 'general process of industrialisation, urbanisation and modernisation'.[115] More specifically, they argue that:

> A shift from rural subsistence economy to an urban market-oriented industrial economy is generally associated with reductions in risks to communicable diseases because of better sanitation in urban areas. At the same time, however, economic growth brings

> with it new health problems. Very high rates of injuries related to motor vehicles, industrial accidents and toxic chemicals (e.g. pesticides) are one consequence of rapid urbanization, industrialization and mechanization of agriculture. Undernutrition may diminish ... only to be replaced by overnutrition with rising risks of death due to obesity, hypertension, atherosclerosis and diabetes. Rising incomes also bring changes in lifestyle including increases in smoking, alcohol use and substance abuse, all of which are expected to increase the risk for chronic diseases.[116]

Many of these arguments can also be found in a recent World Bank report on *The Challenge of Non-Communicable Diseases and Road Traffic Injuries in Sub-Saharan Africa*. In this report, the Bank argued that the growing NCD epidemic in the region has been driven by 'rising incomes', 'rapid urbanisation and changing lifestyle practices'.[117] As the Bank further pointed out, Africa was the victim of its own success and economic development:

> There is a growing optimism about Africa. Since the turn of the century, Africa's growth has been robust, averaging 5–6 per cent GDP growth a year, making important contributions to poverty reduction ... Against this backdrop, [the NCD epidemic] is a growing health challenge for Africa, spurred on in part by its own successes.[118]

The Bank's report is replete with concrete examples of how the rise in NCDs in Africa was linked to economic development, urbanisation and Western lifestyles. So, using the case of circulatory diseases, the report illustrates how the 'types of disease' present in a country or its population 'reflect [this country's] stage of development':

> In countries at the earliest stages of development, circulatory diseases due to nutritional deficiency or infections (such as rheumatic heart disease) predominate. As countries develop, circulatory diseases related to hypertension (such as hemorrhagic stroke) become more common.[119]

And, later in the report, the Bank argues that, when 'people move away from villages' to cities, they lose their 'traditional family or community safety nets' and become exposed to an 'urban environment ... associated with raised blood pressure, blood sugar and body mass index'.[120]

Conclusion

In this chapter, I discussed how postwar modernisation theory has shaped the way epidemiologists imagine the African smoking epidemic. Specifically, I outlined the way international expert networks did not just map tobacco use among Africans using surveys and estimation techniques but also analysed the unfolding of the smoking epidemic on the continent through the lens of modernisation, associating increases in prevalence with economic growth and industrialisation as well as urbanisation and female emancipation. I also pointed out some of the corollaries of using such a framework to make sense of smoking in Africa – the belief that, as the continent modernises, tobacco use will necessarily rise in the same way it has done in the West; the idea that modernity and modernisation are pathogenic; and the failure to examine the role of the tobacco industry in the making of the African smoking epidemic. To finish, I stressed the enduring and pervasive spell that modernisation theory seems to have over epidemiologists, outlining how it continues up to this day to influence the way they understand the African smoking epidemic and other global health issues like the epidemiological transition and the growing chronic disease burden in the region. More generally perhaps, I hope this chapter will encourage historians and social scientists working in the field to explore not just how contemporary epidemiological practices are reconfiguring the field of global health but also how sometimes long-forgotten political and social philosophies like modernisation theory shape epidemiological imaginaries.

Acknowledgements

Many thanks to Megan Vaughan for her insightful comments on how to improve my argument. An earlier version of the chapter was presented at a workshop on Africa and the Epidemiological Imagination held at UCL in September 2018; I thank the organisers and participants for their feedback. The empirical research on which this chapter is based was supported by a Wellcome Trust Society & Ethics Research Fellowship (No. 100556/B/12/Z).

Notes

1 For example, Adams, *Metrics: What Counts in Global Health*; Storeng and Behague, 'Playing the Numbers Game'.
2 For example, Wahlberg and Rose, 'The Governmentalization of the Living'; Reubi, 'Epidemiological Accountability'.

3 For example, Kearns, 'HIV, AIDS and the Global Imaginary'; Reubi, 'A Genealogy of Epidemiological Reason'.
4 Hutt and Burkitt, 'Geographical Distribution of Cancer in East Africa', 719; Doll, 'Foreword'.
5 For example, Baylet et al., 'Conséquences Médicales de la Consommation du Tabac'; Bradshaw and Schonland, 'Smoking, Drinking and Oesophageal Cancer'; Schmidt et al., 'Epidémiologie du Cancer des Bronches'.
6 Reubi and Berridge, 'The Internationalisation of Tobacco Control'.
7 Femi-Pearse, Adeniyi-Jones and Oke, 'Respiratory Symptoms'.
8 Lore, 'Smoking Habits in Kenya I'; Lore and Lwenya, 'Smoking Habits in Kenya II'.
9 Tessier et al., 'Smoking Behaviour'.
10 Schmidt et al., 'Enquête sur la Consommation Tabagique'.
11 Bradshaw and Schonland, 'Oesophageal and Lung Cancers'; Bradshaw and Schonland, 'Smoking, Drinking and Oesophageal Cancer'.
12 For example, Bradshaw and Schonland, 'Smoking, Drinking and Oesophageal Cancer'; Lore, 'Smoking Habits in Kenya I'; Tessier et al., 'Smoking Behaviour'.
13 For example, WHO, *Tobacco or Health: Report by the Programme Committee*; Masironi and Rothwell, 'Tendances et Effets du Tabagisme'; WHO, *Tobacco or Health: A Global Status Report*.
14 Lopez, Collishaw, and Piha, 'A Descriptive Model'; WHO, *Tobacco or Health: A Global Status Report*.
15 Fréour, 'Tobacco Smoking in Africa'.
16 Crofton, 'WHO Technical Advisory Group on Tobacco or Health', paragraph 5.1.
17 Crofton, 'Tobacco and the Third World', 164.
18 Monteiro, 'Smoking and Health in Benin'.
19 WHO, *Tobacco Smoking in the World*, 1.
20 Crofton, 'The Gathering Smoke Clouds', 269.
21 Femi-Pearse, Adeniyi-Jones, and Oke, 'Respiratory Symptoms'.
22 Baylet et al., 'Enquête sur l'Utilisation du Tabac'.
23 Baker, Johnston, and Turner, 'Smoking Habits of Blacks in Industry'; Lore and Lwenya, 'Smoking Habits in Kenya II'.
24 Amonoo-Lartson and Pappoe, 'Prevalence of Smoking in Secondary Schools', 1292; Ball, 'Tobacco Consumption in Africa'.
25 WHO, *Tobacco Smoking in the World*, 15.
26 Wone, Koate, and De Lauture, 'La Lutte Contre le Tabagisme'; WHO, *Tobacco or Health*.
27 Tessier et al., 'Smoking Behaviour'.
28 WHO, *Tobacco or Health: A Global Status Report*, 11.
29 Mackay and Crofton, 'Tobacco', 208.
30 WHO, *Tobacco or Health: A Global Status Report*, 11.
31 Pobee, Larbi, and Kpodonu, 'The Profile of the African Smoker', 227–9.
32 Strebel, Kuhn, and Yach, 'Determinants of Cigarette Smoking', 212.
33 Tessier et al., 'Smoking Behaviour', 98–9.
34 Onadeko and Awotedu, 'Smoking Patterns in Females', 126.
35 Arya and Bennett, 'Smoking Amongst University Students in Uganda', 27; Waldron et al., 'Gender Differences in Tobacco Use', 1272.
36 Kaplan, Carriker, and Waldron, 'Gender Differences in Tobacco Use', 309.
37 Mackay and Crofton, 'Tobacco', 208.
38 Monteiro, 'Le Tabagisme en Milieu Scolaire', 2.
39 Fréour, 'Le Tabagisme', 267–70.
40 Strebel et al., 'Determinants of Cigarette Smoking', 212.
41 Baylet, Diop, and De Medeiros, 'Enquête sur l'Usage du Tabac', 83.
42 Baker et al., 'Smoking Habits', 67.
43 WHO, *Tobacco or Health: A Global Status Report*, 18.
44 Mackay and Crofton, 'Tobacco', 208
45 Cooper, 'Development, Modernization and the Social Sciences'; Ekbladh, *The Great American Mission*.
46 Cooper, 'Development, Modernization and the Social Sciences'.
47 Cited in Arndt, *Economic Development*, 53.
48 Cooper, 'Development, Modernization and the Social Sciences'.
49 Arndt, *Economic Development*.
50 Femi-Pearse, Adeniyi-Jones and Oke, 'Respiratory Symptoms', 57.

51 Femi-Pearse, Adeniyi-Jones and Oke,'Respiratory Symptoms', 57.
52 Gareeboo et al., 'Epidemiological Studies', 249.
53 Bradshaw and Schonland, 'Oesophageal and Lung Cancers', 275.
54 Nostbakken, 'UICC Smoking Control Activities', 170.
55 D'Hondt and Vandewiele, 'Attitudes of Senegalese Schoolgoing Adolescents', 350.
56 Yach, 'Tobacco in Africa', 31–2.
57 Oettlé, 'Cancer in Africa', 393; Burkitt, 'Some Diseases', 275; Taha and Ball, 'Smoking and Africa', 991.
58 Baylet et al., 'Enquête sur l'Usage du Tabac', 40; Wone et al., 'La Lutte Contre le Tabagisme', 245.
59 Oettlé, 'Cancer in Africa', 383; Baylet et al., 'Conséquences Médicales de la Consommation du Tabac', 42.
60 Wone et al., 'La Lutte Contre le Tabagisme', 245; Fréour, 'Le Tabagisme', 269.
61 Baylet et al., 'Conséquences Médicales de la Consommation du Tabac', 40–2; Baylet et al., 'Enquête sur l'Usage du Tabac', 83.
62 McGlashan and Harington, 'Lung Cancer', 346.
63 Fréour, 'Le Tabagisme', 267–8.
64 Waldron, 'Patterns and Causes of Gender Differences in Smoking', 989.
65 Chapman, 'Changes in Adult Cigarette Consumption', 281.
66 Baylet et al., 'Conséquences Médicales de la Consommation du Tabac', 43.
67 Kaplan et al., 'Gender Differences in Tobacco Use', 310.
68 Collishaw and Lopez, 'Prevalence of Cigarette Smoking', 327.
69 Reubi, 'Modernisation, Smoking and Chronic Disease'.
70 Lopez, Collishaw, and Piha, 'Descriptive Model', 245–6.
71 Elegbeleye, 'Bronchial Carcinoma in Nigerians', 61.
72 Diop, Baylt, and Hountondji, 'Le Tabagisme en Afrique', 241.
73 Fréour, 'Le Tabagisme', 267–70.
74 Warner, 'Toward a Global Strategy', 32.
75 Cf. Reubi, 'Modernisation, Smoking and Chronic Disease'.
76 Asma and Pederson, 'Tobacco Control in Africa', 353.
77 Asma and Pederson, 'Tobacco Control in Africa', 353.
78 Ransome-Kuti, 'Tobacco Control in Africa'.
79 Lopez, Collishaw, and Piha, 'Descriptive Model', 245–6.
80 Lopez, Collishaw, and Piha, 'Descriptive Model', 245.
81 Arndt, *Economic Development*; Cooper, 'Development, Modernization and the Social Sciences'; Ekbladh, *The Great American Mission*.
82 Gateff and Lebras, 'Problemes Epidemiologiques', 431.
83 Schmidt et al., 'Cancer des Bronches', 1830.
84 Loubière, 'Facteurs Etiologiques', 34–5.
85 Warner, 'Toward a Global Strategy', 32.
86 Stebbins, 'Transnational Tobacco Companies', 228.
87 Vaughan, *Curing their Ills*, 108. Cf. also: Heaton, *Black Skin, White Coats*, Ch.1.
88 Vaughan, *Curing their Ills*.
89 Vaughan, *Curing their Ills*, 108, 111.
90 Cooper, 'Development, Modernization and the Social Sciences'.
91 Proctor, *The Nazi War on Cancer*, 25.
92 Lalonde, *A New Perspective on the Health of Canadians*, 5; Larsen, 'The Birth of Lifestyle Politics', 212.
93 For example, Muller, *Tobacco and the Third World*; Boesen and Mohele, *The 'Success Story' of Peasant Tobacco Production*; Currie and Ray, 'Going Up in Smoke'.
94 Weisz and Vignola-Gagné, 'The World Health Organization'; Reubi and Berridge, 'Internationalisation of Tobacco Control'.
95 Cited in Centre for Tobacco Control in Africa, *CTCA Synopsis*, 2.
96 Dlamini-Zuma, 'A Comprehensive, Health-Promotion Approach', 831.
97 African Union, *The Impact of Tobacco Use*, 2.
98 Gates Foundation, 'Tobacco Control Strategy Overview'.
99 Uganda Tobacco Control Alliance, *Why Uganda Urgently Needs a Tobacco Control Law*, 1.
100 Blecher and Ross, *Tobacco Use in Africa*, 1–2.
101 Saloojee, 'Tobacco in Africa', 267.

102 International Development and Research Council, 'Best Approaches for Stifling Growth of Non-Communicable Diseases'.
103 Goldsmith and Boyle, 'Women's Empowerment and Tobacco Use', 388.
104 Ibeh and Ele, 'Prevalence of Cigarette Smoking', 335.
105 Lopez, Collishaw, and Piha, 'Descriptive Model'.
106 WHO, *Tobacco Smoking in the World*, 1; WHO, *Tobacco or Health: A Global Status Report*, 11; WHO 2019, 'World Health Statistics'.
107 For example, Femi-Pearse, Adeniyi-Jones, and Oke 'Respiratory Symptoms'; Lore and Lwenya, 'Smoking Habits in Kenya II'; Tessier et al., 'Smoking Behaviour'.
108 Pampel, 'Tobacco Use in Sub-Saharan Africa'; CDC, *Global Adult Tobacco Survey: Nigeria 2012*; CDC, *Global Adult Tobacco Survey: Kenya 2014*; CDC, *Enquête Mondiale sur le Tabagisme chez les Adultes: Sénégal 2015*.
109 Reitsma et al., 'Smoking Prevalence'.
110 Jerven, *Africa: Why Economists Get It Wrong*.
111 For example, WHO AFRO, *Uniting Against NCDs*; World Bank, *The Challenge of Non-Communicable Diseases*.
112 WHO AFRO, *Uniting Against NCDs*, 1–2.
113 WHO AFRO, *Uniting Against NCDs*, 1; WHO AFRO, *The African Regional Health Report*, xviii.
114 Naghavi and Forouzanfar, 'Burden of Non-Communicable Diseases', 95.
115 Frenk et al., 'Health Transition in Middle-Income Countries', 31; Jamison and Mosley, 'Disease Control Priorities', 16–17.
116 Jamison and Mosley, 'Disease Control Priorities', 17.
117 World Bank, *The Challenge of Non-Communicable Diseases*, 2.
118 World Bank, *The Challenge of Non-Communicable Diseases*, 7.
119 World Bank, *The Challenge of Non-Communicable Diseases*, 15.
120 World Bank, *The Challenge of Non-Communicable Diseases*, 26.

Bibliography

Adams, Vincanne (ed.). *Metrics: What Counts in Global Health*. Durham, NC: Duke University Press, 2016.

African Union. *The Impact of Tobacco Use on Health and Socio-Economic Development in Africa*. Addis Ababa: African Union, 2012.

Amonoo-Lartson, R. and Matilda E. Pappoe. 'Prevalence of Smoking in Secondary Schools in the Greater Accra Region of Ghana', *Social Science and Medicine*, 34 (1992): 1291–3.

Arndt, Heinz Wolfgang. *Economic Development: The History of an Idea*. Chicago: University of Chicago Press, 1987.

Arya, O.P. and F.J. Bennett. 'Smoking Amongst University Students in Uganda', *East African Medical Journal*, 47 (1970): 18–28.

Asma, Samira and Linda Pederson. 'Tobacco Control in Africa', *Tobacco Control*, 8 (1999): 353–4.

Baker, M.D., J.R. Johnston, and D.M. Turner. 'Smoking Habits of Blacks in Industry', *South African Medical Journal*, 54 (1978): 67–9.

Ball, Keith. 'Tobacco Consumption in Africa', *Tobacco Control*, 2 (1993): 334.

Baylet, R. et al. 'Enquête sur l'Utilisation du Tabac dans les Centres Coutumiers et en Milieu Urbanisé au Sénégal', *Bulletin de la Société Médicale d'Afrique Noire en Langue Française*, 19 (1974): 36–40.

Baylet, R. et al. 'Recherches sur les Conséquences Médicales de la Consommation du Tabac en Afrique Noire', *Bulletin de la Société Médicale d'Afrique Noire en Langue Française*, 19 (1974): 41–5.

Baylet, R., S. Diop and D. De Medeiros. 'Enquête sur l'Usage du Tabac parmi les Etudiants en Médecine de 4e Année, Faculté de Médecine de Dakar', *Bulletin de la Société Médicale d'Afrique Noire en Langue Française*, 19 (1974): 80–3.

Blecher, Evan and Hana Ross. *Tobacco Use in Africa*. Atlanta, GA: American Cancer Society, 2013.

Boesen, Jannik and A.T. Mohele. *The 'Success Story' of Peasant Tobacco Production in Tanzania*. Uppsala: Scandinavian Institute of African Studies, 1979.

Bradshaw, Evelyn and Mary Schonland. 'Oesophageal and Lung Cancers in Natal African Males in Relation to Certain Socio-Economic Factors', *British Journal of Cancer*, 23 (1969): 275–84.

Bradshaw, Evelyn and Mary Schonland. 'Smoking, Drinking and Oesophageal Cancer in African Males of Johannesburg, South Africa', *British Journal of Cancer*, 30 (1974): 157–63.

Burkitt, Denis. 'Some Diseases Characteristic of Modern Western Civilization', *British Medical Journal*, 1 (1973): 274–8.

CDC. *Global Adult Tobacco Survey: Nigeria 2012 Fact Sheet*. Atlanta, GA: CDC, 2012.

CDC. *Global Adult Tobacco Survey: Kenya 2014 Fact Sheet*. Atlanta, GA: CDC, 2014.

CDC. *Enquête Mondiale sur le Tabagisme chez les Adultes: Sénégal 2015 Fiche d'Information*. Atlanta, GA: CDC, 2015.

Centre for Tobacco Control in Africa. *CTCA Synopsis*. Kampala: CTCA, 2011.

Chapman, Simon. 'Changes in Adult Cigarette Consumption per Head in 128 Countries, 1986–90', *Tobacco Control*, 1 (1992): 281–4.

Collishaw, Neil and Alan Lopez. 'Prevalence of Cigarette Smoking in Developing Countries', *Tobacco Control*, 4 (1995): 327.

Cooper, Frederick. 'Development, Modernization and the Social Sciences in the Era of Decolonization', *Revue d'Histoire des Sciences Humaines*, 10 (2004): 9–38.

Crofton, John. 'The Gathering Smoke Clouds', *International Journal of Epidemiology*, 13 (1984): 269–70.

Crofton, John. 'WHO Technical Advisory Group on Tobacco or Health: An Informal Report'. Unpublished, 1989.

Crofton, John. 'Tobacco and the Third World', *Thorax*, 45 (1990): 164–9.

Currie, Kate and Larry Ray. 'Going Up in Smoke', *Social Science and Medicine*, 19 (1984): 1131–9.

D'Hondt, Walter and Michel Vandewiele. 'Attitudes of Senegalese Schoolgoing Adolescents Towards Tobacco Smoking', *Journal of Youth and Adolescence*, 12 (1983): 333–52.

Diop, S., R. Baylet and H. Hountondji. 'Le Tabagisme en Afrique', *Médecine d'Afrique Noire*, 27 (1980): 237–44.

Dlamini-Zuma, Nkosazana. 'A Comprehensive, Health-Promotion Approach to Tobacco Control', *South African Medical Journal*, 103 (2013): 831.

Doll, Richard. 'Foreword'. In: *Tumors in a Tropical Country*, edited by A.C. Templeton, v–vi. Berlin: Springer, 1973.

Ekbladh, David. *The Great American Mission: Modernization and the Construction of an American World Order.* Princeton, NJ: Princeton University Press, 2011.

Elegbeleye. O. 'Bronchial Carcinoma in Nigerians', *The Journal of Tropical Medicine and Hygiene*, 78 (1975): 59–62.

Femi-Pearse, D., A. Adeniyi-Jones, and A.B. Oke. 'Respiratory Symptoms and their Relationships to Cigarette-Smoking, Dusty Occupations and Domestic Air Pollution', *West African Medical Journal*, June 1973, 57–63.

Frenk, Julio et al. 'Health Transition in Middle-Income Countries', *Health Policy and Planning*, 4 (1989): 29–39.

Fréour, Paul. 'Le Tabagisme Envahit le Tiers-Monde', *Bulletin de l'Académie Nationale de Médecine*, 169 (1985): 267–72.

Fréour, Paul. 'Tobacco Smoking in Africa', *Bulletin of the International Union against Tuberculosis and Lung Disease*, 64 (1989): 9–10.

Gareeboo, Hassam, et al. 'Epidemiological Studies of Smoking in Mauritius'. In: *Tobacco or Health*, edited by B. Durston and K. Jamrozik, 249–52. Perth: Health Department of Western Australia, 1990.

Gateff, G. and J. Lebras. 'Problemes Epidemiologiques des Grandes Villes Africaines', *Médecine d'Afrique Noire*, 28 (1981): 431–2.

Gates Foundation. 'Tobacco Control Strategy Overview', last modified 5 May 2015, http://www.gatesfoundation.org.

Goldsmith, E. and E. Boyle. 'Women's Empowerment and Tobacco Use', *Annals of Global Health*, 82 (2016): 387–8.

Heaton, Matthew. *Black Skin, White Coats: Nigerian Psychiatrists, Decolonization, and the Globalization of Psychiatry.* Columbus, OH: Ohio University Press, 2013.

Hutt, M.S.R. and Denis Burkitt. 'Geographical Distribution of Cancer in East Africa', *British Medical Journal*, 2 (5464) (1965): 719–22.

Ibeh, C. and P. Ele. 'Prevalence of Cigarette Smoking in Young Nigerian Females', *African Journal of Medicine and Medical Science*, 32 (2003): 335–8.

International Development and Research Council. 'Experts Gather to Discuss Best Approaches for Stifling Growth of Non-Communicable Diseases', last modified 10 October 2016, http://www.idrc.ca.
Jamison, Dean T. and W. Henry Mosley. 'Disease Control Priorities in Developing Countries', *American Journal of Public Health*, 81 (1991): 15–22.
Jerven, Morten. *Africa: Why Economists Get It Wrong*. London: Zed, 2015.
Kaplan, Mara, Laura Carriker, and Ingrid Waldron. 'Gender Differences in Tobacco Use in Kenya', *Social Science and Medicine*, 30 (1990): 305–10.
Kearns, Gerry. 'HIV, AIDS and the Global Imaginary'. In: *Global Health and Geographical Imaginaries*, edited by Clare Herrick and David Reubi, 3–21. London: Routledge, 2017.
Lalonde, Marc. *A New Perspective on the Health of Canadians*. Ottawa: Minister of Supply and Services, 1974.
Larsen, Lars Thorup. 'The Birth of Lifestyle Politics'. In: *Governmentality*, edited by U. Brockling, S. Krasmann, and T. Lemke, 201–24. Hoboken, NJ: Taylor and Francis, 2010.
Lopez, Alan, Neil Collishaw, and Tapani Piha. 'A Descriptive Model of the Cigarette Epidemic in Developed Countries', *Tobacco Control*, 3 (1994): 242–7.
Lore, W. 'Smoking Habits in Kenya I', *East African Medical Journal*, 64 (1987): 248–52.
Lore, W. and R. Lwenya. 'Smoking Habits in Kenya II', *East African Medical Journal*, 65 (1988): 71–80.
Loubière, R. 'Facteurs Etiologiques des Cancers en Afrique Intertropicale', *Médecine d'Afrique Noire*, 28 (1981): 31–5.
Mackay, Judith and John Crofton. 'Tobacco and the Developing World', *British Medical Journal*, 22 (1996): 206–21.
Masironi, Robert and Keith Rothwell. 'Tendances et Effets du Tabagisme dans le Monde'. *Rapport Trimestriel de la Statistique Sanitaire Mondiale*, 41 (1986): 228–41.
McGlashan, N.D. and J.S. Harington. 'Lung Cancer 1978–1981 in the Black Peoples of South Africa', *British Journal of Cancer*, 52 (1985): 339–46.
Monteiro, Bruno. 'Smoking and Health in Benin'. Paper presented at the International Conference on Tobacco & Health organised by the WHO and Swaziland Government in Mbabane, Swaziland, 1982.
Monteiro, Bruno. 'Le Tabagisme en Milieu Scolaire à Conakry: Enquête à Réaliser en Mai–Juin, 1992'. Unpublished, 1992.
Muller, Mike. *Tobacco and the Third World*. London: War on Want, 1978.
Naghavi, Mohsen and Mohammad Forouzanfar. 'Burden of Non-Communicable Diseases in Sub-Saharan Africa in 1990 and 2010', *Lancet*, 381 (2013): 95.
Nostbakken, David. 'UICC Smoking Control Activities in Africa'. In: *Tobacco or Health*, edited by B. Durston and K. Jamrozik, 169–78. Perth: Health Department of Western Australia, 1990.
Oettlé, Alfred George. 'Cancer in Africa'. *Journal of the National Cancer Institute*, 33 (1964): 383–439.
Onadeko, B.O. and A.A. Awotedu. 'Smoking Patterns in Females in Higher Institutions in Nigeria'. In: *Abstracts, Fifth World Conference on Smoking and Health, Winnipeg, Canada, 1983*, edited by P. Bonla and F. Wright, 126. Ottawa: Canadian Council on Smoking and Health, 1983.
Pampel, Fred. 'Tobacco Use in Sub-Saharan Africa', *Social Science and Medicine*, 66 (2008): 1772–83.
Pobee, Joe, E.B. Larbi, and J. Kpodonu. 'The Profile of the African Smoker', *East African Medical Journal*, 61 (1984): 227–33.
Proctor, Robert. *The Nazi War on Cancer*. Princeton, NJ: Princeton University Press, 1999.
Ransome-Kuti, Olikoye. 'Tobacco Control in Africa', *WHO Tobacco Alert*, April 1992, 1.
Reitsma, Marissa et al. 'Smoking Prevalence and Attributable Disease Burden in 195 Countries and Territories, 1990–2015', *Lancet*, 389 (2017): 1885–906.
Reubi, David. 'Modernisation, Smoking and Chronic Disease: Of Temporality and Spatiality in Global Health', *Health & Place*, 39 (2016): 188–95.
Reubi, David. 'A Genealogy of Epidemiological Reason: Saving Lives, Social Surveys and Global Population', *BioSocieties*, 13 (2018): 81–102.
Reubi, David. 'Epidemiological Accountability: Philanthropists, Global Health and the Audit of Saving Lives', *Economy & Society*, 47 (2018): 83–110.
Reubi, David and Virginia Berridge. 'The Internationalisation of Tobacco Control, 1950–2010', *Medical History*, 60 (2016): 453–72.

Saloojee, Yussef. 'Tobacco in Africa'. In: *Tobacco and Public Health*, edited by C. Boyle, N. Gray, J. Henningfield, J. Seffrin, and W. Zatonski, 267–77. Oxford: Oxford University Press, 2004.

Schmidt, D. et al. 'Epidémiologie du Cancer des Bronches chez le Noir Africain à Abidjan', *Nouvelle Presse Médicale*, 7 (1978): 1827–30.

Schmidt, D. et al. 'Enquête sur la Consommation Tabagique en Milieu Africain à Abidjan'. *Poumon-Cœur*, 37 (1981): 87–94.

Stebbins, Kenyon Rainer. 'Transnational Tobacco Companies and Health in Underdeveloped Countries', *Social Science and Medicine*, 30 (1990): 227–35.

Storeng, Katerini and Dominique Behague. 'Playing the Numbers Game: Evidence-Based Advocacy and the Technocratic Narrowing of the Safe Motherhood Initiative', *Medical Anthropology Quarterly*, 28 (2014): 260–79.

Strebel, Peter, Louise Kuhn, and Derek Yach. 'Determinants of Cigarette Smoking in the Black Township Population of Cape Town', *Journal of Epidemiology and Community Health*, 43 (1989): 209–31.

Taha, Ahmed and Keith Ball. 'Smoking and Africa', *British Medical Journal*, 280 (1980): 991–3.

Tessier, Jean-Francois, et al. 'Smoking Behaviour and Attitudes of Medical Students towards Smoking and Anti-Smoking Campaigns', *Tobacco Control*, 1 (1992): 95–101.

Uganda Tobacco Control Alliance. *Why Uganda Urgently Needs a Tobacco Control Law*. Kampala: Uganda Tobacco Control Alliance, 2013.

Vaughan, Megan. *Curing their Ills: Colonial Power and African Illness*. Cambridge: Polity, 1991.

Wahlberg, Ayo and Nikolas Rose. 'The Governmentalization of the Living: Calculating Global Health', *Economy & Society*, 44 (2015): 60–90.

Waldron, Ingrid. 'Patterns and Causes of Gender Differences in Smoking'. *Social Science and Medicine*, 32 (1991): 989–1005.

Waldron, Ingrid et al. 'Gender Differences in Tobacco Use in Africa, Asia, the Pacific and Latin America', *Social Science and Medicine*, 27 (1988): 1269–75.

Warner, Kenneth. 'Toward a Global Strategy to Combat Smoking', *Journal of Public Health Policy*, 5 (1984): 28–39.

Weisz, George and Etienne Vignola-Gagné. 'The World Health Organization and the Globalization of Chronic Non-Communicable Disease', *Population and Development Review*, 41 (2015): 507–32.

WHO. *Tobacco Smoking in the World*. Geneva: WHO, 1978.

WHO. *Tobacco or Health: Report by the Programme Committee*. Geneva: WHO, 1985.

WHO. *Tobacco or Health: A Global Status Report*. Geneva: WHO, 1997.

WHO. 2019. 'World Health Statistics Data Visualization Dashboard', http://apps.who.int/gho/data/view.sdg.3-a-data-reg?lang=en.

WHO AFRO. *Uniting Against NCDs*. Brazzaville: WHO AFRO, 2011.

WHO AFRO. *The African Regional Health Report, 2014*. Brazzaville: WHO AFRO, 2014.

Wone, I., P. Koate, and H. De Lauture. 'La Lutte contre le Tabagisme dans une Optique de Santé de Communauté', *Médecine d'Afrique Noire*, 27 (1990): 245–51.

World Bank. *The Challenge of Non-Communicable Diseases and Road Traffic Injuries in Sub-Saharan Africa*. Washington DC: World Bank, 2013.

Yach, Derek. 'Tobacco in Africa', *World Health Forum*, 17 (1996): 29–36.

5

Sugar Consumption and Diabetes

Megan Vaughan

In April 2018 South Africa joined a handful of countries that have introduced a tax on sugar-sweetened beverages.[1] The implementation of the new levy was the culmination of a long campaign by activists, including public health professionals, and the growing evidence, derived from both local and international studies, of the relationship between sugar consumption (particularly sugary sweetened beverages or SSBs) and a range of health conditions. The South African evidence presented in the 2000s showed a marked increase in sugar consumption over the previous two decades and is often viewed as part of a larger 'nutrition transition' in the country occurring since the advent of majority government in 1994. This is in turn linked to the country's current problems of rising rates of obesity (including child obesity), type 2 diabetes and other conditions associated with poor diets.[2] Though the factors behind the increased prevalence of these health conditions are undoubtedly complex, and still the subject of debate, it seems likely that sugar consumption (especially in the form of sweetened beverages) does play a significant role. Without questioning the importance of more recent developments in South Africa, this paper points to a longer history of sugar consumption in the country which is part of the larger story of the commercialisation of the South African food industry and its careful nurturing of a consumer base amongst black communities, both urban and rural.

In two articles published shortly before the implementation of the tax, Alex Myers and his colleagues expressed scepticism about the ability of public policy to be effective against the powerful South African sugar industry.[3] In many ways the story I tell in this chapter echoes those sentiments, but it also demonstrates two other points. Firstly, it shows that type 2 diabetes (or diabetes mellitus) was already becoming a serious health problem for urban African communities in the 1950s and 1960s, indicating that the current debate around the 'nutrition transition' in South Africa needs to be placed in a longer historical context. Secondly it complicates (though does not replace) the picture of conservative race-driven theories highlighted by Diana Wylie in her pioneering work on the history of nutritional science in South Africa.[4] Some medical researchers in apartheid-era South Africa were already sounding the alarm at what is now labelled the 'double burden of malnutrition' – that is, the co-existence within the country, and indeed within communities and families, of undernutrition and overweight/obesity. Though, as Wylie argues, many accounts of African malnutrition were either victim blaming or deeply paternalistic (in some cases maternalistic), other researchers pointed to the role of the food industry and food policy in its creation. One of those was George D. Campbell, whose work on sugar and diabetes in South Africa brought him into direct conflict with the powerful local sugar industry, and whose research contributed to a larger international campaign directed at highlighting the health implications of increased sugar consumption.

It appears that it is in the context of the recent debates on the sugar tax in South Africa, and indeed of sugar consumption globally, that Campbell's work has found a new audience.[5] I first came across Campbell's research as a reference in Gary Taubes' book on sugar.[6] As with the work of John Yudkin, whose *Pure, White and Deadly* was 'rediscovered' in the 2000s,[7] Campbell's early attention to sugar and refined carbohydrates in the diets of African and Indian communities in South Africa now assumes new relevance. This attention emerged directly from his clinical work in Durban in the late 1950s and 1960s, and, as Cummings and Engineer have shown, it later became linked to the work of others studying these issues from an African perspective, as well as that of Peter Cleave, with whom he eventually published a book.[8] Like many of his colleagues working on what would now be called non-communicable diseases (NCDs) in eastern and southern Africa, Campbell did not see their development as part of an inevitable 'transition', as would later be predicted by epidemiological transition theory (see Introduction to this volume). Though his early clinical work led him to view diabetes as a disease of affluence, he later framed it as a disease of urbanisation, in recognition that it was also affecting poorer urban communities. By the 1970s, even this label seemed to him to have become inadequate as he reported on its increasing visibility in rural areas of

South Africa. In Campbell's view, there was nothing inevitable about this development – it was the result of a food industry, and particularly a local sugar industry, actively marketing refined carbohydrates and sugary foods to Africans.[9]

Campbell was born in Durban in 1925 into a family with sugar interests.[10] Despite this, or perhaps because of it, he became a vocal opponent of that industry and of its strategies to increase the volume of the local market for its product, particularly amongst Africans. At the same time, he used his insider status to access sugar industry internal documentation and to conduct research amongst workers on sugar estates.

After war service, medical training in Edinburgh, and research posts in the US and Scotland, Campbell returned to practice in Durban, establishing the first diabetic clinic there in 1958.[11] As he reported in numerous publications and in his 1968 MD thesis for Edinburgh University, the clinic was very quickly overwhelmed with patients.[12] Initially these came mainly from Durban's Indian community, which experienced alarmingly high rates of diabetes.[13] In addition to running this very busy clinic, Campbell researched the aetiology of the disease in this community, and what he saw as the peculiarities of its clinical manifestations. Early onset and severe vascular disease were especially common amongst his Indian patients. In dialogue with researchers in India, he compared rates of diabetes in the communities of origin there with those of the descendants of migrants in Durban. He also compared these urban residents to communities of Indian origin living and working on Natal's sugar estates. Amongst Indian-origin communities, he researched what he called 'connubial diabetes': the simultaneous appearance of diabetic symptoms in husband/wife pairs.[14] Campbell pursued a number of theories (including the 'thrifty gene' hypothesis, which he saw as playing some part),[15] but fairly quickly arrived at the view that the dominant factor at work was the food environment – with refined carbohydrates and sugar as the main culprits.[16] He never wavered from this view and, indeed, as he began to investigate diabetes amongst African communities, it only strengthened.

As more African patients began arriving at the clinic at the King Edward VIII Hospital, Campbell began a longitudinal study in 1959, following 133 of them for nine years.[17] The majority of these patients had moved from rural areas to reside in Durban between 1936 and 1943 ('boom' years in the port city). As Campbell noted, this period also coincided with a dramatic increase in national per capita sugar consumption, from an average of 40lbs per annum in 1936 to over 70lbs in 1943. But in South Africa this average disguised differences between communities, with white consumption leading the way and Indian figures not far behind. Over the postwar years and into the 1970s, Campbell would follow (and critique) the advertising and marketing strategies adopted by the South African sugar industry as it attempted to increase demand and consumption amongst the country's majority African population – not only in urban areas, where sugar was already a fixed feature of the diet, but also in rural areas where it was not.

In the late 1950s most of Campbell's African diabetic patients in the clinic were relatively well off, by African standards, and this he saw as reflecting a more general rise in living standards in postwar urban South Africa, adding that in Durban these were advances made by the Africans' 'own exertions'.[18] He quickly dubbed the disease *Isifo Sikitasi*, or the 'disease of the briefcase', reflecting the relative affluence (and gender) of his first patients. Whilst 20 years previously the majority of patients seen at this 'non-white' hospital had been suffering from infective and deficiency diseases, now they were suffering from these *plus* hypertension, cerebral vascular conditions, peptic ulcer, diabetes and, occasionally, myocardial infarction. Campbell was careful to note that it was really impossible to assess the incidence of diabetes in the Durban African population from attendance at his clinic, which was affected by a number of factors, but it appeared that the disease had been 'inordinately rare' in rural areas but had become 'fairly common' in urban dwellers. Campbell was fluent in siZulu and so able to communicate with his patients directly (a useful clinical tool that he wryly recommended to other South African physicians). Tracking their life histories, he argued that there was a kind of 'incubation' period for diabetes of about 20 years – what he called the 'twenty year rule'.[19] In other words, rural Africans moving to town developed insulin resistance only after a prolonged exposure to an urban diet, and this finding, he discovered, was replicated by research on migrant communities elsewhere in the world. With his African assistants he produced Zulu-language material to help his patients manage their diets, public education leaflets on prevention which were distributed throughout the Durban area, and presented a series of Zulu-language health programmes broadcast on the radio.

In his MD thesis Campbell emphasised the importance of getting to know his patients personally and of an understanding attitude towards their struggles to adhere to dietary advice. 'Bad' diabetics, he wrote, 'are honest and genuine patients who try as hard as they can to carry out the diabetologist's instructions, but they cannot, because they cannot afford a low carbohydrate diet.'[20] Nevertheless, his Zulu-language pamphlet of

'Advice and Admonitions' was, by present-day standards, rather heavy on the admonitions, including the following statements: 'Your gross obesity disturbs me'; 'You are as fat as a pig (or hippo), and 'Fat people die before their time'.[21] Reflecting on the ways in which 'fatness' might be viewed positively by communities in which nutritional abundance was not the norm, he recounted how the messages of his health education material could backfire. For example, a poster on the dangers of obesity contrasted a slim Zulu woman, who was able to climb a hill to her home and still be able to do her housework when she got there, to an overweight Zulu woman who, after climbing the hill with difficulty and perspiring, collapses into a comfortable-looking chair. Over 90 per cent of those interviewed had interpreted the poster as illustrating that the 'fat' lady was rich (which was why she was fat in the first place), and that having reached the top of the hill was 'at liberty to loll in a chair while the servants did the housework'.[22] As this 'misunderstanding' implied, an association between large body size and prosperity was strong amongst Durban's African communities.

As Campbell accumulated more clinical and contextual information from his clinic's African patients, so he formulated a typology of diabetes. In his early attempts at classification, Campbell delineated a small but significant number of 'thin' diabetics. One sub-group of this category, which he described as being of 'peasant' origin, were mainly older (over 60); another was composed of younger patients (under 40) who were insulin dependent.[23] However, over half of the clinic's patients were middle aged and overweight. Women outnumbered men in this category, and since African women were rarely employed in 'white collar' positions, this rather cast doubt on the accuracy of his characterisation of diabetes as the 'disease of the briefcase'. Campbell noted that some of these patients had to travel long distances to and from work (a reflection of apartheid-era urban policy), had little time to cook and ate late at night. Women, he noted, were particularly prone to weight gain when they moved into urban areas – a finding which by the early 1960s was being reflected in research by others in South Africa, and which resonates with present-day data on female overweight and obesity in the country.[24] One study of Durban's Zulu-speaking dwellers, conducted in 1958, and quoted by Campbell, found that nearly 70 per cent of women were overweight by 10 per cent or more and over a third by 25 per cent or more. On average the women were more than 30lbs heavier than their rural counterparts of the same height. The authors also noted that male heights in this urban sample were significantly lower than those of 'rural Zulus' studied in 1927, implying that the urban men of the late 1950s had experienced less favourable nutritional conditions in their infancies and childhoods than had been the case for rural children in the late 1920s. Pointing to the phenomenon which today is often labelled the 'double burden of malnutrition', the authors also noted that alongside overweight and obesity in the urban population, there existed a high prevalence of malnutrition, evidenced by skin and mucosal lesions. This they attributed to the fact that over 50 per cent of calories in the 'typical' diet came from refined maize flour.[25] If Durban's African population was getting heavier by the late 1950s, this was not necessarily the result of better nutrition, and in his clinic Campbell was seeing the consequences.

Dietary change, carbohydrates and refined sugar

In 1950s South Africa, medical research routinely both reflected and provided a 'scientific' rationale for ideologies of race (as described by Pentecost in this volume). But, as is well known, South Africa's community of medical scientists and practitioners also contained more radical thinkers and proponents of 'social medicine'.[26] Campbell did not count himself as one of the latter, but he was highly critical of racial theory when employed as an explanation for susceptibility to diabetes.[27] Though he had noted distinct differences between Durban's Indian and African populations in terms of the clinical manifestations of diabetes, Campbell had early on discarded 'heredity' in favour of 'environment' as the driver of diabetes causation. Foremost amongst the environmental factors he saw operating was the changing diet and the role of the country's powerful food industry in shaping this.

Reflecting his own family's interest in the region's ethnography and history, Campbell dived into a rather speculative longer-term analysis of dietary change in the Natal region.[28] Noting the dominance of the Zulu aristocratic name Dlamini amongst the patients who first arrived at his clinic, Campbell noted from Bryant's 1907 study of Zulu medicine that diabetes (*umxhoboko*) had been known as the 'King's Disease', which 'affected fat people' whose bodies 'get wasted from the inside'.[29] Though at first glance the high diabetic incidence amongst the Dlaminis might look like a hereditary factor at work, Campbell argued that, over the ten years of his practice, he had become convinced that among the Zulu population 'environmental factors have swamped those due to heredity'. He pointed to what he saw as three major changes in the diet of Africans in the Natal region over the previous 100 years. He argued that in the nineteenth century the Zulu people had largely subsisted on animal products (meat and sour milk) but this diet had undergone a major change with the rinderpest epidemic which swept the region in the 1890s, wiping out herds. The 'maize and cereal' era which followed (he dated this 1895–1945) had probably lowered the general resistance of the population to disease, but this was nothing to the detrimental effects of what he called the post-1945 era of 'refined carbohydrates' which had particularly affected urban dwellers. This he characterised as a shift from unrefined carbohydrates to white bread 'of the highest refinement', sugar and sugared foods, and 'a growing now massive ingestion of sweetened soft drinks'.[30] This 'era' had seen the emergence not only of type 2 diabetes, but also of obesity.

Campbell's characterisation of these nutritional 'eras' was certainly rather crude, but he was probably right to surmise that a set of longer-term factors were interacting with more recent shifts in diet and environment to produce what would today be labelled 'metabolic disorders'.[31] His central focus, however, was on what he saw as the dramatic changes of the post-1945 era, particularly for the migrant who moved from a rural to an urban area. For this he drew on a fairly rich body of nutritional survey work conducted in the 1950s, as well as his own observations, including a characteristically South African 'experiment' on his own domestic worker, which would probably not pass an ethics review today. He also compared the results of two dietary surveys – one carried out (1959) in the urban location of Lamontville ('settled' urban dwellers, employed and in family housing) and another in 1952 in a rural area of Northern Natal (Nongoma).[32] The latter community was poor, undernourished and particularly lacking in protein. The members of the former were much better fed, though Campbell noted that malnutrition was still a problem amongst some urban children. Aside from marked differences in animal protein intake and the nature of the cereals consumed (home-prepared maize in the rural area, white bread in the urban one), there was also a large gap in sugar consumption. In Nongoma around 1 per cent of dietary calories derived from sugar, and this was mostly used in the preparation of alcoholic drinks; in Lamontville it constituted 16 per cent of calories.[33] By the late 1950s and early 1960s, rural consumption was beginning to catch up.

Meanwhile in the clinic, Campbell was seeing many more poorer urban residents with diabetes. In his somewhat dystopic 1969 address to the National Association of Scientists, entitled 'Man as an Ecological Animal', Campbell noted the presence of these patients from the 'lowest' social groups, who 'were not, and obviously could not be lavish eaters', but many of whom were 'very fat'.[34] He also cited work by a colleague in

Durban who had found obesity amongst people subsisting on less than 2000 calories a day. He would later underline the importance of these results (and those of comparative studies among the Pima Indians and other groups) in his evidence to the 1973 US Senate Select Committee on Nutrition and Human Needs.[35] It seemed clear to him, through both comparative and longitudinal study, that the most likely causative factor was the urban diet of refined carbohydrates (white bread), sugar and sweetened foods.[36] By his own account, by the mid-60s, he had become a 'massive environmentalist', deriding both those who clung to racial theories of disease causation and the 'rat and test-tube merchants' who confined their research to the laboratory.

In the majority of his publications Campbell made it clear that he did not think it was possible to isolate the physiological effects of sugar consumption from the broader effects of refined carbohydrates.[37] However, this did not stop him from viewing increased sugar intake in South Africa's 'non-white' population as particularly damaging and invidious, especially as this was the result of very deliberate marketing strategies adopted by the South African sugar industry. In a 1965 letter to Cleave he quoted at length from a South African Cane Growers Association internal report, produced by its research and marketing department in 1962.[38] Noting that the market for sugar amongst the white, Indian and 'Coloured' communities of South Africa was nearing saturation point (thanks to 'great advances' in marketing to those communities in the previous 20 years), the researchers turned their attention to the majority 'Bantu' population. Per capita annual consumption by the 'urban Bantu' had reached 85lbs, and 'Although he could eat considerably more than he does, it seems he can hardly afford to do so.' Surveys had shown that the 'urban Bantu' were already spending 40.3 per cent of their income on food 'which is unavoidably carrying insufficient protein' and that 8.1 per cent of that food bill went on sugar (the equivalent figure for Europeans was 6.5 per cent). Without a significant rise in wages, the opportunities to expand urban sugar consumption seemed limited. The research committee turned its attention to the 'outer rural areas', where nearly 60 per cent of the population lived. Rural Africans consumed on average 39lbs of sugar per capita each year, and this represented 31 per cent of the South African sugar market. Because 'these people are so numerous' it was clear that there were potentially large gains to be made by encouraging the consumption of even just one extra pound of sugar per person. Apparently their strategies to do so were effective. In 1964 Campbell was reporting a marked increase in rural consumption, which he said had taken place over the previous three to four years. This included increases in remoter rural areas where transport costs were higher.[39] Campbell was incensed by the marketing strategies of the sugar industry, including its use of the spurious notion of the 'appestat' – an early example of bogus neuroscience that enabled them (in the US and elsewhere) to claim that sugar could be used as a slimming aid. In South Africa however, the 'appestat' was less likely to appeal to African consumers than claims that sugar empowered, strengthened and energised, and this is what the industry emphasised.[40] Campbell stepped up his criticism of the industry from the early 1960s and, in 1965, attacked it directly at South African Medical Congress, resulting in newspaper coverage, including a cartoon (see Figure 5.1 below) depicting himself, which he relished.

But, as is well known, the industry, both locally and internationally, struck back and in particular launched a well-funded attack on artificial sweeteners.[41] In 1967 an editorial in the South African Tongaat Sugar Company's journal, *The Condenser*, asserted that 'Glucose is a nutritious

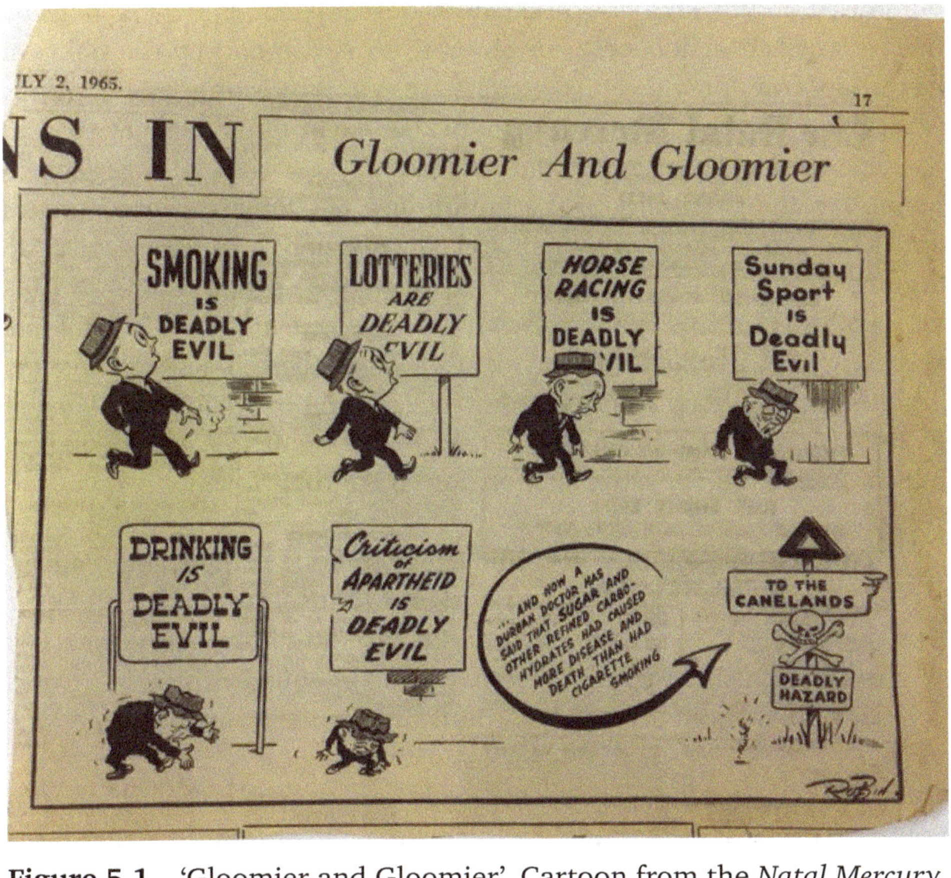

Figure 5.1 'Gloomier and Gloomier', Cartoon from the *Natal Mercury*, 2 July 1965. © Independent News and Media Group, South Africa

food which has a place in the fabric of a modern society', and that 'if the sweetness which sugar provides is habit-forming, this is no reason to condemn its properties'.[42] Supported by the apartheid government, and by a growing industrial market, the South African sugar industry continued to enjoy a boom which had begun in the postwar years and lasted to the slump (helped by sanctions) which began in the mid-1980s.[43] Today, with consumption now plateauing at around four times the WHO-recommended intake, and faced by the possible consequences of the sweetened beverage tax, the South African Sugar Association (SASA) continues to pour doubt on scientific findings and to promote the importance of this 'natural' product to a balanced diet.

By the time of delivering his address on 'Man as an Ecological Animal' in 1969, Campbell had concluded that the members of so-called 'advanced' countries were turning into 'pillars of sugar'. Reflecting a more widespread ecological pessimism, he pointed to the consequences of global overpopulation and the co-existence of malnutrition/starvation with overconsumption. The human race, he argued, was not advancing but poised on the edge of a 'precipitous descent' – as evidenced both by the widespread incidence of degenerative disease and by the political history of the previous 50 years.[44] In an interesting and perhaps prescient twist to his very emphatically environmentalist approach, he suggested that recent scientific evidence on antibiotic resistance pointed to the possibility of the inheritance of acquired characteristics and a rapprochement with Lamarckism.[45] Campbell did not give up arguing against the sugar industry. As we have seen, he defended his views robustly in front of Senator McGovern's hearings in 1973. But it is revealing that in the 1980s he still felt compelled to make the same arguments. In a letter to the editor of the *South African Medical Journal* in 1980, Campbell vigorously objected to the industry's advertising on television and radio, particularly on 'Radio Bantu':

> Particular reservation must be expressed about the slanted advertisements on Radio Bantu. The words *ushukela unamandla* ('sugar has strength' and therefore 'sugar imparts strength') are particularly sinister in this regard, since, whether intended or not, the word *amandla* ('strength') is also synonymous with sexual potency.[46]

Campbell's apparent failure to persuade the medical establishment in South Africa to stand up against the sugar industry hardly comes as a surprise, given what we know about South African political economy and the history of the sugar industry. Campbell's work, however, draws attention to the fact that in South Africa, the penetration of industrialised diets into rural as well as urban African communities goes back much further than the 1990s, when the growing problem of NCDs (combined with HIV) started refocusing attention on nutrition. With the benefit of hindsight, it is also easy to point to the limitations of his work. Because he (initially at least) framed diabetes as primarily a 'disease of the briefcase' and hence of increasing affluence, he may have paid less attention to the question of undernutrition in the communities from which his patients originated. At the same time as Campbell carried out his research on diabetes, a number of his South African colleagues were engaged in work on what was perceived, by some at least, as the scandal of widespread protein/calorie malnutrition.[47] As we now know from developmental origins of health and disease (DOHAD) theory, these two forms of malnutrition may in some individuals be directly related – the underweight infant may be predisposed to central obesity, insulin resistance and diabetes as an adult, as well as other conditions normally associated with increased affluence.[48] There are hints of this in some of his own research, and also in the work by others on obesity that he cites, but he does not make the connection himself. In some ways his work, perceptive though it was, is also an early example of the ways in which specialisation in what are now called NCDs can limit our understanding of disease environments. Campbell did note that many of his patients suffered from multiple morbidities, but his clinical and research focus was on their diabetic condition. Recent work in South Africa and elsewhere points to the complex relationship between infectious and 'non-communicable' conditions, and to the importance of addressing them within one frame, as well as to the challenges of multimorbidity within the 'non-communicable' category of diseases.[49]

A tentative conclusion

The historical framework of 'transition', a version of modernisation theory, has been widely critiqued from the perspective of sub-Saharan Africa for some time. Given what we know about the uneven effects of capitalism on the continent and the impact of different forms of colonialism (some of which quite consciously inhibited 'modernisation'), it is not surprising that the epidemiological version of this framework should also prove less than satisfactory. In much colonial health research on the continent, new disease patterns were frequently attributed to the inability of Africans to 'adapt' to modern life and were sometimes explicitly linked to racial theory. This intellectual history left a marked hangover – the ground between universalism and difference was a narrow one, inflected by the history of racism. Present-day Global Health institutions have, I think, inherited these tensions. As has been often noted, the 'universal' human body of biomedicine is in fact modelled on the bodily experience of European and North American populations, and deviations from this norm are frequently racialised.[50] The current use made of the theory of epidemiologic transition to explain the rising prevalence of what are now called non-communicable conditions probably obscures as much as it illuminates. It is undeniable that demographic changes and rapid urbanisation have a profound influence on patterns of disease. However, these effects are not usefully thought of as the consequences of 'transition'. We need a less linear and more environmentally grounded theory of change that pays attention to the inheritance of longer histories of infectious disease, nutrition, economic change and environmental pollution, as well as to the (sometimes unintended) consequences of medical interventions, particularly those directed at infant and child health. Critically, as much global research on NCDs demonstrates, we need to appreciate the ways in which what are so frequently still termed 'diseases of affluence' have in fact come to dominate the lives of the world's poorest communities.[51] As Campbell's diabetes work in the 1950s and 60s demonstrated, the active marketing of unhealthy foodstuffs in South Africa could transform a 'disease of the briefcase' to one of much wider concern within a generation.

Notes

1 Research for this paper was generously supported by an Investigator Award from the Wellcome Trust: Award No. 170510. I am extremely grateful to Keith Breckenridge and Catherine Burns for their advice and archival leads in South Africa and to the archivists of the Wellcome Library for their advice. Particular thanks go to Professor Catherine Campbell and her family, who gave me permission to quote from George D. Campbell's correspondence with Peter Cleave, held in the Wellcome Library, and for generously sharing her insights into her father's work and life with me.

2 Republic of South Africa, National Department of Health, 'Strategy for the Prevention and Control of Obesity'; Republic of South Africa, National Department of Health, 'Strategic Plan for the Prevention and Control of Non-Communicable Diseases'; Republic of South Africa, Department of National Treasury, 'Taxation of Sugar Sweetened Beverages'; Steyn and Temple, 'Evidence to Support a Food-based Dietary Guideline'; Kruger et al., 'Obesity in South Africa'; Rouquest-Ross, Vink, and Sigge., 'Food Consumption Changes'; Cois and Day, 'Obesity Trends'.

3 Myers et al., 'Sugar and Health in South Africa'; Myers et al., 'The History of the South African Sugar Industry'.

4 Wylie, *Starving on a Full Stomach*.

5 Brian Williams, 'Letter to the Editor'.

6 Taubes, *The Case Against Sugar*, 156–7.

7 Yudkin, *Pure, White and Deadly*. A revised edition of Yudkin's book was published in 1986. Though working on similar lines, Campbell did not agree with many of Yudkin's arguments.
8 Cummings and Engineer, 'Denis Burkitt'; Cleave, Campbell, and Painter, *Diabetes*.
9 This view is echoed by more recent commentators on the role of the food industry in the production of malnutrition and obesity: Ledger, *An Empty Plate*; Greenberg, 'Corporate Power in the Agro-Food System'.
10 George D. Campbell, 1925–98. He was a direct descendant of Sir Marshall Campbell (1848–1917), a settler, who was a pioneer of the sugar industry in Natal, and he mentions this connection in his correspondence with Peter Cleave: Wellcome Library, Correspondence of Peter Cleave and G.D. Campbell. According to his family, the Campbells of Natal were divided into two 'wings': one represented by the commercial sugar interests, the other by public service and intellectual pursuits. George D. Campbell was firmly in the second camp. See also Cummings and Engineer, 'Denis Burkitt'.
11 Campbell had a number of other medical interests. As a result of his work (1956–7) in the medical isotopes unit at the University of Edinburgh, he was one of the first to warn of the damaging effects of thalidomide. In Durban, in addition to being an expert on diabetes, he was also known as an expert on shark attacks, and published on this subject. Later in his career he worked in a number of rural hospitals in South Africa and also earned a reputation for his research on mycotoxins.
12 Campbell and McKechnie, 'Recent Observations on Zulu and Natal Indian Diabetics'; Campbell, 'Diabetes in Asians and Africans'; Campbell, 'Some Observations'; Campbell, 'Zulu Diabetic'.
13 Campbell did not regard the type 1/type 2 distinction as useful but he was mostly referring to what other researchers would call diabetes mellitus, or type 2. This is a larger discussion.
14 Campbell, 'Connubial Diabetes'.
15 Neel, 'Diabetes Mellitus'.
16 However, Campbell did find that cane cutters could consume vast amounts of sugar (both refined sugar in their rations and raw sugar cane) without apparently developing glycosuria. He put this down to the extremely hard physical labour they performed and their consequent energy expenditure. He also experimented on marine animals, attempting to induce glycosuria.
17 The methodology is discussed in detail in Campbell's MD thesis, 'Zulu Diabetic'.
18 On rising living standards in the postwar period and African consumption see Ross, 'The Politics of Household Budget Studies'; Posel, 'Getting Inside the Skin of the Consumers'.
19 Campbell, 'Zulu Diabetic', 47.
20 Campbell, 'Zulu Diabetic', 104.
21 Campbell, 'Zulu Diabetic', Appendix 2. See also, Campbell and Lugg, *Handbook to Aid*.
22 Campbell, 'Zulu Diabetic', 107.
23 On the 'thin diabetic' phenotype in South Asia and its history see Solomon, *Metabolic Living*.
24 Campbell, 'Zulu Diabetic', 53; Slome et al., 'Weight, Height and Skinfold Thickness'; Chesler, 'A Study of Attitudes'; Gradige et al., 'The Role of Lifestyle'.
25 Slome et al., 'Weight, Height and Skinfold Thickness', 507. Slome and his colleagues were using US norms against which to measure obesity and overweight – a practice which is of course open to question and might have skewed their results. On malnutrition in South Africa at this time see Wylie, *Starving on a Full Stomach*, especially Chapter 7.
26 Marks, 'South Africa's Early Experiment'; Digby and Sweet, 'Social Medicine'.
27 He expressed this very clearly when giving evidence to the US Senate's Select Committee on Nutrition and Human Needs in 1973, when he was pressed on the question by the Chair, Senator McGovern. The transcript was consulted in the Wellcome Library, London, PP/TLC/E2.
28 Campbell, 'Zulu Diabetic', 27–32. Campbell was related to Killie Campbell (1881–1965), a well-known Africana collector. Her collection was bequeathed to the University of Natal. Several other members of the family also took an interest in African history and ethnography.
29 Bryant, *A Description of Native Foodstuffs*. Campbell also included in his thesis a Zulu Royal Family tree onto which he marked each known case of diabetes or *umxhoboko*. He found this disease to be particularly associated with King Mphande (reign 1840–72), who 'was so obese that he could not walk and had to be dragged around on ox-skins or a small cart'. Campbell compared this sedentary stay-at-home king to his famously militant and physically fit predecessors, Shaka and Dingaan. Clearly much of this has to be viewed through the lens of

Shaka mythology, though Campbell has at least some evidence to support it. Campbell, 'Zulu Diabetic', 44.

30 Campbell also drew on the work of Halley Stott of the Valley Trust, who had collected data in 1958 showing a distinct shift to refined carbohydrates and processed foods even in this rural area: Stott, 'The Valley Trust Socio-Medical Project', 51–5 and Appendix A(a).

31 Wells, *The Metabolic Ghetto*.

32 Campbell, 'Zulu Diabetic', 32–3. The surveys Campbell was referring to were Gampel's 1959 study of Lamontville location, just south of Durban, conducted for the Institute of Family, Health and Community Planning at the University of Natal, and Brinton and Drysdale's 1952 survey of 'peasant groups' in Northern Zululand, published in the *Journal of Social Research*, volume 13. I have not been able to consult either of these studies.

33 He would later argue that when sugar constituted 20 per cent of calorie intake, this was a tipping point for diabetes.

34 Campbell, 'Man as an Ecological Animal'.

35 Wellcome Library, London, PP/TLC/C/1/11, Box 14.

36 This wider comparative work was published in 1969 with Peter Cleave: T. L. Cleave and G. D. Campbell, *Diabetes, Coronary Thrombosis and the Saccharine Disease*. Cleave and Campbell later fell out rather dramatically over issues of authorship, as is evident from their correspondence. See also Cummings and Engineer, 'Denis Burkitt'.

37 This was one source of his and Cleave's disagreement with the work of Yudkin, author of *Pure, White and Deadly*.

38 Wellcome Library, PP/TLC/C/1/11, Box 14. Campbell to Cleave, 6 February 1965 and Campbell to Cleave, 21 April 1965.

39 Wellcome Library, PP/TLC/C/1/11, Box 14. Campbell to Cleave, 28 December 1964.

40 Wellcome Library, PP/TLC/C/1/11, Box 14. Campbell to Cleave, 13 January 1965.

41 When Campbell went to give evidence to the US Senate Select Committee on Nutrition and Human Needs in 1973 he was pressed on the question of the safety of artificial sweeteners. In the course of this questioning he revealed that he was being paid by Coca-Cola to carry out research on sugar substitutes. Wellcome Library, PP/TLC/E2:

'McGovern: What about soft drinks?
Campbell: I must declare an interest here, because I am actually in the employ of Coca-Cola as a consultant in synthetic sweeteners and I would hate to prejudice my very pleasurable association with this company, but I think that soft drinks are the biggest villains of all, because they are the things that start the children off.'

42 Campbell had family connections with the Tongaat company and carried out research on their plantations. Tongaat Sugar Company, *The Condenser*.

43 Myers et al., 'History of South African Sugar Industry'.

44 Here he cited the Holocaust, Stalin's purges and, referring to the Partition of India, 'the sanguine manner in which the British Labour Party imposed Apartheid upon India'. Tellingly, he did not mention the South African architects of apartheid itself and the consequences of the apartheid regime for African health. Wellcome Library, PP/TLC/C/1/11, Box 14. Campbell, 'Man as an Ecological Animal'.

45 This seems to anticipate the insights of epigenetics, now playing a central part in the understanding of disease causation, and influential in South Africa; see Pentecost in this volume and Pentecost, 'The First One Thousand Days'.

46 Campbell and Jackson, 'Sugar for Energy'; Campbell, 'Sugar Has Become the Opium of the People'.

47 Wylie, *Starving on a Full Stomach*.

48 Barker, 'The Origins of the Developmental Origins Theory'.

49 Oni and Unwin, 'Why the Communicable/Non-Communicable Disease Dichotomy Is Problematic'; Mendenhall and Norris, 'When HIV is Ordinary and Diabetes New'; Moran-Thomas, *Traveling with Sugar*; Lalkhen and Mash, 'Multimorbidity in Noncommunicable Diseases'.

50 Lock and Nguyen, *An Anthropology of Biomedicine*; Vaughan, 'Conceptualising Metabolic Disorder'; Solomon, *Metabolic Living*; Yates-Doerr, *The Weight of Obesity*.

51 Stuckler and Siegel, *Sick Societies*; Patel, *Stuffed and Starved*.

Bibliography

Barker, David J. 'The Origins of the Developmental Origins Theory', *Journal of Internal Medicine*, 261 (2007): 412–17.

Bryant, A. T. *A Description of Native Foodstuffs and Their Preparation*. Pietermaritzburg: Natal Government, 1907.

Campbell, G. D. 'Connubial Diabetes and the Possible Role of "Oral Diabetogens"', *British Medical Journal*, 1 (1961): 1538–9.

Campbell, G. D. 'Some Observations upon 4000 African and Asian Diabetics Collected in Durban between 1958 and 1962', *East African Medical Journal*, 40 (1963): 267–76.

Campbell, G. D. 'Diabetes in Asians and Africans in and around Durban', *South African Medical Journal*, 37 (1963): 1195–208.

Campbell, G. D. 'The Zulu Diabetic'. MD Thesis, University of Edinburgh, 1968.

Campbell, G. D. 'Man as an Ecological Animal': Guest Lecture, National Association of Scientists (Eastern Province Branch), 10 March 1969. Wellcome Library, London: PP/TLC/C/1/11, Box 14.

Campbell, G. D. 'Sugar Has Become the Opium of the People', *Nutrition and Health*, 10 (1995): 93–104.

Campbell, G. D. and W. P. Jackson. 'Sugar for Energy: Misleading Advertising', *South African Medical Journal*, (1980): 767.

Campbell, G. D. and H. C. Lugg. *Handbook to Aid in the Treatment of Zulu Patients*. Durban: University of Natal Press, 1961.

Campbell, G. D. and J. McKechnie. 'Recent Observations on Zulu and Natal Indian Diabetics in Durban', *South African Medical Journal*, 35 (1961): 1008–11.

Chesler, Julia. 'A Study of Attitudes and Knowledge Concerning Obesity in an Urban African Community', *South African Journal of Nutrition*, 35 (1961): 129–31.

Cleave, T. L. and G. D. Campbell. *Diabetes, Coronary Thrombosis and the Saccharine Disease*. Bristol: John Wright, 1969.

Cois, Annibale and Candy Day. 'Obesity Trends and Risk Factors in the South African Adult Population', *BMC Obesity*, 2 (2015): 42.

Cummings, J.H. and A. Engineer. 'Denis Burkitt and the Origins of the Dietary Fibre Hypothesis', *Nutrition Research Reviews*, 31 (2018): 1–15.

Digby, Anne and Helen Sweet. 'Social Medicine and Medical Pluralism: The Valley Trust and Botha's Hill Health Centre, South Africa, 1940s to 2000', *Social History of Medicine*, 25 (2012): 425–45.

Gradige, Philippe et al. 'The Role of Lifestyle and Psycho-Social Factors in Predicting Changes in Body Composition in Black South African Women', *PLoS One*, 10, no. 7 (2015), doi: 10/1371/journal.pone.0132914.

Greenberg, Steven. 'Corporate Power in the Agro-Food System and South Africa's Consumer Environment', Working Paper 32, Institute for Poverty, Land and Agrarian Studies, University of Western Cape, 2016.

Kruger, S. et al. 'Obesity in South Africa: Challenges for Government and Health Professionals', *Public Health Nutrition*, 8, no. 5 (2005): 491–500.

Lalkhen, H. and R. Mash. 'Multimorbidity in Noncommunicable Diseases in South African Primary Health Care', *South African Medical Journal*, 105 (2015): 134–8.

Ledger, Tracy. *An Empty Plate: Why We Are Losing the Battle for Our Food System, Why It Matters and How We Can Win It Back*. Auckland Park: Jacana Media, 2016.

Lock, Margaret and Vin-Kim Nguyen. *An Anthropology of Biomedicine*. Chichester: Wiley-Blackwell, 2010.

Marks, Shula. 'South Africa's Early Experiment in Social Medicine: Its Pioneers and Politics', *American Journal of Public Health*, 87 (1997): 452–9.

Mendenhall, Emily and Shane Norris. 'When HIV is Ordinary and Diabetes New: Remaking Suffering in a South African Township', *Global Public Health*, 10 (2015): 1–14.

Moran-Thomas, Amy. *Traveling with Sugar: Chronicles of a Global Epidemic*. Berkeley, CA: University of California Press, 2019.

Myers, Alex, et al. 'Sugar and Health in South Africa: Potential Challenges to Leveraging Policy Change', *Global Public Health*, 12 (2015): 1–18.

Myers, Alex, et al.. 'The History of the South African Sugar Industry Illuminates Deeply Rooted Obstacles for Sugar Reduction Anti-Obesity Interventions, *African Studies*, 76 (2017): 475–90.

Neel, James V. 'Diabetes Mellitus: A "Thrifty" Genotype rendered Detrimental by "Progress"?', *American Journal of Human Genetics*, 14, no. 4 (1962): 353–62.

Oni, Tolullah and Nigel Unwin. 'Why the Communicable/Non-Communicable Disease Dichotomy is Problematic for Public Health Control Settings: Implications of Multimorbidity for Health Systems in an Era of Health Transition', *International Health*, 7 (2015): 390–9.

Patel, Raj. *Stuffed and Starved: From Farm to Fork: The Hidden Battle for the World Food System*. Revised edition. New York: Melville House, 2012.

Pentecost, Michelle. 'The First One Thousand Days: Epigenetics in the Age of Global Health' in *The Palgrave Handbook of Biology and Society*, edited by M. Meloni et al., 269–94. Basingstoke: Palgrave Macmillan, 2018.

Posel, Deborah. 'Getting Inside the Skin of the Consumers: Race, Market Research and the Consumerist Project in Apartheid South Africa', *Itinerario*, 42 (2018): 12–138.

Republic of South Africa, National Department of Health. *Strategic Plan for the Prevention and Control of Non-Communicable Diseases, 2013–2017*. Pretoria: National Department of Health, 2013.

Republic of South Africa, National Department of Health. *Strategy for the Prevention and Control of Obesity, 2015–2020*. Pretoria: National Department of Health, 2015.

Republic of South Africa, Department of National Treasury. *Taxation of Sugar Sweetened Beverages Policy Paper*. Pretoria: Department of National Treasury, 2016.

Ross, Robert. 'The Politics of Household Budget Studies in South Africa', *History in Africa*, 43 (2016): 205–28.

Rouquest-Ross, L. C., N. Vink, and G. O. Sigge. 'Food Consumption Changes in South Africa since 1994', *South African Journal of Science*, 111 (2015), doi: 10.17159/sajs.2015/20140354.

Slome, C. et al. 'Weight, Height and Skinfold Thickness of Zulu Adults in Durban', *South African Medical Journal*, 34 (1960): 505–9.

Solomon, Harris. *Metabolic Living: Food, Fat and the Absorption of Illness in India*. Durham, NC: Duke University Press, 2016.

Steyn, N. P. and N. J. Temple. 'Evidence to Support a Food-Based Dietary Guideline on Sugar Consumption in South Africa', *BMC Public Health*, 12 (2012): 502.

Stott, Halley Harwin. 'The Valley Trust Socio-Medical Project for the Production of Health in a Less Developed Rural Area'. MD Thesis, Edinburgh University, 1976.

Stuckler, David and Karen Siegel. *Sick Societies: Responding to the Global Challenge of Chronic Disease*. Oxford: Oxford University Press, 2011.

Taubes, G. *The Case Against Sugar*. London: Portobello Books, 2017.

Tongaat Sugar Company, *The Condenser*, 5, no. 5 (1967): 14–19.

Vaughan, Megan. 'Conceptualising Metabolic Disorder in Southern Africa: Biology, History and Global Health', *Biosocieties*, 14 (2019): 123–42.

Wells, J. *The Metabolic Ghetto: An Evolutionary Perspective on Nutrition, Power Relations and Chronic Disease*. Cambridge: Cambridge University Press, 2016.

Wellcome Library, Archival Collections, MSS. PP/TLC/C/11, Box 14. Correspondence of Peter Cleave with G.D. Campbell.

Williams, Brian. 'Letter to the Editor', *Mail and Guardian*, 11 May 2018: https://mg.co.za/article/2018-05-11-00-letters-to-the-editor-may-11-to-17, last accessed 6 December 2019.

Wylie, Diana. *Starving on a Full Stomach: Hunger and the Triumph of Cultural Racism in Modern South Africa*. Charlottesville, VA: University of Virginia Press, 2001.

Yates-Doerr, Emily. *The Weight of Obesity: Hunger and Global Health in Postwar Guatemala*. Oakland, CA: University of California Press, 2015.

Yudkin, J. *Pure, White and Deadly*. London: Davis-Poynter, 1972.

Part 2

6

Africa and Chronic Disease: Rechecking the Effectiveness of Measures

Kafui Adjaye-Gbewonyo

The global health community has gradually been turning its attention toward chronic non-communicable diseases (NCDs) in low- and middle-income countries (LMICs).[1] However, as Sanuade explains in the next chapter, the lack of well-established NCD surveys, disease registries, cohort studies and complete health facility data has meant that the data available to understand chronic NCDs, their risk factors and appropriate interventions in these settings are limited. There have been recent attempts to fill in these data gaps. The World Health Organization (WHO) has implemented World Health Surveys, Stepwise Approach to Surveillance (STEPS) and the longitudinal Study on Global Ageing and Adult Health (SAGE). Countries such as South Africa have conducted National Health and Nutrition Examination Surveys. The INDEPTH Network of Health and Demographic Surveillance Sites has been implementing verbal autopsy methods to measure causes of death. Nevertheless, questions remain about the validity and accuracy of some of the survey instruments being used to measure chronic diseases in population surveillance.

Firstly, many survey instruments designed to diagnose chronic conditions in non-clinical settings were originally developed and validated in Europe or the United States. Thus, they may not be as valid in other cultural settings. In addition, even for measures that were developed and tested for global use, one must still consider the extent to which they capture the phenomena they intend to measure. Of course, as anthropologists of global health often note, the exercise of trying to measure and quantify human experience is in itself fraught with many complexities and problems and results in reducing people's lives to numbers. We may therefore lose important nuances in the process. Nevertheless, in this era of governance and global health, measuring disease burden is necessary for allocating scarce resources and justifying evidence-based use of these resources. Thus, creating valid and meaningful instruments for measuring disease and ill health is critical.[2]

In this chapter, I give a brief overview of how validity is assessed and then present two case studies of self-reported, symptom-based measures relating to chronic NCDs. The first case is of a scale that measures what may be considered a 'mental' health phenomenon, namely depression/depressive symptoms measured by the Center for Epidemiologic Studies of Depression (CES-D) scale. The second case is of an instrument that measures what may be described as a 'physical' health phenomenon, namely angina pectoris (or chest pain due to coronary heart disease) measured by the Rose Angina Questionnaire (RAQ). While these are two seemingly different health issues, as becomes evident below, the links between physical and emotional pain are often strong and the divide between 'mental' and 'physical' may in some ways be viewed as artificial.[3]

This chapter reviews questions, concerns and data about the validity of these scales primarily from a measurement perspective. Thus, assuming that the health constructs of 'depression' and 'angina' are meaningful in African contexts, how can we assess the validity of these instruments for measuring the occurrence of these health phenomena in African settings? There is of course another question of equal or greater concern – that of whether these health constructs, as presently defined, are themselves valid in various African societies. This is a question that this chapter will only touch on briefly, but which has been widely debated, particularly in relation to global mental health.[4]

Assessing validity

From the standpoint of scales – survey instruments used to measure underlying constructs – validity is one of what are referred to as the psychometric properties of a scale. As its name implies, the term 'psychometric' refers to psychological measurement and psychometrics is a branch of psychology that focusses on the quantitative measurement of the mind through instruments such as scales.[5] Scales are designed as a series of questions or items that all intend to measure a single latent construct or underlying variable (for example, depression).[6] The psychometric properties of a scale include measures of its validity (or whether the scale indeed measures the construct it is designed to measure) and reliability (how consistently the scale measures the construct and reproduces the results when there is no real change). A scale must be reliable in order to be valid, but reliability alone does not ensure validity.[7]

There are a number of different types of validity to consider when assessing an instrument. These include face validity, criterion-related validity, content validity and construct validity. 'Face validity' refers to how well the scale appears to measure the latent construct on its face – in other words whether the scale, when looked at, appears to measure what it intends to measure. However, the concept of face validity has been criticised by some scholars for being ambiguous.[8] Criterion-related validity assesses the scale's predictive capability or how well the scale or instrument compares to a 'gold standard' such as a clinical diagnosis. It is typically measured with a correlation coefficient, or area under the curve, and can also use predictive values.[9] Content validity refers to how well an instrument captures or represents the full content and all dimensions of a construct. This is often assessed using expert evaluations or using factor analysis.[10] Factor analysis is a technique which examines how the different items in a scale group together. This is done in order to identify different dimensions of the scale/construct and can help to examine whether the scale reliably measures all the dimensions of a construct as intended. In addition, by comparing factor analyses of responses to a scale in different samples, one can also examine whether the items group into similar factors (or dimensions) in these populations and therefore measure the same underlying constructs, or if they differ across populations.[11]

Finally, construct validity examines the relationship between the scale and other variables in order to assess whether the scale behaves in a way that one would theoretically expect it to behave. For example, you can assess *convergent* construct validity by looking at the association between the scale and other variables that are expected to be related in some way (either positively or negatively/inversely) to the latent construct the scale measures. You can assess *discriminant* construct validity by looking at the association between the scale and other variables that you would not expect to be related at all to the underlying construct it measures (that is, variables that are independent of the construct).[12]

In addition to the qualities of reliability and validity, there are other considerations that must be made to establish *measurement equivalence* in cross-cultural research.[13] Sweetland, Belkin and Verdeli note that it is important to establish five types of equivalences:

1) linguistic equivalence, such that translations retain meaning across cultures;
2) content equivalence, such that each scale item corresponds to phenomena that are experienced across cultures;
3) conceptual equivalence, such that the same latent construct is being measured across cultures;
4) technical equivalence, such that the methods used to measure the construct or administer the instrument are comparable across cultures; and
5) cultural equivalence, such that the results can be interpreted across cultures.[14]

Some of these factors are not often considered in global population-health research, where more attention has been paid to validating instruments by assessing criterion-related validity and content validity without much explicit consideration of the conceptual, technical and content equivalences of the instruments cross-culturally. In the next sections, I examine measures of validity for two survey instruments of chronic disease phenomena.

Case study 1: Depression

Culture and symptomatology in the measurement of depression

Depression is one of the leading causes of morbidity worldwide, according to estimates from the Global Burden of Disease.[15] While global data on clinical diagnoses of depression are likely to be incomplete due to low healthcare utilisation, several global and national population surveys attempt to measure depression and depressive symptoms using psychometric scales. The Africa region has often been found to have lower rates of reported depression and depressive symptoms in population surveys.[16] However, it is increasingly believed that rates of depression in Africa may be higher than previously recognised because of under-diagnosis.[17] It is clear for example that the way in which symptoms of depression are experienced or manifest themselves differs across cultural settings.[18] In fact, a significant body of research suggests that culture impacts the way in which mental illness is experienced and expressed.[19] Often though, how we define 'culture' is not made explicit and the term is frequently used merely to refer to 'cultural groups' or categories. Therefore, additional work to specify the components of 'culture' that may matter for psychological wellbeing, whether they include values, psychological perspectives (individualism versus collectivism), and so on, may strengthen this body of evidence.[20] Here, I use the term 'culture' broadly to refer to the value systems, orientations, beliefs, psychological perspectives and practices of groups linked by their history, geography or socioeconomic position.

In addition to recognising that the symptoms and manifestation of depression may differ across cultures, one may also question whether the concept of 'depression' is in fact universal, or is rather an example of a 'pseudo-etic syndrome' – one which is culture-bound but is assumed to be universal and is consequently imposed on other cultures through measurement and treatment.[21] In other words, there may not always be conceptual equivalence in the sense that the conditions or disorders that are present in a given society may not exactly correspond to 'depression'; these conditions, as well as depression itself, may be specific to that culture. Questions such as these have been raised among scholars in the field of transcultural psychiatry. In addition, some have argued that psychology and psychiatry in the global North have tended to pathologise distress as illness rather than viewing it as a product of social conditions; this biomedical framing, derived from a specific Western European cultural context, is being pushed and exported to other parts of the world.[22] Furthermore, as Ingleby notes, symptoms that may be viewed as abnormal in some circumstances may sometimes also be normal reactions under abnormal or adverse circumstances. Thus, instruments that assess symptoms without considering the contexts in which the symptoms occur may incorrectly diagnose psychological disorders and inflate their prevalence (or may alternatively result in under-reporting symptom severity since this assessment may be relative to the hardships to which one is accustomed).[23] Some research has suggested for example that many societies use a situational model of depression, viewing depressive symptoms as normal reactions to difficult life situations, rather than using the biological and psychological models common in Europe and America that view depression as a disease caused by the biology or personality of individuals.[24]

To address some of these issues, some scholars have increasingly turned to 'psychological distress' in order to encompass a range of symptoms and cultural responses of common mental disorders, rather than focusing on specific *Diagnostic Statistical Manual of Mental Disorders* (DSM) conditions from North America.[25] Similarly, some anthropologists have focussed on the idioms of distress in various cultures which also include symptoms of distress that may not always be considered pathological. For example, 'thinking too much' has been identified as an idiom of distress in many cultures.[26] Nevertheless, in the global mental health arena, mood disorders such as depression have generally been accepted as being common to all cultures, unlike conditions such as post-traumatic stress disorder which are more contested.[27] However, this is an issue where perhaps further discussion is warranted.

Assuming that something resembling 'depression' *is* a universal construct (which will be assumed throughout the analysis below), the emphasis on feelings of sadness to define depression may contribute to under-reporting, since most people around the world experience physical or somatic symptoms with depression.[28] Patel and Stein note that research in Africa and elsewhere has shown that the core symptoms of common mental disorders, which include depression and anxiety, present similarly in most societies.[29] Somatic symptoms (such as tiredness and weakness, body pain, sleep problems and so on) are the most commonly reported symptoms in Africa as in other parts of the world. While it was previously believed that the psychological distress of depression was felt as somatic symptoms in African and other 'non-Western' societies, Patel and Stein argue that, in fact, psychological symptoms *are* experienced by most people in 'non-Western' populations but they are often not reported without being asked about.[30] However, a 1999 study by Fullerton and Ormel observed that 11 per cent of patients diagnosed with depression in several countries reported no psychological symptoms even when asked explicitly about them.[31] Nevertheless, the specific characteristics and content of both cognitive and somatic symptoms have been found to differ, in some cases, in African and other communities compared to Western European communities. For example, studies of symptoms of mental disorders in Nigeria and Zimbabwe revealed some symptoms that did not resemble those used in biomedical classifications of mental disorders. These included sensations such as heat or heat in the head, a trembling tongue, crawling or turning in the head, moving under the skin, and so on.[32] In addition, the models used to explain common mental disorders also show some differences in many African societies compared to Western European societies. Specifically, there is generally a heavier emphasis on supernatural causes as one of the many explanations for these conditions in some African contexts compared to European ones.[33]

Aside from potential differences in the symptomatology and explanatory models for depression, there may also be issues with technical equivalence or the validity of the *methods* used to administer psychometric instruments. Familiarity with using Likert scales and self-assessments, for instance, can be affected by the literacy levels, formal educational attainment, socioeconomic status and cultural values of those to whom the instruments are being administered.[34]

Several psychometric instruments have been developed to measure depression. Those commonly used in research were developed predominantly among European and North American populations. These include the Beck Depression Inventory, the nine-item Patient Health Questionnaire (PHQ-9), the Mini-International Neuropsychiatric Interview (MINI) and the Hamilton Rating Scale for Depression, among others.[35] In the following section, I will examine the use of the Center for Epidemiological Studies Depression scale (CES-D) in African contexts. Although scales such as the PHQ-9 are becoming more widely used, the CES-D was designed specifically for use in epidemiological studies in the general population and in primary care.[36] And, as discussed below, a short-form version of the CES-D was adopted by Statistics South Africa for use in a national longitudinal survey on economics and wellbeing in South Africa – the National Income Dynamics Study (NIDS) – which was conducted from 2008 to 2017.[37] Consequently, there have been several studies analysing depression and depressive symptoms in South Africa based on the CES-D, while its validity in this context seems less well evaluated. The section below explores the literature relating to the validity of the CES-D and its derivatives in Africa.

Development and validation of the Center for Epidemiological Studies Depression scale (CES-D)

The CES-D was developed by the National Institute of Mental Health in Maryland, USA and first published in 1977.[38] The original scale included 20 items asking about the occurrence of a variety of recognised symptoms of depression over the past week (see Table 6.1 below) on a Likert scale:

- Rarely or none of the time (less than 1 day);
- Some or a little of the time (1–2 days);
- Occasionally or a moderate amount of time (3–4 days);
- Most or all of the time (5–7 days).

Scores can range from 0 (no depressive symptoms) to 60 (worst depressive symptoms) and generally scores of 16 or higher have been used to identify depression cases.[39] Since the development of the CES-D, short-form versions have also been developed, validated and/or used in variety of populations, including a 10-item version known as the CES-D-10.[40]

In the original report on the CES-D, the psychometric properties of the scale were judged to be good and the scale reportedly performed well

Table 6.1 Center for Epidemiologic Studies of Depression (CES-D) Scale Items[47]

	CES-D Item	**Item also appears in CES-D-10**
1	I was bothered by things that usually don't bother me.	Yes
2	I did not feel like eating; my appetite was poor.	No
3	I felt that I could not shake off the blues even with family or friends.	No
4	I felt that I was just as good as other people.	No
5	I had trouble keeping my mind on what I was doing.	Yes
6	I felt depressed.	Yes
7	I felt that everything I did was an effort.	Yes
8	I felt hopeful about the future.	Yes
9	I thought my life had been a failure.	No
10	I felt fearful.	Yes
11	My sleep was restless.	Yes
12	I was happy.	Yes
13	I talked less than usual.	No
14	I felt lonely.	Yes
15	People were unfriendly.	No
16	I enjoyed life.	No
17	I had crying spells.	No
18	I felt sad.	No
19	I felt that people dislike me.	No
20	I could not get 'going'.	Yes

among different US demographic groups.[41] However, concerns were raised that some of the items were biased among certain demographic groups, such as among people who were elderly, black and women, though not all of the concerns have been substantiated.[42] A 2015 meta-analysis of validation studies for the CES-D concluded that it had good accuracy as a screening tool to identify people for further clinical assessment; however, the authors did not recommend using it as a stand-alone diagnostic measure for depression.[43]

In the US, where the CES-D was developed, studies using factor analysis to determine the content validity of the scale have generally found the CES-D to have four factors or dimensions, namely: depressed mood, somatic effects, interpersonal problems and diminished positive affect.[44] However, results have varied in some ethnic minority samples where three-factor or two-factor structures fit the data better.[45] For example, a recent study of a 12-item version of the CES-D in a sample of black American men found that two main factors (dimensions) emerged – interpersonal negative affect and diminished positive affect. Unlike the four-factor model, depressed mood and interpersonal problems did not emerge as separate dimensions in this sample.[46] As we will see below, similar observations have been made in some African samples.

Assessing validity of the CES-D in African contexts

Postconflict and refugee populations

Like much of the research on psychological distress conducted in LMICs, a number of studies validating the CES-D in African samples have been conducted among refugees or survivors of conflict. The validity and factor structure of the CES-D were examined in studies among survivors of the Rwandan genocide and Eritrean refugees in Ethiopia.[48] In the Ethiopian study, the authors found the scale to have high reliability and there was high agreement among experts on the relevance of the translated items in the scale (a measure of content validity).[49] In both studies, the authors found that a two-factor structure best fits the data from their samples. One factor represented depressive symptoms or negative affect, including somatic, psychological and interpersonal symptoms combined. The other dimension consisted of the questions relating to positive affect. These results show that there may be conceptual differences in depressive symptomatology in these post-conflict African samples compared to the four-factor model observed in the general US population. This suggests that there are either cultural differences in the expression and manifestation of depression or other variables differentially affecting responses to the scale in these samples. As authors Getnet and Alem conclude, this illustrates the social construction of depression.[50]

Moreover, in their Rwandan sample, Lacasse and colleagues also observed interesting findings regarding the item 'I felt like everything was an effort', which loaded slightly onto the positive affect dimension although it was negatively associated with the other items in that factor. The authors interpreted this result as suggesting that respondents in this sample may be viewing the 'effort' item in a positive light rather than in a negative one.[51] (The study of black American men mentioned above interestingly also found issues with the 'effort' item in the scale.)[52] Thus, more consideration of the interpretation of this item may be needed.

In terms of construct validity, while there was evidence of convergent validity in the study among Eritrean refugees since depressive symptoms as measured by the CES-D were associated with other variables as expected (for example, pre-migration and post-migration living difficulties, post-traumatic stress disorder, emotion-oriented coping and alcohol use), an unusual finding was that mean CES-D scores were similar among men and women, being slightly higher among the men.[53] Depression and depressive symptoms are generally known to be higher among women.[54] However, given that this is a refugee sample, there may be unique factors contributing to the pattern of depressive symptoms here, such as differing exposures to stressors among refugee men and women compared to in the general population. This underscores why psychometric instruments such as the CES-D should take context into account; it also highlights the limitations of using primarily refugee or vulnerable populations to validate scales for psychological distress in Africa.

Use of the CES-D in South Africa

In South Africa, the CES-D and its short-form versions have been used in several studies. Sweetland's review reported on two studies testing the criterion-related validity of the CES-D against the Mini International Neuropsychiatric Interview (MINI) as the gold standard in samples of individuals with HIV and/or TB in South Africa and Uganda. In the South African study, the authors selected the MINI as a 'gold standard' because it was developed to correspond to diagnoses based on the DSM fourth edition (DSM-IV) and International Classification of Diseases 10th revision (ICD-10). It had also been validated against the DSM third edition revisions (DSM-III-R) and used as a 'gold standard' in several other validation studies around the world. However, one might question the validity of the 'gold standards', often produced in Europe and North America[55] (not to mention the diagnoses themselves, as discussed earlier).

Both the South African and Ugandan studies found the CES-D to be fairly sensitive in detecting true positive cases, with between 70 and 80 per cent of individuals identified as depressed using the CES-D also being classified as depressed using the MINI.[56] Specificity (detection of true negatives) was lower, however, in the South African HIV+ sample, with only around 60 per cent of those identified as non-cases (not depressed) with the CES-D also identified as non-cases with the MINI.[57]

Interesting findings were also observed linguistically in the South African sample. Given that the CES-D was developed in the English language in the United States, which has a European-based dominant culture, one might expect it to perform best in other European-origin populations and languages. However, in this sample, although the CES-D did perform better (had higher sensitivity and specificity) among Afrikaans speakers than among Xhosa speakers, it also performed better among Afrikaans speakers than English speakers.[58] This leaves interesting questions for research about how both the CES-D and the 'gold standard' MINI – which was developed jointly by European and American practitioners[59] – are identifying depression in these populations. It also highlights the need for appropriate translation of these scales into local languages and cultural contexts.

The validity of the CES-D in South African samples can also be assessed by examining its construct validity or relationship to other variables. Hamad and colleagues interviewed low-income adults in Cape Town, Durban and Port Elizabeth. They found that higher CES-D scores (that is, greater depressive symptoms) were associated with lower educational attainment and subjective social status as well as with less income stability and with more household members.[60] These relationships confirm theoretical assumptions based on social determinants of health as well as previous research that predicts greater depression among those of lower socioeconomic status.[61] In addition, depression as determined by the CES-D was more prevalent among the women in the sample than the men,[62] again confirming previous research and theory from social determinants of health which show depressive symptomatology to be higher among women.[63] Furthermore, white respondents had lower depressive symptoms compared to black African respondents. Given South Africa's history of colonialism and apartheid, which has produced enduring racial hierarchies, with white South Africans at the top and black South Africans at the bottom of this hierarchy, this result could also be viewed as following expected patterns that depression is associated with marginalisation.[64] Thus, in this sample, the CES-D appears to be performing in expected ways suggesting that, on the whole, it may be at least somewhat valid in measuring a general construct related to depression. It should be noted, however, that the cities in which this validation study was conducted differ in many ways from other parts of the country, such as rural and peri-urban areas. Thus, we cannot assume from this study that the findings observed here would be similar in those contexts.

A short-form version of the CES-D, the CES-D-10, has also been used in South Africa's National Income Dynamics Study (NIDS).[65]

Research using these data gives clues into the construct validity of the CES-D in South Africa as well, by allowing for analyses of its relationship with other variables.[66] Plus, because the NIDS uses national samples, assessments of validity in these samples may be more representative than those discussed above using the full CES-D in smaller samples. In studies using the NIDS, depressive symptoms measured by the CES-D-10 again produced expected associations with a number of variables, thereby demonstrating convergent construct validity. CES-D-10 scores (depressive symptoms) were positively associated with: lower socio-economic status, being female, unemployment, older age, being from the black/African population group and being single.[67] Furthermore, adolescent children of parents scoring high for depression on the CES-D-10 also had a significantly higher likelihood of CES-D-10 depression compared to those whose parents did not have depression. This finding likewise shows evidence of convergent validity according to theories of intergenerational transmission of depression.[68]

Other South African studies have also employed short-form versions of the CES-D and, similarly, found expected relationships with indicators of socioeconomic status, employment, cognitive function and adverse life events, again demonstrating construct validity of these short-form CES-D scales.[69] However, a proper validation study of the CES-D-10 translated into Zulu, Xhosa and Afrikaans was only published in 2017 by Baron and colleagues in a Cape Town sample.[70] They found the CES-D-10 in this sample to be correlated with other measures of depression that had been previously validated in South Africa, such as the PHQ-9 and World Health Organization Disability Assessment Schedule (WHODAS). They also found the CES-D-10 to have high criterion-related validity in their sample by achieving reasonable sensitivity and specificity in diagnosing depression compared to the MINI. When it came to content validity, an exploratory factor analysis suggested a two-factor model in the Xhosa and Zulu samples, with one factor consisting of negative affect and somatic symptoms and the other factor consisting of the positive affect items,[71] similar to what was observed with the full CES-D in the Rwandan and Eritrean refugee samples.[72] However, in their Afrikaans sample, the data were best explained by a single-factor model, suggesting a unidimensional construct of depression consisting of negative affect and somatic symptoms. The differences observed between the three linguistic groups show that even within South Africa, the experience and expression of depression and the idioms used to describe it differ across the various ethnic groups.[73]

Summary

In summary, there have been few published studies directly validating the CES-D in African samples. While most of the studies discussed here have reported on the reliability of the CES-D and CES-D-10, fewer studies assess the content validity and particularly the criterion-related validity in these African contexts.[74] Therefore, one is most often left with inferring the construct validity of the scales by examining their relationships with other variables reported in the research studies using the scales. Nevertheless, those results, as well as the few findings on the sensitivity of the CES-D compared to other accepted diagnostic criteria for major depressive episodes (like the MINI), provide some hope that the CES-D may be picking up meaningful information regarding depression in some African contexts. The factor analysis studies also give interesting results, revealing that two main dimensions or expressions of depression as measured by the CES-D appear in several of the African samples; these are negative affect (which in these samples includes and is not separate from somatic expressions and interpersonal problems) and diminished positive affect. This finding suggests some differences in how depression symptoms may be viewed and expressed in these African populations compared to the general US population in which the CES-D was originally developed.

However, much of the data presented here come from South Africa. Given the vast diversity of cultures and contexts in Africa, we cannot necessarily assume that results observed in South African validation studies would hold elsewhere on the continent. In addition, as Sweetland and others note, the standard statistical validation methods used in research such as those described above (for example, criterion-related validity) have meant that the studies have resorted to comparing the scales to other diagnostic measures that were also developed in non-African settings. Few studies have attempted to validate these scales against local conceptions of depression,[75] though some cultural validation work has been done on the PHQ-9.[76] Doing so, however, would be critical to establishing validity in specific African contexts. And, although this would not facilitate the comparison of standardised global measures and diagnoses of depression, it would address the question of whether the CES-D measure correlates with local ideas of depression and psychological distress, which is in itself an important question, given that these conditions may not be understood in universal ways.

Thus, when it comes to the CES-D and perhaps other depression instruments, the words of Hill and colleagues regarding mental health research may be instructive: 'health researchers should not dismiss inquiries into mental health for fear that symptoms will differ too much across cultures. It is possible to meaningfully translate these concepts into the local idiom and thereby shed light onto emotional questions that would otherwise remain in the dark.'[77] Still, locally derived measures may be most appropriate to assess depression epidemiology in various settings. Paying attention to the context in which symptoms of distress may occur – the social, economic and political circumstances surrounding these symptoms – may also improve the utility of scales used to measure psychological distress.

Case study 2: Angina pectoris

In theory, assessing chronic diseases of the 'body' seems more straightforward than assessing mental illness. This is because there are often 'objective' and observable physical markers used to diagnose conditions like cardiovascular diseases, lung diseases and cancer whereas, for many mental illnesses, such biomarkers do not exist.[78] However, in most parts of the world, people do not regularly access healthcare services and, when they do, screening for conditions that they have not presented for may not be standard practice. Furthermore, human and financial resources to take diagnostic services to community members are limited. Therefore, to measure the prevalence of certain chronic conditions at the population level, symptom-based questionnaires have been developed for use in surveys. Like the psychometric scales for mental illness, determining the presence of a physical ailment using a questionnaire also requires that the questionnaire is valid, is understood as intended by those responding to it and is measuring what was meant to be measured. The section below reviews attempts to validate in African settings one such questionnaire that was developed to measure angina pectoris (angina), or chest pain that is a symptom of coronary heart disease. As becomes evident, measuring a symptom such as pain is also not always a straightforward task.

Development, use and validation of the Rose Angina Questionnaire

Angina pectoris is caused by ischemia, or the blockage or narrowing of blood vessels in the heart, typically from atherosclerosis or the build-up of plaque. Angina is a sign of coronary heart disease, a form of cardiovascular disease (CVD), and manifests itself through symptoms of pain in the chest (left side) on exertion that resolves while resting or with medication.[79]

The Rose Angina Questionnaire (RAQ) was developed in 1962 by British epidemiologist Geoffrey Rose as part of a measure of ischaemic heart disease in men. The questionnaire was adopted by the WHO and, in 1977, it was adapted for self-administration.[80] The items in the questionnaire are shown in Figure 6.1 below. The RAQ can be used to diagnose 'definite' angina by meeting all the criteria (exertional chest pain on the left side, left arm or sternum that requires one to stop or slow down and that resolves while resting or with medication) or to diagnose 'possible' angina (chest pain on exertion only, without the need to satisfy other criteria).[81]

LONDON SCHOOL OF HYGIENE CHEST PAIN QUESTIONNAIRE
(Version for self-administration)

PART A

(a) **Have you ever had any pain or discomfort in your chest?**
1. ☐ Yes 2. ☐ No (Go to C)

(b) **Do you get this pain or discomfort when you walk uphill or hurry?**
1. ☐ Yes 2. ☐ No (Go to B)

(c) **Do you get it when you walk at an ordinary pace on the level?**
1. ☐ Yes 2. ☐ No

(d) **When you get any pain or discomfort in your chest what do you do?**
1. ☐ Stop
2. ☐ Slow down
3. ☐ Continue at the same pace

(e) **Does it go away when you stand still?**
1. ☐ Yes 2. ☐ No

(f) **How soon?**
1. ☐ 10 minutes or less
2. ☐ More than 10 minutes

(g) **Where do you get this pain or discomfort?**
Mark the place(s) with X on the diagram.

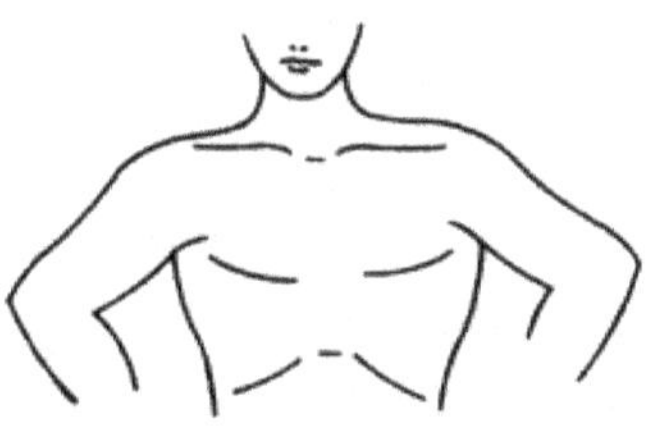

PART B

Have you ever had a severe pain across the front of your chest lasting for half an hour or more?
1. ☐ Yes 2. ☐ No

PART C

(a) **Do you get a pain in either leg on walking?**
1. ☐ Yes 2. ☐ No (Go to next question)

(b) **Does this pain ever begin when you are standing still or sitting?**
1. ☐ Yes 2. ☐ No

(c) **Do you get this pain in your calf (or calves)?**
1. ☐ Yes 2. ☐ No

(d) **Do you get it when you walk uphill or hurry?**
1. ☐ Yes 2. ☐ No

(e) **Do you get it when you walk at an ordinary pace on the level?**
1. ☐ Yes 2. ☐ No

(f) **Does the pain ever disappear while you are still walking?**
1. ☐ Yes 2. ☐ No

(g) **What do you do if you get it when you are walking?**
1. ☐ Stop
2. ☐ Slow down
3. ☐ Continue at same pace

(h) **What happens to it if you stand still?**
1. ☐ Usually continues more than 10 minutes
2. ☐ Usually disappears in 10 minutes or less

DEFINITIONS OF POSITIVE CLASSIFICATIONS

A. *Angina* 'Yes' to a and b, 'stop' or 'slow down' to d, 'yes' to e, '10 minutes or less' to f. Site must include *either* sternum (any level) *or* L. anterior chest and left arm. GRADE 1='no' to c, GRADE 2='yes' to c.
B. *Possible infarction* 'Yes' in this section.
C. *Intermittent claudication* 'Yes' to a, 'no' to b, 'yes' to c and d, 'no' to f, 'stop' or 'slow down' to g, and 'usually disappears in 10 minutes or less' to h. GRADE 1='no' to e, GRADE 2='yes' to e.

Figure 6.1 Rose Questionnaire for self-administration. © BMJ Publishing Group Ltd

In Europe, the RAQ has undergone several validation studies and has been found to be somewhat predictive of future coronary heart disease in some studies,[82] though it appears that it is specifically the questions on exertional chest pain that are predictive of coronary heart disease while the remaining questions may be redundant.[83] However, debates about the validity of the RAQ persist. For example, the questionnaire has generally been found to be highly specific in detecting true negative cases (between 80 per cent and 95 per cent) but not very sensitive in detecting true positive cases of angina (between 19 per cent and 83 per cent).[84] This might be because it is not necessarily able to distinguish chest pain due to ischaemic heart disease from more general chest pain.[85] In the UK where the RAQ was developed, there are also indications of potential issues with cross-cultural validity; the RAQ has been found to perform inconsistently and to be less sensitive among some Asian ethnic minority groups.[86]

Nevertheless, the questionnaire has been adapted and used widely in epidemiological studies globally. Items based on the questionnaire were included in the World Health Survey (WHS), which was implemented in 70 countries. It is reported that a validation study was initially done in seven countries in order to validate the WHS's symptom-based chronic disease measures against gold standard diagnoses.[87] A version of the RAQ also continues to be used in the Study on Global Ageing and Adult Health (SAGE).[88] The Global Burden of Disease study found the RAQ's definite angina diagnosis to be the most reliable standard to use for their purposes, resulting in less overestimation in population studies than self-reports of a doctor's diagnosis of angina.[89] Thus, there appears to be some utility in using the RAQ to estimate ischaemic heart disease at the population level, in the absence of other reliable measures.

Some of the results observed in global WHS studies using the RAQ have followed expected patterns; RAQ-diagnosed angina rates increased among those who were overweight or obese and among those who were older, both risk factors for heart disease.[90] However, in a 2012 study analysing the WHS from 41 countries, Hosseinpoor and colleagues observed some unexpected findings.[91] They found angina as diagnosed by RAQ to be the most prevalent non-communicable disease/symptom examined in the study. The fact that angina was more prevalent than NCDs such as arthritis, asthma, diabetes and depression raises some questions about the RAQ's validity, potentially suggesting that it could be leading to false positives. Angina was also more prevalent among the poor and less educated, countering some of the assumptions informed by the theory of epidemiological transition that NCDs may still be diseases of the rich in LMICs.[92] Nevertheless, increasing evidence is suggesting a link between NCDs and poverty globally, calling into question some of the predictions implied by epidemiological transition theory.

Another intriguing finding in the WHS studies was that the age-standardised prevalence of angina was higher in women (around 15 per cent) than in men (around 10 per cent). Male sex has traditionally been considered a risk factor for ischaemic heart disease, particularly before age 60, and sequelae of angina, such as myocardial infarction (MI) (heart attack), as well as mortality from coronary heart disease and MI are generally higher among men than women.[93] However, other studies both in high-income and low- and middle-income countries have similarly observed higher prevalence of RAQ-diagnosed angina among women, which has raised questions about the RAQ's validity among women.[94] It is possible that differences in the definition of angina used, for example 'definite' angina (satisfies all Rose criteria) versus 'possible' angina (only exertional pain criterion used) could explain some of these discrepancies.[95] Victorian-era research on angina also described 'pseudo angina', referring to anginal pain without coronary heart disease, as being more common in women.[96] This gender paradox in angina versus other ischemic heart disease outcomes leaves several unanswered questions: has there been an underdiagnosis of ischaemic heart disease in women in clinical settings? Is the RAQ performing differently or measuring different things in men and women? Are disease symptoms manifesting differently across the sexes? These are epidemiological questions whose answers have not yet been identified and which complicate efforts to validate the RAQ.

Other concerns raised about the RAQ are that the questions might be interpreted in terms of psychological or emotional pain rather than physical pain. For example, some believe that non-Western cultures tend to experience depression more commonly through somatic symptoms which could therefore lead to greater reporting of symptoms such as chest pain and discomfort that may be interpreted as angina.[97] So, as mentioned previously, the 'mind' versus 'body' distinction may not always be so clear, which has implications for how we measure both angina and depression in surveys. Not only are there issues of physical pain potentially being a symptom of psychological distress, but mental and physical disorders are often comorbid. Thus, depression may increase risk for cardiovascular complications while cardiovascular disease may increase risk for depression.[98] Below, I assess research using the RAQ in Africa to attempt to address issues of its validity in African settings.

Assessing the validity of the RAQ in African contexts

Published validation studies of the RAQ in African countries are difficult to find although the questionnaire has been used in several African studies. Some studies have observed higher than expected rates of angina and other CVD symptoms and outcomes when using the RAQ in sub-Saharan Africa. Though such a result could suggest that ischaemic heart disease is more prevalent in Africa than previously assumed, it has also led some to believe that the RAQ may not be as valid in this region.[99]

To help get at some of the questions of cross-cultural validity of the RAQ, I tried to ascertain respondents' understandings and interpretations of the SAGE version of the RAQ in a selection of interviews and focus group discussions that formed part of a larger pilot study on family histories of chronic disease in coastal Ghana. This was in a sense a crude attempt to measure the face validity of the survey. The questionnaire was read and questions were asked about it in three focus group discussions of variable size and socioeconomic background (14 participants, 8 participants, 4 participants), two intergenerational interviews each consisting of three people and two individual interviews, all in the Greater Accra area. These were either conducted in English or were orally translated to local languages. Participants had been recruited purposively for the broader study and were largely older adults. Men were under-represented in the sample.

Participants generally understood the RAQ questions as asking about physical pain. For example, a female participant in an English-language focus group of middle-class older adults specifically made reference to this type of pain being indicative of a heart attack. However, the discussions and interviews themselves had generally included topics relating to health and chronic diseases such as hypertension, diabetes and other health issues; thus, participants may have already been primed by these discussions to view the questionnaire in this light. Respondents generally denied having experienced the angina symptoms described in the questionnaire, which may also provide some assurance that it is not overdiagnosing in this sample.

However, other physical health symptoms were also raised in response to the RAQ questions. A couple of interviewees who were asthmatic discussed discomfort in the chest and tiredness on exertion due to asthma symptoms rather than heart symptoms. Thus, further research may want to explore how individuals with asthma respond to the questionnaire in different settings. A number of the participants, being older adults, also tended to bring up pain on exertion that they experienced in other parts of the body, such as in the legs and knees, and pain related to arthritis as well as general tiredness and breathlessness. In addition, in one of the focus group discussions conducted in a local language among a lower socioeconomic stratum, a respondent asked whether they were referring to heart palpitations/rapid beating while another respondent began talking about pain from heartburn. While issues of translation may have contributed to the misinterpretation, the reference to heartburn is an important one to consider given that gastrointestinal conditions such as gastro-oesophageal reflux disease can also cause chest pain.[100] Another male participant in the group (who was also slightly younger and had more formal education than many of the women) responded that the questions were not asking about heartburn but about pain in the chest when climbing a hill.

In general though, most respondents in this small selection of interviews and discussions made reference to physical pain on exertion and emotional issues were not mentioned. Overall, many of the respondents felt that the questions were clear and understandable, particularly in the English-language discussions. A woman in the middle-class group did comment, however, that the question on what happens to the pain when you stand still did not seem to follow from the previous question, since 'stand still' was not given as an option for what one does when the pain occurs. While this was just an informal and unsystematic attempt to assess comprehension of the RAQ in a small non-representative sample of participants as part of a study on other topics, it does suggest avenues for more structured validation research and, at the same time, gives some indication that there may be some level of comprehension of the RAQ in this setting.

A more formal assessment of the validity of the RAQ was conducted by Ajuluchukwu and Mbakwem in Nigeria.[101] Patients in a cardiac outpatient clinic presenting with chronic chest pain were administered both the RAQ and an electrocardiogram (ECG). More than three-quarters of the more than 200 patients had been referred with a diagnosis of angina. However, the authors found that only 7 per cent of those presenting with chest pain had angina as diagnosed by the RAQ (including that the pain was relieved within less than 10 minutes of stopping or resting, but excluding the location of pain question). Many of the patients had ECG abnormalities. However, no ECG features were statistically associated with RAQ angina diagnosis.[102] The lack of association between RAQ angina and ECG features in this sample seems a bit problematic in terms of assessing validity of the RAQ. But there is no universally recognised gold standard diagnosis for angina and therefore the ECG may not necessarily be the best standard for determining criterion-related validity.[103] Moreover, the sample size was small, which may have limited the power to detect differences; and the study used a clinical sample of all those presenting with chest pain for the comparison group, rather than a general population sample. On the plus side, the fact that only 7 per cent of those presenting with chest pain had angina as diagnosed by the RAQ does give some assurance that the RAQ is not indiscriminately classifying all those with chest pain as having angina. The authors conclude that many of the patients may have had non-cardiac chest pain, although they were referred as cardiac patients and there may therefore be overdiagnosis of angina by doctors compared to the RAQ. However, an alternative possibility that the RAQ may be underdiagnosing angina in some patients should also be acknowledged. Nevertheless, given the generally low prevalence of ischaemic heart disease in Nigeria, the authors concluded that the RAQ was useful for detecting angina in their setting.[104]

My preliminary examination of the RAQ in Ghana and Ajuluchukwu and Mbakwem's study in Nigeria give an incomplete picture of the validity of the RAQ in African settings. Given the shortage of published validation studies of the RAQ in Africa, we have to resort to examining the relationship between RAQ diagnoses of angina and variables with which angina should in theory be related in order to assess convergent construct validity. Such variables may include established risk factors for angina and ischaemic heart disease such as body mass index (BMI), age, smoking, blood pressure, diabetes and alcohol consumption as well as other co-morbid conditions such as anxiety and depression.[105]

Some support for the convergent construct validity of the RAQ comes from studies examining the association between angina and depression, which has previously been linked to coronary heart disease. Loerbroks and colleagues found that the odds of angina as diagnosed by the RAQ were much higher among those with depression in a pooled sample of 18 African countries in the WHS.[106] Studies using SAGE data similarly found a significant positive association between depression and angina as diagnosed by the SAGE version of the RAQ in South Africa, while accounting for other factors. However, this was not observed in the Ghana samples, which in one case actually displayed an inverse association.[107] Thus, further investigation may be required to explore this inconsistency.

Mixed results have also been observed in terms of the relationship between angina diagnosed by the RAQ and other co-morbid conditions and risk factors for angina/ischaemic heart disease in African samples.

In the Research on Obesity and Diabetes among African Migrants (RODAM) study in Ghana, Cole and colleagues observed that respondents who had long sleep (over eight hours) had a higher prevalence of CVD as diagnosed by the Rose questionnaire than those who slept normal or short hours, but this relationship was not statistically significant when adjusting for other factors.[108]

In a study using the age 50+ samples in the six participating SAGE countries, including Ghana and South Africa,[109] the prevalence of angina increased with age as expected, except in the South African sample. Adequate fruit and vegetable consumption was only associated with a lower prevalence of angina in the Ghana sample and while angina was more prevalent among those with diabetes in South Africa, the association with diabetes was not significant in the Ghanaian sample. In the South African sample, having ever consumed alcohol was associated with increased RAQ angina, but this was not the case in the Ghana sample, where the relationship between alcohol consumption and RAQ angina seemed to trend in the opposite direction. Similarly, many of the other presumed risk factors for CVD such as hypertension, smoking and BMI were not statistically associated with angina in the samples examined, including in Ghana and South Africa. Moreover, those with high or moderate physical activity actually had a higher prevalence of angina, though this was not statistically significant and could be an indication that they were merely more likely to detect chest pain on physical exertion if they were doing more physical exertion. Thus, the observations made in this study in terms of the associations between angina and established risk and protective factors do not provide much consistent support for the convergent construct validity of the RAQ in the Ghana and South African surveys, nor in some of the other countries examined.

Similarly, Gaziano and colleagues found mixed results in terms of the RAQ's association with established risk factors for angina in their rural South African sample. Risk factors like age followed established patterns with RAQ angina, indicating a level of convergent validity, but behavioural risk factors had less consistent variation. For example, smoking was not independently associated with RAQ after controlling for other metabolic risk factors such as cholesterol and blood pressure.[110] This could however be explained by the fact that the effects of smoking on angina may have been mediated by changes in these metabolic factors and already accounted for in their models. Nevertheless, the results of these studies leave questions about the convergent validity of the RAQ in Ghanaian and South African samples.

Summary

The evidence and discussions above leave much to be desired in terms of determining the validity of the RAQ in African and other settings. Positive RAQ responses have been found to be associated with much greater risk for CVD.[111] However, some of the inconsistent and unexpected results seen in population studies using the RAQ in African and other countries suggest that we either need to reassess the validity of the RAQ in certain populations or reassess our understanding of the epidemiology of ischaemic heart disease. In particular, the relationship between RAQ symptoms and gender deserves further attention, as well as the lack of consistent relationships between RAQ-diagnosed angina and a number of assumed behavioural and metabolic risk factors for coronary heart disease in African samples such as in the Ghana and South Africa SAGE. Additional research may help to clarify what the RAQ is measuring and expand our knowledge about the development and presentation of ischaemic heart disease in different settings and among different population groups. In addition, while the RAQ seemed to be fairly well understood as referring to physical rather than emotional pain in a crude assessment I conducted among a small sample of coastal Ghanaians, the discussions with respondents did raise some issues for consideration, including distinguishing cardiac chest pain on exertion from chest pain and discomfort due to other non-cardiac physical conditions such as asthma and gastrointestinal disease. All in all, it seems clear that further and more systematic attempts to validate the RAQ and similar measures in African countries are greatly needed.

Conclusions

The CES-D and RAQ are just two examples of chronic-disease-related survey instruments that are in use in African populations. Reviewing results from studies implementing these instruments in African samples reveals that, while these measures may be useful in detecting meaningful health differences, they do not necessarily perform similarly across populations. The CES-D studies give some confidence in the validity of the CES-D for measuring depressive symptoms in African contexts, but the studies also demonstrate the social construction of depression in that the dimensions and symptoms may vary and group together differently in different populations. Furthermore, the validity of the construct of 'depression' as a whole across cultures perhaps has still to be established more definitively. Thus, local idioms of distress may prove more useful.

The results from the RAQ studies seem to leave some questions regarding its validity for detecting ischaemic heart disease in African and non-African settings, though a number of researchers acknowledge its usefulness. Therefore, additional validation studies of the RAQ and its adaptations in different settings, examining not only construct validity but also content and criterion-related validity and using both quantitative and qualitative methods, would be beneficial.

These two case studies of chronic disease measures demonstrate the importance of cross-cultural validation of survey instruments to measure disease, illness and wellness for global use. There have been some methods suggested by authors such as Sweetland and colleagues and Luyt to improve the validity of instruments and scales in different settings.[112] These include using mixed methods approaches for validation and allowing flexibility in the interview or survey process, in order for respondents to ask questions and get clarification on the intended meanings of the questions. In addition, the use of rapid ethnographic methods such as free listing and card sorting can be used to identify and group culturally relevant symptoms and adapt existing measures to the local context.[113] Some of this work is being done for measures of psychological distress, for example.[114] The dilemma, however, lies in the conflict between generating measures that can be compared across time and place – which is often desired when studying the epidemiology of disease and health transitions – versus generating results that are context specific and therefore potentially more applicable and meaningful in certain settings but not necessarily comparable across populations. Each type of measure serves different purposes and further collaboration between epidemiologists and other social scientists may help to determine how best to balance these competing priorities.

Notes

1 I would like to thank Dr Rochelle Burgess (UCL) and Dr Marlee Tichnor (University of Edinburgh) for their comments on an earlier draft of this paper. I would also like to acknowledge Professor Megan Vaughan, Dr Olutobi Sanuade and Dr Marissa Mika for their feedback. This work was supported by the Wellcome Trust-funded Chronic Disease in Sub-Saharan Africa Project led by Professor Megan Vaughan.

2 Adams, 'Metrics of the Global Sovereign', 19–54; Crystal Biruk, *Cooking Data*.

3 Fernando, 'The Roads Less Traveled'.

4 Fernando, 'The Roads Less Traveled'; Summerfield, 'How Scientifically Valid is the Knowledge Base?'.

5 Jones and Thissen, '1 a History and Overview of Psychometrics'; Bech, *Clinical Psychometrics*.

6 DeVellis, *Scale Development*.
7 DeVellis, *Scale Development*, 59.
8 DeVellis, *Scale Development*, 71.
9 DeVellis, *Scale Development*, 61–3; Baron, Davies, and Lund, 'Validation of the 10-Item Centre'.
10 DeVellis, *Scale Development*, 59–61.
11 Lacasse et al., 'The Factor Structure of the CES-D'.
12 DeVellis, *Scale Development*, 64–70.
13 Luyt, 'A Framework for Mixing Methods'.
14 Sweetland, Belkin, and Verdeli, 'Measuring Depression'; Fernando, 'The Roads Less Traveled'.
15 Kassebaum et al., 'Global, Regional and National Disability-Adjusted Life-Years'; Patel and Stein, 'Common Mental Disorders'.
16 Loerbroks et al., 'The Association of Depression and Angina Pectoris'; Hill and de Menil, 'Women's Self-Reported Mental Health'; Patel and Stein, 'Common Mental Disorders'.
17 Sweetland, Belkin, and Verdeli, 'Measuring Depression'; Hill and de Menil, 'Women's Self-Reported Mental Health'; Patel and Stein, 'Common Mental Disorders'.
18 Loerbroks et al., 'The Association of Depression and Angina Pectoris'; Sweetland, Belkin, and Verdeli, 'Measuring Depression'.
19 Lacasse et al., 'The Factor Structure of the CES-D'; Akyeampong, Hill and Kleinman (eds.), *The Culture of Mental Illness*; Patel and Stein, 'Common Mental Disorders'.
20 Karasz and Singelis, 'Qualitative and Mixed Methods Research'; Fernando, 'The Roads Less Traveled'; Mills and Fernando, 'Globalising Mental Health'.
21 Fernando, 'The Roads Less Traveled'.
22 Mills and Fernando, 'Globalising Mental Health'.
23 Ingleby, 'How "Evidence-Based" Is the Movement for Global Mental Health?'.
24 Karasz, Garcia, and Ferri, 'Conceptual Models of Depression'.
25 Familiar et al., 'Exploring Psychological Distress'.
26 Kaiser et al., 'Thinking Too Much'.
27 Fernando, 'The Roads Less Traveled'.
28 Patel and Stein, 'Common Mental Disorders'; Fernando, 'The Roads Less Traveled'.
29 Patel and Stein, 'Common Mental Disorders'.
30 Patel and Stein, 'Common Mental Disorders'.
31 Fernando, 'The Roads Less Traveled'.
32 Patel and Stein, 'Common Mental Disorders'.
33 Patel and Stein, 'Common Mental Disorders'.
34 Sweetland, Belkin and Verdeli, 'Measuring Depression'; Patel and Stein, 'Common Mental Disorders'.
35 Maust et al., 'Psychiatric Rating Scales'.
36 Vilagut et al., 'Screening for Depression'.
37 National Income Dynamics Study, 'What Is NIDS?'.
38 Radloff, 'The CES-D Scale'.
39 Vilagut et al., 'Screening for Depression'.
40 Bjorgvinsson et al., 'Psychometric Properties of the CES-D-10'; Cole et al., 'Development and Validation of a Rasch-Derived CES-D Short Form'; Zhang et al., 'Validating a Shortened Depression Scale'; Adams et al., 'Factor Analysis of the CES-D 12'; Briggs et al., 'Validation of the 8-Item Centre'.
41 Radloff, 'The CES-D Scale'.
42 Cole et al., 'Test of Item-Response Bias'; Berkman et al., 'Depressive Symptoms'; Gallo, Anthony, and Muthen, 'Age Differences in Symptoms of Depression'; Adams et al., 'Factor Analysis of the CES-D 12'.
43 Vilagut et al., 'Screening for Depression'.
44 Lacasse et al., 'The Factor Structure of the CES-D'; Berkman et al., 'Depressive Symptoms'; Getnet and Alem, 'Validity of the Center for Epidemiologic Studies Depression Scale'; Radloff, 'The CES-D Scale'.
45 Lacasse et al., 'The Factor Structure of the CES-D'.
46 Adams et al., 'Factor Analysis of the CES-D 12'.
47 Radloff, 'The CES-D Scale'; Andresen et al., 'Screening for Depression in Well Older Adults'.
48 Lacasse et al., 'The Factor Structure of the CES-D'; Getnet and Alem, 'Validity of the Center for Epidemiologic Studies Depression Scale'.

49 Getnet and Alem, 'Validity of the Center for Epidemiologic Studies Depression Scale'.
50 Getnet and Alem, 'Validity of the Center for Epidemiologic Studies Depression Scale'.
51 Lacasse et al., 'The Factor Structure of the CES-D'.
52 Adams et al., 'Factor Analysis of the CES-D 12'.
53 Getnet and Alem, 'Validity of the Center for Epidemiologic Studies Depression Scale'.
54 Martini et al., 'New Women-Specific Diagnostic Modules'.
55 Sweetland, Belkin, and Verdeli, 'Measuring Depression'.
56 Sweetland, Belkin, and Verdeli, 'Measuring Depression'; Myer et al., 'Common Mental Disorders'.
57 Myer et al., 'Common Mental Disorders'.
58 Myer et al., 'Common Mental Disorders'.
59 Sheehan et al., 'The Mini International Neuropsychiatric Interview'.
60 Hamad et al., 'Social and Economic Correlates of Depressive Symptoms'.
61 Adjaye-Gbewonyo et al., 'Income Inequality and Depressive Symptoms'; Berkman, Kawachi, and Glymour (eds.), *Social Epidemiology*; Hill and de Menil, 'Women's Self-Reported Mental Health'; de-Graft Aikins, 'Mental Illness and Destitution in Ghana'; Patel and Stein, 'Common Mental Disorders'; Lorant et al., 'Socioeconomic Inequalities in Depression'; Dohrenwend et al., 'Socioeconomic Status and Psychiatric Disorders'.
62 Hamad et al., 'Social and Economic Correlates of Depressive Symptoms'.
63 Adjaye-Gbewonyo et al., 'Income Inequality and Depressive Symptoms'; Hill and de Menil, 'Women's Self-Reported Mental Health'; Patel and Stein, 'Common Mental Disorders'; Berkman et al., 'Depressive Symptoms'; Martini et al., 'New Women-Specific Diagnostic Modules'.
64 Patel and Stein, 'Common Mental Disorders'.
65 National Income Dynamics Study, 'What Is NIDS?'.
66 Alaba and Chola, 'The Social Determinants of Multimorbidity'; Meffert et al., 'Increase of Perceived Frequency of Neighborhood Domestic Violence'; Adjaye-Gbewonyo et al., 'Income Inequality and Depressive Symptoms'; Adjaye-Gbewonyo et al., 'High Social Trust'; Tomita, Labys, and Burns, 'Depressive Symptoms Prior to Pregnancy'; Tomita and Burns, 'A Multilevel Analysis of Association between Neighborhood Social Capital and Depression'; Burns, Tomita, and Lund, 'Income Inequality'; Tomita, Labys, and Burns, 'A Multilevel Analysis of the Relationship between Neighborhood Social Disorder and Depressive Symptoms'.
67 Adjaye-Gbewonyo et al., 'Income Inequality and Depressive Symptoms'; Adjaye-Gbewonyo et al., 'High Social Trust'; Tomita and Burns, 'A Multilevel Analysis of Association between Neighborhood Social Capital and Depression'; Tomita, Labys, and Burns, 'A Multilevel Analysis of the Relationship between Neighborhood Social Disorder and Depressive Symptoms'; Burns, Tomita, and Lund, 'Income Inequality'; Hill and de Menil, 'Women's Self-Reported Mental Health'; Patel and Stein, 'Common Mental Disorders'; Baron, Davies, and Lund, 'Validation of the 10-Item Centre'; Hughes and Waite, 'Health in Household Context'.
68 Eyal, Burns, and Geel, 'The Intergenerational Transmission of Depression'.
69 Folb et al., 'Socioeconomic Predictors and Consequences of Depression'; Humphreys et al., 'Cognitive Function in Low-Income and Low-Literacy Settings'; Payne et al., 'Adverse Life Events and Late-Life Wellbeing'.
70 Baron, Davies, and Lund, 'Validation of the 10-Item Centre'.
71 Baron, Davies, and Lund, 'Validation of the 10-Item Centre'.
72 Lacasse et al., 'The Factor Structure of the CES-D'; Getnet and Alem, 'Validity of the Center for Epidemiologic Studies Depression Scale'.
73 Baron, Davies, and Lund, 'Validation of the 10-Item Centre'.
74 Myer et al., 'Common Mental Disorders'; Getnet and Alem, 'Validity of the Center for Epidemiologic Studies Depression Scale'; Lacasse et al., 'The Factor Structure of the Ces-D'; Baron, Davies, and Lund, 'Validation of the 10-Item Centre'.
75 Sweetland, Belkin, and Verdeli, 'Measuring Depression and Anxiety'; Fernando, 'The Roads Less Traveled'.
76 Kohrt et al., 'Detection of Depression in Low Resource Settings'.
77 Hill and de Menil, 'Women's Self-Reported Mental Health'.
78 Ingleby, 'How "Evidence-Based" Is the Movement for Global Mental Health?'.
79 Wee, Burns, and Bett, 'Medical Management of Chronic Stable Angina'; Peterson, 'The Burden of Angina Pectoris'.

80 Rose, McCartney, and Reid, 'Self-Administration of a Questionnaire on Chest Pain'; Hanna, Hunt, and Bhopal, 'Using the Rose Angina Questionnaire Cross-Culturally'; Leng and Fowkes, 'The Edinburgh Claudication Questionnaire'.
81 Fischbacher et al., 'The Performance of the Rose Angina Questionnaire'.
82 Achterberg et al., 'Prognostic Value of the Rose Questionnaire'; Graff-Iversen, Selmer, and Løchen, 'Rose Angina Predicts'; Rahman et al., 'Rose Angina Questionnaire'; Rose, McCartney, and Reid, 'Self-Administration of a Questionnaire on Chest Pain'; Fischbacher et al., 'The Performance of the Rose Angina Questionnaire'.
83 Lawlor, Adamson, and Ebrahim, 'Performance of the WHO Rose Angina Questionnaire'; Bodegard et al., 'Possible Angina Detected by the WHO Angina Questionnaire'; Graff-Iversen, Selmer, and Løchen, 'Rose Angina Predicts'; Fischbacher et al., 'The Performance of the Rose Angina Questionnaire'.
84 Fischbacher et al., 'The Performance of the Rose Angina Questionnaire'; Liu et al., 'Global Variability in Angina Pectoris'.
85 Hotopf, 'Rose Questionnaire Is Not What It Seems'.
86 Hanna and Bhopal, 'Assessing Cultural and Linguistic Appropriateness of the Rose Angina Questionnaire'; Hanna, Hunt, and Bhopal, 'Using the Rose Angina Questionnaire'; Rahman et al., 'Rose Angina Questionnaire'; Fischbacher et al., 'The Performance of the Rose Angina Questionnaire'.
87 Moussavi et al., 'Depression, Chronic Diseases and Decrements in Health'.
88 World Health Organization, 'Health Statistics and Information Systems'.
89 Forouzanfar et al., 'Assessing the Global Burden of Ischemic Heart Disease'.
90 Liu et al., 'Global Variability in Angina Pectoris'.
91 Hosseinpoor et al., 'Socioeconomic Inequality in the Prevalence of Noncommunicable Diseases'.
92 Moran et al., 'The Epidemiology of Cardiovascular Diseases in Sub-Saharan Africa'; Forouzanfar et al., 'Assessing the Global Burden of Ischemic Heart Disease'; Hosseinpoor et al., 'Socioeconomic Inequality in the Prevalence of Noncommunicable Diseases'.
93 Hosseinpoor et al., 'Socioeconomic Inequality in the Prevalence of Noncommunicable Diseases'; Forouzanfar et al., 'Assessing the Global Burden of Ischemic Heart Disease'; HEART UK, 'Risk Factors for Coronary Heart Disease'.
94 Chaturvedi, McKeigue, and Marmot, 'Relationship of Glucose Intolerance to Coronary Risk'; Wilcosky, Harris, and Weissfeld, 'The Prevalence and Correlates of Rose Questionnaire Angina'; Quashie et al., 'Prevalence of Angina and Co-Morbid Conditions'; Peterson, 'The Burden of Angina Pectoris'; Fischbacher et al., 'The Performance of the Rose Angina Questionnaire'; Gaziano et al., 'Cardiometabolic Risk'; Hemingway et al., 'Prevalence of Angina in Women Versus Men'.
95 Forouzanfar et al., 'Assessing the Global Burden of Ischemic Heart Disease'.
96 Ajuluchukwu and Mbakwem, 'Evaluation of Chest Pain'; Ockene et al., 'Unexplained Chest Pain'.
97 Loerbroks et al., 'The Association of Depression and Angina Pectoris'; Chaturvedi, 'Ethnicity as an Epidemiological Determinant'; Cole et al., 'Sleep Duration'.
98 Loerbroks et al., 'The Association of Depression and Angina Pectoris'; Rumsfeld and Ho, 'Depression and Cardiovascular Disease'; Hare et al., 'Depression and Cardiovascular Disease'.
99 Moran et al., 'The Epidemiology of Cardiovascular Diseases in Sub-Saharan Africa'; Forouzanfar et al., 'Assessing the Global Burden of Ischemic Heart Disease'; Webb, Rheeder, and Van Zyl, 'Diabetes Care and Complications'.
100 Ford, Suares, and Talley, 'Meta-Analysis'.
101 Ajuluchukwu and Mbakwem, 'Evaluation of Chest Pain'.
102 Ajuluchukwu and Mbakwem, 'Evaluation of Chest Pain'.
103 Fischbacher et al., 'The Performance of the Rose Angina Questionnaire'.
104 Ajuluchukwu and Mbakwem, 'Evaluation of Chest Pain'.
105 Medalie and Goldbourt, 'Angina Pectoris among 10,000 Men'; Khot et al., 'Prevalence of Conventional Risk Factors'; Greenland et al., 'Major Risk Factors'; Kannel et al., 'Factors of Risk'.
106 Loerbroks et al., 'The Association of Depression and Angina Pectoris'.
107 Brinda et al., 'Health, Social and Economic Variables'; Quashie et al., 'Prevalence of Angina and Co-Morbid Conditions'.
108 Cole et al., 'Sleep Duration'.

109 Quashie et al., 'Prevalence of Angina and Co-Morbid Conditions'.
110 Gaziano et al., 'Cardiometabolic Risk'.
111 Liu et al., 'Global Variability in Angina Pectoris'; Fischbacher et al., 'The Performance of the Rose Angina Questionnaire'.
112 Sweetland, Belkin, and Verdeli, 'Measuring Depression and Anxiety'; Luyt, 'A Framework for Mixing Methods'.
113 Sweetland, Belkin, and Verdeli, 'Measuring Depression and Anxiety'.
114 Familiar et al., 'Community Perceptions of Mental Distress'.

Bibliography

Achterberg, Sefanja, et al. 'Prognostic Value of the Rose Questionnaire: A Validation with Future Coronary Events in the Smart Study', *European Journal of Preventive Cardiology*, 19 (1) (2012): 5–14.

Adams, Leslie B. et al. 'Factor Analysis of the CES-D 12 among a Community Sample of Black Men', *American Journal of Men's Health*, 13 (2) (2019), doi.org/10.1177/1557988319834105.

Adams, Vincanne. 'Metrics of the Global Sovereign'. In *Metrics: What Counts in Global Health*, edited by Vincanne Adams, 19–54. Durham, NC: Duke University Press, 2016.

Adjaye-Gbewonyo, Kafui et al. 'Income Inequality and Depressive Symptoms in South Africa: A Longitudinal Analysis of the National Income Dynamics Study', *Health & Place*, 42 (2016): 37–46.

Adjaye-Gbewonyo, Kafui, et al. 'High Social Trust Associated with Increased Depressive Symptoms in a Longitudinal South African Sample', *Social Science & Medicine*, 197 (2018): 127–35.

Ajuluchukwu, J. N. A. and Amam C. Mbakwem. 'Evaluation of Chest Pain in Ambulatory Patients in Lagos, Using the Rose Questionnaire and Resting Electrocardiogram', *Nigerian Quarterly Journal of Hospital Medicine*, 12 (1) (2004): 60–5.

Akyeampong, Emmanuel, Allan G. Hill, and Arthur Kleinman (eds.). *The Culture of Mental Illness and Psychiatric Practice in Africa*. Bloomington, IN: Indiana University Press, 2015.

Alaba, Olufunke and Lumbwe Chola. 'The Social Determinants of Multimorbidity in South Africa', *International Journal for Equity in Health*, 12 (2013): 63.

Andresen, Elena M. et al. 'Screening for Depression in Well Older Adults: Evaluation of a Short Form of the CES-D (Center for Epidemiologic Studies Depression Scale)', *American Journal of Preventive Medicine*, 10 (1994): 77–84.

Baron, Emily C., Thandi Davies, and Crick Lund. 'Validation of the 10-Item Centre for Epidemiological Studies Depression Scale (CES-D-10) in Zulu, Xhosa and Afrikaans Populations in South Africa', *BMC Psychiatry*, 17 (1) (2017): 6.

Bech, Per. *Clinical Psychometrics.* Chichester: Wiley-Blackwell, 2012.

Berkman, Lisa F. et al. 'Depressive Symptoms in Relation to Physical Health and Functioning in the Elderly', *American Journal of Epidemiology*, 124 (3) (1986): 372–88.

Berkman, Lisa F., Ichiro Kawachi, and Maria M. Glymour (eds.). *Social Epidemiology*, 2nd edition. Oxford: Oxford University Press, 2014.

Biruk, Crystal. *Cooking Data: Culture and Politics in an African Research World.* Durham, NC: Duke University Press, 2018.

Bjorgvinsson, Thröstur et al. 'Psychometric Properties of the CES-D-10 in a Psychiatric Sample', *Assessment* 20 (4) (2013): 429–36.

Bodegard, Johan et al. 'Possible Angina Detected by the WHO Angina Questionnaire in Apparently Healthy Men with a Normal Exercise ECG: Coronary Heart Disease or Not? A 26 Year Follow up Study', *Heart*, 90 (6) (2004): 627–32.

Briggs, Robert et al. 'Validation of the 8-Item Centre for Epidemiological Studies Depression Scale in a Cohort of Community-Dwelling Older People: Data from the Irish Longitudinal Study on Ageing (TILDA)', *European Geriatric Medicine*, 9 (1) (2018): 121–6.

Brinda, Ethel M. et al. 'Health, Social and Economic Variables Associated with Depression among Older People in Low and Middle Income Countries: World Health Organization Study on Global Ageing and Adult Health', *The American Journal of Geriatric Psychiatry*, 24 (12) (2016): 1196–208.

Burns, Jonathan K. Andrew Tomita, and Crick Lund. 'Income Inequality Widens the Existing Income-Related Disparity in Depression Risk in Post-Apartheid South Africa: Evidence from a Nationally Representative Panel Study', *Health & Place*, 45 (2017): 10–16.

Chaturvedi, Nish. 'Ethnicity as an Epidemiological Determinant – Crudely Racist or Crucially Important?', *International Journal Epidemiology*, 30 (5) (2001): 925–7.

Chaturvedi, Nish, Paul M. McKeigue, and Michael G. Marmot. 'Relationship of Glucose Intolerance to Coronary Risk in Afro-Caribbeans Compared with Europeans', *Diabetologia*, 37 (8) (1994): 765–72.

Cole, Helen V. et al. 'Sleep Duration Is Associated with Increased Risk for Cardiovascular Outcomes: A Pilot Study in a Sample of Community Dwelling Adults in Ghana', *Sleep Medicine*, 34 (2017): 118–25.

Cole, Jason C. et al. 'Development and Validation of a Rasch-Derived CES-D Short Form', *Psychological Assessment*, 16 (4) (2004): 360–72.

Cole, Stephen R. et al. 'Test of Item-Response Bias in the CES-D Scale: Experience from the New Haven Epese Study', *Journal of Clinical Epidemiology*, 53 (2000): 285–9.

de-Graft Aikins, Ama. 'Mental Illness and Destitution in Ghana: A Social-Psychological Perspective'. In *The Culture of Mental Illness and Psychiatric Practice in Africa*, edited by Emmanuel Akyeampong, Allan G. Hill, and Arthur Kleinman, 112–43. Bloomington, IN: Indiana University Press, 2015.

DeVellis, Robert F. *Scale Development: Theory and Applications*, 3rd edition. Thousand Oaks, CA: Sage Publications, 2012.

Dohrenwend, Bruce P. et al. 'Socioeconomic Status and Psychiatric Disorders: The Causation-Selection Issue', *Science*, 255 (5047) (1992): 946–52.

Eyal, Katherine C., Justine C. Burns, and Jennifer A Geel. 'The Intergenerational Transmission of Depression in South African Adolescents: A Cross-Sectional Longitudinal Study'. Version 2 SALDRU Working Paper Number 200. Cape Town: SALDRU, UCT, 2018.

Familiar, Itziar et al. 'Community Perceptions of Mental Distress in a Post-Conflict Setting: A Qualitative Study in Burundi', *Global Public Health*, 8 (8) (2013): 943–57.

Familiar, Itziar et al. 'Exploring Psychological Distress in Burundi during and after the Armed Conflict', *Community Mental Health Journal*, 52 (1) (2016): 32–8.

Fernando, Gaithri A. 'The Roads Less Traveled: Mapping Some Pathways on the Global Mental Health Research Roadmap', *Transcultural Psychiatry*, 49 (3–4) (2012): 396–417.

Fischbacher, Colin M. et al. 'The Performance of the Rose Angina Questionnaire in South Asian and European Origin Populations: A Comparative Study in Newcastle, UK', *International Journal of Epidemiology*, 30 (5) (2001): 1009–16.

Folb, Naomi et al. 'Socioeconomic Predictors and Consequences of Depression among Primary Care Attenders with Non-Communicable Diseases in the Western Cape, South Africa: Cohort Study within a Randomised Trial', *BMC Public Health*, 15 (2015): 1194.

Ford, Alexander C., Nicole C. Suares, and Nicholas J. Talley. 'Meta-Analysis: The Epidemiology of Noncardiac Chest Pain in the Community', *Alimentary Pharmacology & Therapeutics*, 34 (2) (2011): 172–80.

Forouzanfar, Mohammad H. et al. 'Assessing the Global Burden of Ischemic Heart Disease, Part 2: Analytic Methods and Estimates of the Global Epidemiology of Ischemic Heart Disease in 2010', *Global Heart*, 7 (4) (2012): 331–42.

Gallo, Joseph J., James C. Anthony, and Bengt O. Muthen. 'Age Differences in Symptoms of Depression: A Latent Trait Analysis', *Journal of Gerontology: Psychological Sciences*, 49 (6) (1994): 251–64.

Gaziano, Thomas A. et al. 'Cardiometabolic Risk in a Population of Older Adults with Multiple Co-Morbidities in Rural South Africa: The HAALSI (Health and Aging in Africa: Longitudinal Studies of INDEPTHCommunities) Study', *BMC Public Health*, 17 (1) (2017): 206.

Getnet, Berhanie and Atalay Alem. 'Validity of the Center for Epidemiologic Studies Depression Scale (CES-D) in Eritrean Refugees Living in Ethiopia', *BMJ Open*, 9 (5) (2019): e026129.

Graff-Iversen, Sidsel, Randi Selmer, and Maja-Lisa Løchen. 'Rose Angina Predicts 23-Year Coronary Heart Disease Mortality in Women and Men Aged 40–49 Years', *Heart*, 94 (4) (2008): 482–6.

Greenland, Philip et al. 'Major Risk Factors as Antecedents of Fatal and Nonfatal Coronary Heart Disease Events', *The Journal of the American Medical Association*, 290 (7) (2003): 891–7.

Hamad, Rita et al. 'Social and Economic Correlates of Depressive Symptoms and Perceived Stress in South African Adults', *Journal of Epidemiology & Community Health*, 62 (6) (2008): 538–44.

Hanna, Lisa C. and Raj Bhopal. 'Assessing Cultural and Linquistic Appropriateness of the Rose Angina Questionnaire in Three Ethnic Groups, in Migrant Health in Europe: International Conference on Differences in Health and Health Care Provision', *Ethnicity & Health*, 9 (Supplement 1) (2004): S6–S21.

Hanna, Lisa C., Sonja M. Hunt, and Raj S. Bhopal. 'Using the Rose Angina Questionnaire Cross-Culturally: The Importance of Consulting Lay People When Translating Epidemiological Questionnaires', *Ethnicity & Health*, 17 (3) (2012): 241–51.

Hare, D. L. et al. 'Depression and Cardiovascular Disease: A Clinical Review', *European Heart Journal*, 35 (21) (2014): 1365–72.

HEART UK – The Cholesterol Charity. 'Risk Factors for Coronary Heart Disease (CHD)', 23 June 2014, https://www.heartuk.org.uk/downloads/health-professionals/factsheets/risk-factors-for-chd.pdf.

Hemingway, Harry et al. 'Prevalence of Angina in Women Versus Men: A Systematic Review and Meta-Analysis of International Variations across 31 Countries', *Circulation*, 117 (12) (2008): 1526–36.

Hill, Allan G. and Victoria de Menil. 'Women's Self-Reported Mental Health in Accra, Ghana'. In *The Culture of Mental Illness and Psychiatric Practice in Africa*, edited by Emmanuel Akyeampong, Allan G. Hill, and Arthur Kleinman, 186–203. Bloomington, IN: Indiana University Press, 2015.

Hosseinpoor, Ahmad Reza et al. 'Socioeconomic Inequality in the Prevalence of Noncommunicable Diseases in Low- and Middle-Income Countries: Results from the World Health Survey', *BMC Public Health*, 12 (2012): 474.

Hotopf, Matthew. 'Rose Questionnaire Is Not What It Seems', *The British Medical Journal*, 325 (7359) (2002): 337.

Hughes, Mary Elizabeth and Linda J. Waite. 'Health in Household Context: Living Arrangements and Health in Late Middle Age', *Journal of Health and Social Behavior*, 43 (1) (2002).

Humphreys, Glyn W. et al. 'Cognitive Function in Low-Income and Low-Literacy Settings: Validation of the Tablet-Based Oxford Cognitive Screen in the Health and Aging in Africa: A Longitudinal Study of an INDEPTH Community in South Africa (HAALSI)', *The Journals of Gerontology Series B Psychological Sciences and Social Sciences*, 72 (1) (2017): 38–50.

Ingleby, David. 'How "Evidence-Based" Is the Movement for Global Mental Health?', *Disability and the Global South*, 1 (2) (2014): 203–26.

Jones, Lyle V. and David Thissen. '1 a History and Overview of Psychometrics', *Handbook of Statistics*, 26 (2006): 1–27.

Kaiser, Bonnie N. et al. '"Thinking Too Much": A Systematic Review of a Common Idiom of Distress', *Social Science & Medicine*, 147 (2015): 170–83.

Kannel, William B. 'Factors of Risk in the Development of Coronary Heart Disease – Six-Year Follow-up Experience: The Framingham Study', *Annals of Internal Medicine*, 55 (1) (1961): 33–50.

Karasz, Alison, Nerina Garcia, and Lucia Ferri. 'Conceptual Models of Depression in Primary Care Patients: A Comparative Study', *Journal of Cross-Cultural Psychology*, 40 (6) (2009): 1041–59.

Karasz, Alison and Theodore M. Singelis. 'Qualitative and Mixed Methods Research in Cross-Cultural Psychology: Introduction to the Special Issue', *Journal of Cross-Cultural Psychology*, 40 (6) (2009): 909–16.

Kassebaum, Nicholas J. et al. 'Global, Regional, and National Disability-Adjusted Life-Years (Dalys) for 315 Diseases and Injuries and Healthy Life Expectancy (Hale), 1990–2015: A Systematic Analysis for the Global Burden of Disease Study 2015', *Lancet*, 388 (10053) (2016): 1603–58.

Khot, Umesh N. et al. 'Prevalence of Conventional Risk Factors in Patients with Coronary Heart Disease', *The Journal of the American Medical Association*, 290 (7) (2003): 898–904.

Kohrt, Brandon A. et al. 'Detection of Depression in Low Resource Settings: Validation of the Patient Health Questionnaire (Phq-9) and Cultural Concepts of Distress in Nepal', *BMC Psychiatry*, 16 (2016): 58.

Lacasse, Justin J. et al. 'The Factor Structure of the CES-D in a Sample of Rwandan Genocide Survivors', *Social Psychiatry and Psychiatric Epidemiology*, 49 (3) (2014): 459–65.

Lawlor, Debbie A., Joy Adamson, and Shah Ebrahim. 'Performance of the WHO Rose Angina Questionnaire in Post-Menopausal Women: Are All of the Questions Necessary?', *Journal of Epidemiology & Community Health*, 57 (7) (2003): 538–41.

Leng, Gareth C. and F. Gerald R. Fowkes. 'The Edinburgh Claudication Questionnaire: An Improved Version of the WHO/Rose Questionnaire for Use in Epidemiological Surveys', *Journal of Clinical Epidemiology*, 45 (10) (1992): 1101–9.

Liu, Longjian et al. 'Global Variability in Angina Pectoris and Its Association with Body Mass Index and Poverty', *American Journal of Cardiology*, 107 (5) (2011): 655–61.

Loerbroks, Adrian et al. 'The Association of Depression and Angina Pectoris across 47 Countries: Findings from the 2002 World Health Survey', *European Journal of Epidemiology*, 29 (7) (2014): 507–15.

Lorant, Vincent et al. 'Socioeconomic Inequalities in Depression: A Meta-Analysis', *American Journal of Epidemiology*, 157 (2) (2003): 98–112.

Luyt, Russell. 'A Framework for Mixing Methods in Quantitative Measurement Development, Validation and Revision', *Journal of Mixed Methods Research*, 6 (4) (2011): 294–316.

Martini, Julia et al. 'New Women-Specific Diagnostic Modules: The Composite International Diagnostic Interview for Women (CIDI-Venus)', *Archives of Women's Mental Health*, 12 (5) (2009): 281–9.

Maust, Donovan et al. 'Psychiatric Rating Scales', *Handbook of Clinical Neurology*, 106 (2012): 227–37.

Medalie, Jack H. and Uri Goldbourt. 'Angina Pectoris among 10,000 Men', *The American Journal of Medicine*, 60 (6) (1976): 910–21.

Meffert, Susan M. et al. 'Increase of Perceived Frequency of Neighborhood Domestic Violence Is Associated with Increase of Women's Depression Symptoms in a Nationally Representative Longitudinal Study in South Africa', *Social Science & Medicine*, 131 (2015): 89–97.

Mills, China and Suman Fernando. 'Globalising Mental Health or Pathologising the Global South? Mapping the Ethics, Theory and Practice of Global Mental Health', *Disability and the Global South*, 1 (2) (2014): 188–202.

Moran, Andrew et al. 'The Epidemiology of Cardiovascular Diseases in Sub-Saharan Africa: The Global Burden of Diseases, Injuries and Risk Factors 2010 Study', *Progress in Cardiovascular Diseases*, 56 (3) (2013): 234–9.

Moussavi, Saba et al. 'Depression, Chronic Diseases and Decrements in Health: Results from the World Health Surveys', *Lancet*, 370 (2007): 851–8.

Myer, Landon et al. 'Common Mental Disorders among HIV-Infected Individuals in South Africa: Prevalence, Predictors and Validation of Brief Psychiatric Rating Scales', *AIDS Patient Care and STDs*, 22 (2) (2008): 147–58.

National Income Dynamics Study. 'What Is NIDS?', last modified 2019, http://www.nids.uct.ac.za/about/what-is-nids.

Ockene Ira S. et al. 'Unexplained Chest Pain in Patients with Normal Coronary Arteriograms: A Follow-Up Study of Functional Status', *The New England Journal of Medicine*, 303 (22) (1980): 1249–52.

Patel, Vikram and Dan J. Stein. 'Common Mental Disorders in Sub-Saharan Africa: The Triad of Depression, Anxiety and Somatization'. In *The Culture of Mental Illness and Psychiatric Practice in Africa*, edited by Emmanuel Akyeampong, Allan G. Hill, and Arthur Kleinman, 50–72. Bloomington, IN: Indiana University Press, 2015.

Payne, Collin F. et al. 'Adverse Life Events and Late-Life Wellbeing: Risk and Resilience in an Aging Post-Apartheid South African Cohort'. Population Association of America 2019 Annual Meeting, Austin, TX, 12 April 2019.

Peterson, Eric. 'The Burden of Angina Pectoris and Its Complications [Corrected]', *Clinical Cardiology*, 30 (2) Supplement 1 (2007): I10–15.

Quashie, Nekehia T. et al. 'Prevalence of Angina and Co-Morbid Conditions among Older Adults in Six Low- and Middle-Income Countries: Evidence from Sage Wave 1', *International Journal of Cardiology*, 285 (2019): 140–6.

Radloff, Lenore Sawyer. 'The CES-D Scale', *Applied Psychological Measurement*, 1 (3) (1977): 385–401.

Rahman, Muhammad A. et al. 'Rose Angina Questionnaire: Validation with Cardiologists' Diagnoses to Detect Coronary Heart Disease in Bangladesh', *Indian Heart Journal*, 65 (1) (2013): 30–9.

Rose, Geoffrey, P. McCartney, and D. D. Reid. 'Self-Administration of a Questionnaire on Chest Pain and Intermittent Claudication', *Journal of Epidemiology & Community Health*, 31 (1) (1977): 42–8.

Rumsfeld, John S. and P. Michael Ho. 'Depression and Cardiovascular Disease: A Call for Recognition', *Circulation*, 111 (3) (2005): 250–3.

Sheehan, David V. et al. 'The Mini International Neuropsychiatric Interview (M.I.N.I.): The Development and Validation of a Structured Diagnostic Psychiatric Interview for DSM-IV and ICD-10', *Journal of Clinical Psychiatry*, 59 (Supplement 20) (1998): 22–33.

Summerfield, Derek. 'How Scientifically Valid Is the Knowledge Base of Global Mental Health?', *The British Medical Journal*, 336 (7651) (2008): 992–4.

Sweetland, Annika C., Gary S. Belkin, and Helena Verdeli. 'Measuring Depression and Anxiety in Sub-Saharan Africa', *Depression and Anxiety*, 31 (3) (2014): 223–32.

Tomita, Andrew and Jonathan K. Burns. 'A Multilevel Analysis of Association between Neighborhood Social Capital and Depression: Evidence from the First South African National Income Dynamics Study', *Journal of Affective Disorders*, 144 (1–2) (2013): 101–5.

Tomita, Andrew, Charlotte A. Labys, and Jonathan K. Burns. 'Depressive Symptoms Prior to Pregnancy and Infant Low Birth Weight in South Africa', *Maternal and Child Health Journal*, 19 (10) (2015): 2179–86.

Tomita, Andrew, Charlotte A. Labys, and Jonathan K. Burns. 'A Multilevel Analysis of the Relationship between Neighborhood Social Disorder and Depressive Symptoms: Evidence from the South African National Income Dynamics Study', *American Journal of Orthopsychiatry*, 85 (1) (2015): 56–62.

Vilagut, Gemma et al. 'Screening for Depression in the General Population with the Center for Epidemiologic Studies Depression (CES-D): A Systematic Review with Meta-Analysis', *PLoS One*, 11 (5) (2016): e0155431.

Webb, Elizabeth M., Paul Rheeder, and Danie G. Van Zyl. 'Diabetes Care and Complications in Primary Care in the Tshwane District of South Africa', *Primary Care Diabetes*, 9 (2) (2015): 147–54.

Wee, Yong, Kylie Burns, and Nicholas Bett. 'Medical Management of Chronic Stable Angina', *Australian Prescriber*, 38 (4) (2015): 131–6.

Wilcosky, Timothy, Robin Harris, and Lisa Weissfeld. 'The Prevalence and Correlates of Rose Questionnaire Angina among Women and Men in the Lipid Research Clinics Program Prevalence Study Population', *American Journal of Epidemiology*, 125 (3) (1987): 400–9.

World Health Organization. 'Health Statistics and Information Systems: Sage Waves 0, 1, 2 & 3', last modified 2019, https://www.who.int/healthinfo/sage/cohorts/en/, accessed 22 May 2019.

Zhang, Wendy et al. 'Validating a Shortened Depression Scale (10 Item CES-D) among HIV-Positive People in British Columbia, Canada', *PLoS One*, 7 (7) (2012): e40793.

7

NCDs and Chronic Diseases in Ghana

Olutobi Sanuade

> Uncertain inputs multiplied by uncertain weights yield estimates that are even more uncertain (Cooper et al., 1998)

Introduction

In Ghana, there is evidence showing that chronic non-communicable diseases (NCDs) are emerging conditions and many studies have made this claim. This assertion is based on epidemiological transition theory which posits that, as a society modernises, the pattern of disease shifts from infectious to chronic non-communicable diseases. But is there a transition going on in Ghana or are studies making this claim trying to fit their data into the epidemiological transition model? To what extent can we say that the patterns of disease have changed in Ghana considering the weak nature of disease surveillance in the country? The focus of this chapter is not to argue whether or not there is a transition going on in Ghana, but rather to evaluate the data used in making knowledge about NCD and chronic disease epidemics in the country in a way that helps to rethink epidemiological transition logic.

The Centers for Disease Control and Prevention (CDC) defines epidemiological surveillance as the 'ongoing systematic collection, analysis, and interpretation of health data essential to the planning, implementation and evaluation of public health practice closely integrated with the timely dissemination of these data to those who need to know.'[1] Monitoring the trends of a disease for appropriate dissemination is a range of processes and, without the completion of these processes, prevention and control measures developed for that particular disease may be grossly misleading.

Due to the growing need to make use of evidence-based statistical measures for global health, attempts have been made to estimate variations in the burden of non-communicable diseases (NCDs) and chronic diseases in different continents across the world. In view of this, there have been several efforts to provide regional statistics on the burden of NCDs and chronic diseases to understand changing health challenges facing people across the world in order to develop appropriate intervention strategies.[2] While those in High-Income Countries (HICs) have adequate epidemiological surveillance systems in place to monitor the burden of these diseases, many Low- and Middle-Income Countries (LMICs), particularly in sub-Saharan Africa (SSA), do not have this system in place. However, several models have been developed to provide estimates of the burden of NCDs and chronic diseases for these regions.

The Institute for Health Metrics and Evaluation (IHME) at the University of Washington spearheaded the data collection on the 2016 global burden of disease (GBD) and this is regarded as the most comprehensive worldwide observational epidemiological study to date.[3] This organisation compiles data on diseases and injuries in different countries using vital registration systems, surveys, censuses and scientific publications. These data are then input into models to estimate various health statistics for a wide range of diseases, disabilities and risk factors; however, some of these estimates have been critiqued on statistical and ethical grounds. For countries with sparse data, models draw strength from data in other countries in the region to produce estimates.[4] According to Christopher Murray, the director of the organisation, IHME has contributed to global health by 'inventing new tools for identifying causes of death, documenting global health expenditures, and creating new ways of measuring health challenges, to help policymakers and donors determine how best to help people live longer, healthier lives'.[5] Rather than presenting actual records of disease occurrence, IHME prioritises metrics and modelled estimates and many criticisms have been raised about this. According to Rachel Parks, although the actual practice of IHME could be different, 'its rhetoric privileges mathematical calculations over human needs'.[6] Cooper and colleagues also pointed out that the reported GBD estimates for many of the countries in sub-Saharan Africa were based on records from South Africa alone, which account for only 1 per cent of the sub-Saharan population covered by vital registration.[7]

Despite the limitations of the GBD, it has generated a database for illnesses and injuries causing deaths and disabilities worldwide. In the absence of national disease registries in many countries, the GBD is often the only source of information providing national estimates on the burden for several conditions. In addition, the GBD has also developed widely used health metrics. For instance, one of the metrics used in estimating the burden of disease in a population and in formulating health policies globally is the disability-adjusted life year (DALY). The DALY was developed from the World Bank's Disease Control Priorities project and popularised through the GBD project led by Christopher Murray.[8,9] The goal was to attach numerical values to various health conditions and disabilities to create a health metric that will combine both morbidity (that is, years of life lived with disability) and mortality (that is, years of life lost) into a single value. The DALY therefore creates a standard way of quantifying the impact of diseases and risk factors on human health in order to help inform how resources should be spent. Even though the DALY attempts to both measure the global burden of disease and to guide the allocation of resources,[10] it fails to provide a measure for resource allocation because it does not account for differentials in resource availability.[11]

Based on the assumption of DALYs, the premature death of a 50-year-old man, for example, should contribute equally to estimates of the global burden of disease irrespective of whether he lives in an urban poor community in Ghana or a wealthy suburb of London. This assumption has been challenged by Becker and colleagues, who said that these two deaths are different because the individuals have different access to resources and might be fulfilling different roles in their communities and families.[12] Allotey and colleagues also conducted an empirical investigation of the context and severity of paraplegia in Australia and Cameroon. They found that, even though paraplegia shares similar clinical manifestations in the two countries, the impact of the condition was more likely to be fatal in Cameroon compared to Australia due to differences in contextual factors.[13] Their conclusion was that the underlying assumption of DALYs ignores context in the assessment of the burden of disease and consequently risks exacerbating inequalities by undervaluing the burden of disease in less-developed countries.

In addition, Anand and Hanson argued that, since DALYs are based on baseline measurements from HICs, the differential found between these populations and those of LMICs measures the 'burden of disease and underdevelopment, and not that of disease alone'.[14] Although recent incarnations of the GBD have calculated the disability weights used to compute DALYs, using responses from survey participants in several countries, there is still uncertainty as to whether these reflect the global population.[15]

Further, ethical concerns have been raised regarding DALYs because of the unequal valuing of life. Particularly, commentators argue that DALYs are constructed in such a way that deaths of people who are old, sick or disabled contribute less to the burden of disease.[16] What this means is that if a person who is expected to live to 70 years gets an NCD or a chronic disease that cuts his/her life short by a year, so that this person dies at 69 years, (s)he has lost 1 year of life. By design, this is treated as less severe compared to the death of another person who dies from this same condition at age 35 years, meaning that that (s)he has lost 35 years of life. It is possible therefore that, for the mortality aspect of DALYs, many commentators may see this as a fair way of accounting for how much of an impact a condition has on human health by looking at how much life is lost to this condition. Nevertheless, this still indicates that deaths in old age are valued less, and this is an ethical question to grapple with. A lot of the controversy, however, may come with the disability aspect of DALYs because of the weighting system and the complexity of this. This unequal valuing of life has been contended by researchers and disabled activists who said that the lives of people with life-long disabilities should be valued equally to those with no disabilities. Hammer argued further that DALYs are implemented according to an economic model that does not depict how the world works.[17] Hence, developing policies based on this kind of estimate can potentially affect millions of lives. In addition, the notion of putting a price on life has been criticised because DALYs confuse the economic value of human beings with the actual value of their lives.[18]

Despite the various critiques of DALY,[19] it is still widely used in developing health policies globally, perhaps because no better metric has emerged. Writing on the role of metrics in the new political regimes of global health, Vincanne Adams has argued that, even though metrics can be seen as a good thing because they counteract political power, they are not unproblematic. This is because it is difficult to find a metric that can serve as a universal standard. She argues that new metrics make new kinds of sovereignty possible. Vincanne Adams referred to this sovereignty as a 'flexible assemblage of data production, number crunching, and scale-up profit sourcing that [...] orchestrates biopolitical health interventions so that they work within capitalism's terms and limits and so that they serve the global architecture of neoliberal debt and profit economies'.[20] Based on current evidence, the DALY has not satisfactorily served as an appropriate universal standard; however, it has persisted because of 'the new, economically justified biomedical sovereignty that it helped to usher in, as the major source of power changed from politics to economics'.[21]

Therefore, even though the IHME has provided extensive information and projections on causes of deaths and injuries, the challenges with DALYs and other health metrics have the possibility of impeding the goals of global health. In 2016, Ghana Ministry of Health (MOH) brought together a group of health experts and development partners in the country in three separate workshops to evaluate the validity of the 2013 GBD for the country.[22] The aim of these workshops was to ensure that the GBD estimates for Ghana are based on the best available information and accepted by health experts as valid, credible and authoritative to assist in planning and formulating health policies. IHME used over 230 sources of published data in Ghana to construct the estimates for diseases and injuries. These Ghanaian experts evaluated 13 out of the top 20 diseases and injuries and found that all the GBD estimates for Ghana were reasonable, except the estimates for tuberculosis (TB), stroke and glaucoma which were underestimated.

Even though there were few contradictions between the IHME and the Ghana MOH estimates, the conclusion drawn by these experts was that the estimates provided by IHME were satisfactory for planning purposes in Ghana and that these estimates provide a reliable view of the larger picture of health needs in the country. This is quite an interesting conclusion considering the fact that the vital registration system in the country is poor, many deaths and births are not recorded, the health care system is not accessible by many Ghanaians, and the true estimates of basic health indices such as death rates or causes of deaths are unknown. One challenge with the conclusion drawn by Ghana MOH is that evaluating the first 13 top burden of disease conditions out of all the diseases and injuries in Ghana is not enough to make a generalisation for all diseases in the country. Also, out of the three main categories of goals for health systems, which include improving aggregate health status; improving equity and reducing poverty; and improving individual welfare, DALYs can only reasonably address the goal of improving aggregate health status.[23] Hence, extrapolating the data on DALYs and other health metrics to mirror the health needs of Ghanaians and developing health plans based on these estimates is inappropriate. Since estimates are as good as the data upon which they are built, this chapter assesses the three main sources of data (that is, hospital records, community survey and national survey) used in estimating and monitoring the burden of NCDs and chronic diseases in Ghana and comments on other potential sources of information (such as Health and Demographic Surveillance Systems and census).

Data used in making knowledge about the burden of non-communicable and chronic diseases

Hospital record system

In November 2017, while I was collecting some data on critical histories of chronic diseases in Ghana, I had an interesting interaction with Professor Paul Nyame, a Ghanaian medic who has been involved in epidemiological studies in a few countries in Africa and Western Asia.[24] One of the questions I asked was if he would share his experiences regarding hospital record systems in Ghana. He mentioned that in the 1970s, the hospital record system in Ghana was intact and it was easy for medical doctors to pull records on different diseases. However, towards the end of 1970s, the record system at the Korle Bu Teaching Hospital (KBTH) broke down due to economic difficulties in the country.

As a result of the global and domestic economic crises of the 1970s, Ghana's economy witnessed a contraction from late 1970s to early 1980s. This economic crisis created a situation where some hospital staff started using the same medical folders[25] for different patients. That is, once a patient did not visit the hospital for a while, the medical folder of that patient was given to a new patient. This created a situation where the medical records of some of the existing patients were completely lost and it was difficult to monitor the medical histories of these patients. When doctors became aware of this, some of them told their patients to go home with their folders to avoid this confusion. Since then, Prof. Nyame told me, the hospital record system in the country has not been completely reliable. During my fieldwork in Ghana, I was at the KBTH and observed that some patients receiving treatment at the hospital still take their folders home. Not only is it possible for patients to lose their folders along with their medical histories, it also means that information about such patients may not exist in the hospital record. Hence, using this kind of hospital data for disease estimates needs to take this omission into account. Even if accurate hospital records are kept, the representativeness of the health facility data is limited by the types of people who access healthcare. Particularly, it has been observed that in many parts of the world, the characteristics of those who use healthcare facilities tend to be different from the general population as a whole. For instance, those who use healthcare facilities usually have higher socioeconomic status and tend to differ by other personal characteristics (for example, age distribution, gender composition, severity of disease, etc.) compared to the general population. So, even if health facility data are well maintained, they can only give a picture of the health of select segments of the population.

Even though hospital admissions are usually selective in relation to personal characteristics, severity of disease, associated conditions and admission policies that vary from hospital to hospital, many hospitals in Ghana still lack improved diagnostic tools, experience congestion and shortage of tools for detecting and diagnosing NCDs and chronic diseases.[26] This consequently leads to high rates of misdiagnosis/underdiagnosis, wrong treatments and different health complications. Empirical research has shown challenges of misdiagnosis in breast cancer and stroke in the country. Regarding breast cancer, Clegg-Lamptey and colleagues showed that previous hospital/medical consultation is a major cause of delay in presentation for breast cancer diagnosis in Ghana.[27] This creates a situation where a benign lump may have spread significantly before a patient is properly diagnosed. In addition, Sarfo and colleagues showed that many of the stroke cases prior to 2008 at Komfo Anokye Teaching Hospital (KATH) could not be classified because of the unavailability of a CT scan.[28] This suggests that, prior to 2008, there may have been a lot of stroke misdiagnoses that could not be accounted for in the second largest tertiary hospital in Ghana. Since the actual number of stroke cases is not known prior to 2008, and given the improvement in diagnosis, it would be easy, although wrong, to assume that stroke cases at the hospital are increasing.

Further, the current structure of the healthcare system in Ghana is such that there are more health facilities available for infectious disease diagnosis and treatment than for NCDs and chronic diseases. Kushitor and Boatemaa particularly showed that, out of the 220 health facilities across Ghana, diagnosis and treatment for malaria between 2007 and 2011 was more accessible than diagnosis and treatment for NCDs such as diabetes and hypertension. One of the reasons for this is that the diagnostic tools for infectious diseases were more available at the health facilities than tools such as blood pressure (BP) monitors and glucometer.[29] Without the availability of diagnostic tools for NCDs and chronic diseases in a health facility, it is basically impractical to monitor the burden of these conditions in such a facility.

In order to strengthen the national disease surveillance system, Ghana adopted the Integrated Disease Surveillance and Response (IDSR) system in 2002 and implemented it nationwide to improve the disease surveillance system.[30] Although the number of diseases required for reporting increased, from 23 in 2002 to 43 in 2011, this system has prioritised communicable diseases such as cholera, diarrhoea, measles, malaria, HIV/AIDs, tuberculosis and so on, and is also crippled with incompleteness and omission of data. Even where data on these communicable diseases were available, they were not often analysed and disseminated so that action could be taken at the local level.

In 2009, software called 'District Health Management Information System (DHMIS)' was developed by Ghana Health Service through collaboration with the University of Oslo in Norway. This software was developed to collect, collate, transmit and analyse routine health service data (from both public and private health facilities) in all the 170 districts in Ghana.[31] There is a claim that DHMIS has led to significant improvements in data collection, reporting and analysis and has strengthened the country's health systems. Nevertheless, many health facilities do not submit their reports on time. Even if there is a timely submission by all the health facilities in the country, the underlying challenges of the hospital record system in Ghana may still feed wrong data into the DHMIS; this will only yield more uncertain estimates.

Community surveys

Community surveys are also an important way to generate data on the burden of NCDs and chronic diseases. One of the benefits of community surveys (especially those that are designed to be representative) is that, since they are done in the community, households and members are selected from different strata of the population in a probabilistic manner. As a result, they can give a better picture of the population and can be used to create population-level estimates in a way that health facility data often cannot. Nevertheless, they are faced with limitations such as omission of people as well as the quantity and quality of clinical information that can be collected.

On 30 April 2014, while I was collecting part of my PhD data on the lived experience of stroke in three poor urban communities in Accra, my research assistant and I had an interesting encounter with one of the community residents. After we finished interviewing a stroke survivor and her caregiver, Mrs Akweley approached us quietly and told us that she had a daughter living with stroke. She asked us to come over to her house to check on her 31-year-old daughter called Beatrice. When we got to the house and she took us to the room where Beatrice has been staying, I was shocked and astounded. This was because this house had been part of the three rounds of Urban Poverty and Health Survey conducted by the Regional Institute for Population Studies (RIPS). This survey was carried out at 18–20-month intervals in 2010 (June), 2011 (December) and 2013 (September), with households and individuals in three low-resource communities in Accra. One of the questions asked during the survey was for the head of the household to list the household members that have been diagnosed with any non-communicable disease. Even though three rounds of survey had been collected in these communities, this household had never reported anyone with stroke despite the fact that Beatrice had been inside the house since we started the survey. When we probed further on why Beatrice had never been listed as someone living with a non-communicable disease, Mrs Akweley told us that they were uncomfortable disclosing the disease status of Beatrice because of the shame and stigma that comes with taking care of a young person with stroke. This made me realise how many people like Beatrice may have been 'uncounted' among people living with NCDs or chronic diseases during community surveys due to socio-cultural reasons.

Based on the results of this longitudinal survey, stroke prevalence in these communities was 0.4 per cent (3 stroke survivors) in 2010, 1.1 per cent (12 stroke survivors) in 2011 and 2.3 per cent (18 stroke survivors) in 2013. Although it seems the stroke prevalence rates were increasing, the number of stroke cases reported in the three rounds of the survey was too small compared to the number of stroke cases that I saw during various research engagements in these communities over three years. In these communities, research showed that hypertension prevalence was 28.3 per cent. Among those with hypertension, 7.4 per cent were aware of their condition, 4.0 per cent were on antihypertensive medications and 3.5 per cent had their blood pressure controlled.[32] Since hypertension is a major cause of stroke in Ghana,[33] the low levels of hypertension awareness, treatment and control in these communities perhaps indicate under-reporting of stroke cases.

National surveys

The only national survey in Ghana which captured eight different NCDs and chronic diseases and their risk factors is the WHO Study on Global AGEing and Adult Health (SAGE). SAGE is part of a Longitudinal Survey Programme in WHO's multi-country studies unit and gathers data on NCDs and chronic conditions (that is, stroke, angina pectoris, diabetes mellitus, osteoarthritis, chronic lung disease, asthma, depression and hypertension), health services coverage, health care utilisation, subjective well-being and quality of life, and social networks.[34] This survey compiles nationally representative information on the health and well-being of adults in six countries (China, Ghana, India, Mexico, Russian Federation and South Africa) and has provided a lot of information on older adult health. Despite the laudable achievements of SAGE, one of the challenges with this survey is that there are usually delays in data sharing which consequently lead to delays in analysis, interpretation and in informing policies. For instance, SAGE Wave 1 was carried out between 2007 and 2008 while Waves 2 and 3 were expected to be implemented in 2013 and 2015, respectively. It was not until 2014/2015 that the Wave 2 data were collected in Ghana and even now, the data are not available for public use. The implication of this is that before policies could be developed based on the findings from this survey, many things may have changed in the country. This delay in timely analysis may inadvertently misguide policies.

Another major national dataset in Ghana is the Demographic and Health Survey which is usually collected every five years. From the inception of the survey in 1988 until 2008, the main focus was on fertility, family planning, infant and child mortality, maternal and child health, and nutrition. However, some information on variables that may be risk factors for NCDs, such as body mass index, tobacco use, and alcohol consumption was collected in recent Demographic and Health Surveys (DHS).[35] In 2014, the Government of Ghana, through the joint efforts of the Ghana Statistical Service (GSS), the Ghana Health Service (GHS), and the National Public Health Reference Laboratory (NPHRL), decided to collect specialised data on blood pressure in the 2014 Ghana Demographic and Health Survey (GDHS). The reason for this was to monitor the hypertension status of Ghanaians and to come up with intervention strategies that can reduce the burden of the condition in the country. Although this is a laudable effort by the government to monitor the non-communicable disease burden in the country, it is limited to hypertension only. Nonetheless, this effort suggests improvement in the effort of the government and donor agencies to improve surveillance on hypertension in the country. It also implies that increasing attention is being paid to NCDs and chronic conditions in Ghana.

Health and demographic surveillance systems

In the 1940s, Health and Demographic Surveillance Systems (HDSSs) was set up in SSA to monitor fertility, mortality, migration and other health and socioeconomic indicators within a defined population over time.[36] As at 2011, a total of 30 HDSS sites have been established in SSA. An HDSS collects data prospectively and longitudinally on a district and generates empirical evidence for health policy making. There are three HDSS sites in Ghana and these are located in three ecological zones (Navrongo, Kintampo and Dodowa).

The Navrongo Health and Demographic Surveillance System (NHDSS) site is located in the Kassena-Nankana District of the Upper East region of Ghana and was established in 1993 by the Navrongo Health Research Centre.[37] The NHDSS monitors the health and demographic dynamics of the two Kassena-Nankana districts of northern Ghana and also evaluates the morbidity and mortality impact of health and social interventions.[38] The NHDSS has particularly gathered data on the following: longitudinal health and demographic data for over two decades; maternal and child health; malaria epidemiology including malariometric features of the area; other biological measures such as carriage, outbreaks and surveillance of the meningococcal meningitis, respiratory infections in children, neglected tropical diseases, micronutrient deficiencies, and safety, immunogenicity, pharmacokinetics of drugs and vaccines, immunology, genomics and genetics biomarkers, and adult NCD-related mortality.

Kintampo Health Research Centre (KHRC) was established in 1994 and it is situated in the middle belt of Ghana in the Bono East (formerly Brong Ahafo) Region.[39] Priority research areas of this centre include communicable diseases with specific focus on malaria, tuberculosis and HIV/AIDS; sexual and reproductive health; maternal, neo-natal and child health; mental health; NCDs such as hypertension and cancer,[40] health systems, mental health and healthcare financing.[41] One core research focus of KHRC is community engagement activities which are usually carried out before, during and after each research project.

The Dodowa Health Research Centre (DHRC) began operation as a Health and Demographic Surveillance System site in 2005. It is located in the south-eastern part of Ghana and covers two peri-urban districts (Shai-Osudoku and Ningo-Prampram districts) of the Greater Accra Region. DHRC generates research evidence of public health importance nationally.[42] The Centre has focused largely on malaria research since its inception but has expanded its research scope to other areas such as maternal, neo-natal and child health, sanitation and health, tuberculosis, neglected tropical disease (NTD), social protection and NCD-related adult mortality.

These three surveillance sites, set up to monitor new health threats, track population changes through fertility, mortality and migration, and monitor the effect of policy interventions on communities, provide incredible opportunities to monitor patterns and trends of NCDs and chronic disease burden in Ghana. Nevertheless, they have not been fully exploited to generate enough data on this research area. The focus of these research centres on NCD-related mortality was popularised by the International Network for the Continuous Demographic Evaluation of Populations and their Health (INDEPTH) which was established in 1998. INDEPTH is a global network, set up to provide a more complete picture of the health status of communities in 19 LMICs in Africa, Asia and Oceania.[43] The INDEPTH Network was founded to facilitate the linkage of existing HDSSs through a focused network and allows researchers from the HDSS sites to jointly collect data and compare findings through working groups formed around specific research agendas. Since the 2000s, many of the INDEPTH sites (working with HDSSs across Africa and Asia) have been collecting longitudinal data on cause of death, including several NCD-related causes of death, using verbal autopsy methods.[44] This has provided important information on adult NCD-specific mortality including neoplasms, metabolic, cardiovascular, respiratory, abdominal, neurological and other NCDs, corresponding to WHO 2012 verbal autopsy standard.[45] For instance, their analysis showed that the proportions of adult NCD mortality (for over 15 years), in the districts covered by Navrongo Health and Demographic Surveillance System and Dodowa Health Research Centre, were 40.9 per cent and 28.3 per cent, respectively. Exploiting the data generated by these HDSS sites may help to monitor the trends and patterns of NCDs and chronic diseases in Ghana and may serve as examples for expanding the surveillance sites to other Ghanaian communities. In addition, these sites may help to develop capacity for NCDs and chronic diseases management and control at community level in Ghana.

Census data

A final potential source of information relating to NCDs and chronic conditions in Ghana is the census. Ghana was the first independent country in SSA to undertake a census.[46] Eleven censuses have been conducted in the country to date; six were carried out before independence in 1957 (that is in 1891, 1901, 1911, 1921, 1931 and 1948) and five have been conducted since independence (that is in 1960, 1970, 1984, 2000 and 2010).[47] The type of data collected in censuses in the country has varied considerably over the years. For instance, minimal data were collected for planning purposes during the pre-independence censuses. From the 1960 census and subsequent censuses in the country, data on basic demographic, geographic and socioeconomic characteristics were included in the questionnaires. During the 2010 Population and Housing Census, five additional modules were added to the questionnaire relating to disability, emigration, information and communication technologies, maternal mortality and agriculture.

Generally, many censuses in Ghana were characterised by low reliability and serious undercounting. Historically, Ghana's population figures were consistently shaped by people's distrust of the state. There were occasions where people were unwilling to cooperate during censuses due to ignorance, socio-cultural factors and fear of taxation.[48] For instance, during the first census in 1891, the proposed use of census data for taxation purposes triggered people's distrust and this elicited different forms of resistance leading to under-enumeration. In 1921, when there was a suspicion that the census would be used for imposition of the poll tax, some people went into hiding to avoid being counted.[49] Other challenges that have limited the reliability of census figures in Ghana include boundary disputes regarding demarcation areas and during actual enumeration of the population; inconsistencies in the timing of the census; shortage of census questionnaires; and logistical problems such as inadequate funds to procure necessary equipment, inadequate storage space to store all completed questionnaires and inadequate office space to accommodate data processing activities.[50]

Despite the challenges of censuses in Ghana, it is still considered as the largest source of information about the entire population. According to the United Nations, 'census data should be used for policymaking, planning and administration, research, business, electoral boundary delimitation and sampling frame for surveys'.[51] In Ghana, some institutions such as the Electoral Commission, National Health Insurance Authority and the National Identification Authority had made use of census figures to guide their activities. Censuses have also been used as sampling frames for major national surveys in the country, including the Ghana Demographic and Health Surveys and the Ghana Living Standard Surveys. So, to what extent has the census been or can it be utilised to generate evidence for NCDs and chronic diseases in Ghana?

In Ghana's 2010 Population and Housing Census (PHC), questions were included regarding overall disability status with specific focus on sight, hearing or speech impairments, physical disabilities, emotional disabilities and mental disabilities.[52] Continued and expanded collection of information on the disability status of Ghanaians may provide useful information in monitoring types of disability in the country. Regular assessments of disability status, as in several other African countries, may allow Ghana to monitor changing patterns of disability over time and how these vary by socioeconomic status and region. Given that in theory censuses survey the entire population, the Ghana Statistical Service (GSS) may explore what additional health information could be gained through the census while respecting the privacy and time of individuals. For instance, information on the severity of disability may be measured in subsequent censuses in Ghana, just like some other countries in sub-Saharan Africa have done.

The disability question asked in the Ghana 2010 census only allows members of the population to be classified as disabled or not disabled. Nevertheless, South Africa (2011) and Tanzania (2012) included severity of disability in their censuses and the categories included 'no difficulty', 'some difficulty' and 'a lot of difficulty'.[53] These categories can give an idea on impact of disability. Further, in addition to collecting information on the types of disability, the GSS may include information on causes of disability in the census, as has been done in Ethiopia, Lesotho, Liberia, Uganda, Rwanda and so on. For example, in the Rwanda 2012 PHC, questions were asked on causes of disability and the responses included congenital diseases/illness, injury/accident, war/mines and genocide. With this information, it is possible to stratify types of disability by causes, which is important for policy interventions. Even though this may be expensive and complicated, the fact that this has been done in some other sub-Saharan African countries means that it is achievable.

Conclusion

This chapter shows that, although there have been several efforts to improve surveillance and measurement of NCDs and chronic diseases in Ghana, there is still room for improvement. The current overview of the situation in Ghana indicates that the Ghana Ministry of Health now relies on the IHME estimates of the Ghana burden of disease, but the question remains as to whether useful policy decisions can be made while there are caveats to the validity of the burden-of-disease measures. Perhaps, rather than depending solely on external sources or agencies to develop models or estimates that will be used to measure the health of Ghanaians, joint collaborations to improve disease surveillance systems, quality of care and efficiency in delivery of care in the country should be promoted. While modelled health estimates are useful, they are based on assumptions which may not reflect the reality on the ground. Hence, they should not be substitutes for collecting quality data. Policymakers and researchers in the country need to have a constant reminder of what Cooper and colleagues said, that 'uncertain inputs multiplied by uncertain weights yield estimates that are even more uncertain.'[54] In order to avoid wasted efforts, there should not be an alternative to investment in good data. Until data that correspond with modelled estimates are available in Ghana, it is highly recommended that the GBD estimates and projections for the country should be used with caution and not be completely relied upon to inform policies.

In the meantime, caution should be taken while interpreting data on NCDs and chronic diseases, especially data retrieved from health facilities. To enhance interpretations of current data available in the country, interdisciplinary approaches which bring epidemiologists, demographers, historians and psychologists together should be adopted. This will help to better make sense of the existing data in the country. Previous workshops on disease surveillance in Ghana have mainly involved epidemiologists and public health researchers. Coupled with this, most of the research on NCDs and chronic diseases until the early 2000s had been carried out by medics. There is a need to bring in more social scientists and pure sciences in NCD and chronic disease debates in Ghana. This may provide an interesting multifaceted approach to monitor the burden of NCDs and chronic diseases in the country. Also, the different data sources should be interpreted independently but combined in a way that tells interesting stories about the epidemiological landscape of Ghana. For instance, hospital data should not be extrapolated to the population because this will be fundamentally flawed. Furthermore, the importance of strengthening the healthcare system to enhance the success of the DHMIS cannot be overemphasised. Measures that improve access to care and address broader societal issues such as health inequalities and poverty are needed.

Notes

1 I would like to thank Professor Paul Nyame (former Rector, Ghana College of Physicians and Surgeons) and Dr Frank Ankobea (President, Ghana Medical Association) for their insights on the epidemiological transition and history of hospital record system in Ghana. I am sincerely grateful to Professor Megan Vaughan, Professor Ama de-Graft Aikins and Dr Kafui Adjaye-Gbewonyo for their comments on an earlier draft of this paper. This work was fully supported by the Wellcome Trust-funded project on 'Chronic Disease in Sub-Saharan Africa' led by Professor Megan Vaughan (Award No. 106534).

2 Murray and Lopez, 'Measuring Global Health'.

3 *Lancet*, 'Global Burden of Disease 2016'.

4 IHME, 'Global Burden of Disease'.
5 IHME, 'Director's Statement', last modified 11 December 2018.
6 Parks, 'The Rise, Critique and Persistence of the DALY'.
7 Cooper et al., 'Disease Burden in Sub-Saharan Africa'.
8 Maldonado and Morira, 'Metrics in Global Health'.
9 Murray, 'Quantifying the Burden of Disease'.
10 Anand and Hanson, 'Disability-Adjusted Life Years'.
11 Parks, 'The Rise, Critique and Persistence of the DALY'.
12 Becker et al., 'The Unique Challenges of Mental Health and MDRTB'.
13 Allotey et al., 'The DALY, Context and the Determinants of the Severity of Disease'.
14 Anand and Hanson, 'Disability-Adjusted Life Years'.
15 Haagsma et al., 'Assessing Disability Weights'; Nord, 'Uncertain Ties'.
16 Parks, 'The Rise, Critique and Persistence of the DALY'.
17 Hammer and Berman, 'Ends and Means'.
18 Parks, 'The Rise, Critique and Persistence of the DALY'.
19 Reidpath et al., 'Measuring Health in a Vacuum'; Anand and Hanson, 'Disability-Adjusted Life Years'; Parks, 'The Rise, Critique and Persistence of the DALY'.
20 Adams, 'Metrics of the Global Sovereign'.
21 Parks, 'The Rise, Critique and Persistence of the DALY'.
22 Ghana Ministry of Health, 'Burden of Disease Study – 2016'.
23 Hammer and Berman, 'Ends and Means'; Parks, 'The Rise, Critique and Persistence of the DALY'.
24 Professor Paul Nyame, an older medic, gained his medical degree in 1966 and worked with the University of Ghana Medical School for about 30 years. He was interviewed in November 2017 at the Secretariat of the Ghana College of Physicians and Surgeons.
25 For a new patient seeking treatment in a health facility in Ghana, (s)he will be asked to get a paper folder where all his/her medical records/tests will be kept. While some hospitals do keep their patients' folders, some allow patients to take their folders home.
26 de-Graft Aikins et al., 'Chronic Non-Communicable Diseases'; Kushitor and Boatemaa, 'The Double Burden of Disease'.
27 Clegg-Lamptey, Dakubo, and Attobra, 'Why Do Breast Cancer Patients Report Late?'.
28 Sarfo et al., 'Trends in Stroke Admission'.
29 Kushitor and Boatemaa, 'The Double Burden of Disease'.
30 Adokiya et al., 'The Integrated Disease Surveillance'.
31 Ghana Ministry of Health, 'Rolling out a Nationwide Web-Based District Health Information System'.
32 Awuah et al., 'Prevalence, Awareness, Treatment and Control of Hypertension'.
33 Sanuade and Agyemang, 'A Review of Stroke in Ghana'.
34 Biritwum et al., 'Ghana Study on Global AGEing'.
35 Ghana Statistical Service, '2014 Ghana Demographic and Health Survey'.
36 Yazoume et al., 'Health and Demographic Surveillance Systems'.
37 Oduro et al., 'Profile of the Navrongo Health and Demographic Surveillance System'.
38 INDEPTH Network, 'Better Health Information for Better Health Policy – Navrongo Health Research Centre'.
39 INDEPTH Network, 'Better Health Information for Better Health Policy – Kintampo Health Research Centre'.
40 Dosoo et al., 'Prevalence of Hypertension in the Middle Belt of Ghana'; Nyame et al., 'Capacity and Readiness'.
41 INDEPTH Network, 'Better Health Information for Better Health Policy – Kintampo Health Research Centre'.
42 INDEPTH Network, 'Better Health Information for Better Health Policy – Dodowa Health Research Centre'.
43 Ng et al., 'Using the INDEPTH HDSS to Build Capacity'; Akuse et al., 'Do Different HDSS Surveillance Systems Result in Different Quality of Pregnancy Outcome Data?'; INDEPTH Network, 'Better Health Information for Better Health Policy'.
44 INDEPTH Network Secretariat, 'Developing and Validating a Standardized Verbal Autopsy Tool'.
45 Streatfield et al., 'Adult Non-communicable Disease Mortality'; World Health Organization, 'Verbal Autopsy Standards'.

46 Serra, 'Hail the Census Night'.
47 Ghana Statistical Service, '2010 Population & Housing Census'.
48 Gold Coast Census Office, 'Report on the Census'; Gold Coast Census Office, *Census Report, 1921*.
49 Serra, 'Hail the Census Night'; Gold Coast Census Office, 'Report on the Census'; Gold Coast Census Office, *Census Report, 1921*.
50 Ghana Statistical Service, '2010 Population & Housing Census'.
51 United Nations, 'Principles and Recommendation for Population and Housing Censuses'.
52 Minnesota Population Center, 'Integrated Public Use Microdata Series'.
53 Minnesota Population Center, 'Integrated Public Use Microdata Series'; Cooper et al., 'Disease Burden in Sub-Saharan Africa'.
54 Cooper et al., 'Disease Burden in Sub-Saharan Africa'.

Bibliography

Adams, Vincanne. 'Metrics of the Global Sovereign: Numbers and Stories in Global Health'. In *Metrics: What Counts in Global Health*, edited by Vincanne Adams, 20–54. Durham, NC: Duke University Press, 2016.

Adokiya, Martin N. et al. 'The Integrated Disease Surveillance and Response System in Northern Ghana: Challenges to the Core and Support Functions', *BMC Health Services Research*, 15 (2015): 1–11.

Akuze, Joseph et al. On behalf of the INDEPTH Network–ENAP metrics study team. 'Do Different HDSS Surveillance Systems Result in Different Quality of Pregnancy Outcome Data?'. 28th International Population Conference of the International Union for the Scientific Study of Population (IUSSP). Cape Town, 2017.

Allotey, Pascale et al. 'The DALY, Context and the Determinants of the Severity of Disease: An Exploratory Comparison of Paraplegia in Australia and Cameroon', *Social Science & Medicine*, 57 (2003): 949–58.

Anand, Sudhir and Kara Hanson. 'Disability-Adjusted Life Years: a Critical Review', *Journal of Health Economics*, 16 (1997): 685–702.

Awuah, Ralphael Baffour et al. 'Prevalence, Awareness, Treatment and Control of Hypertension in Urban Poor Communities', *Journal of Hypertension*, 32 (2014): 1203–10.

Becker, Anne et al. ' The Unique Challenges of Mental Health and MDRTB: Critical Perspectives on Metrics of Disease Burden'. In *Reimagining Global Health: An Introduction*, edited by Paul Farmer, Yong J. Kim, Arthur Kleinman, and Matthew Basilicao, 209–41. Berkeley, CA: University of California Press, 2013.

Biritwum, Richard B. et al. 'Ghana Study on Global AGEing and Adult Health (SAGE), Wave 1: The Ghana National Report 2013', last modified 4 June 2019, https://www.researchgate.net/publication/277305927_Ghana_Study_on_global_AGEing_and_adult_health_SAGE_Wave_1_National_Report.

Centers for Disease Control, 'CDC's Vision for Public Health Surveillance in the 21st Century', *Morbidity and Mortality Weekly Report*, 61 (2012): 1–44.

Clegg-Lamptey, Joe, Jonathan Dakubo, and Y.N. Attobra. 'Why Do Breast Cancer Patients Report Late or Abscond during Treatment in Ghana? A Pilot Study', *Ghana Medical Journal*, 43 (2009): 127–31.

Cooper, Richard S. et al. 'Disease Burden in Sub-Saharan Africa: What Should We Conclude in the Absence of Data', *Lancet*, 351 (1998): 208–10.

de-Graft Aikins et al. 'Chronic Non-Communicable Diseases and the Challenge of Universal Health Coverage: Insights from Community-Based Cardiovascular Disease Research in Urban Poor Communities in Accra, Ghana', *BMC Public Health*, 14 (2014): S3.

Dosoo, David Kwame et al. 'Prevalence of Hypertension in the Middle Belt of Ghana: A Community-Based Screening Study', *International Journal of Hypertension*, 2019.

Ghana Ministry of Health. 'Rolling out a Nationwide Web-Based District Health Information System, DHIMS2 – The Ghana Experience', last modified 12 December 2012, https://www.researchgate.net/profile/Anthony_Ofosu/project/DHIS2-roll-out-in-Ghana/attachment/57f2259508aeb9635636f95c/AS:413037094817792@1475487125868/download/ROLLING+OUT+A+NATIONWIDE+WEB+APPLICATION.pdf?context=ProjectUpdatesLog.

Ghana Ministry of Health. 'Ghana Burden of Disease Study 2016', last modified 12 December 2018, http://www.healthdata.org/acting-data/understanding-%E2%80%98big-picture%E2%80%99-can-lead-healthier-population-ghana.
Ghana Statistical Service. '2010 Population & Housing Census: National Analytical Report', last modified 18 May 2020, https://statsghana.gov.gh/gssmain/fileUpload/pressrelease/2010_PHC_National_Analytical_Report.pdf.
Ghana Statistical Service. '2014 Ghana Demographic and Health Survey', last modified 14 March 2019, http://www.statsghana.gov.gh/docfiles/publications/Ghana_DHS_2014-KIR-6_April_2015.pdf.
Gold Coast Census Office. 'Report on the Census of the Gold Coast Colony for the Year 1891', *National Archives of Ghana (NAG), Accra, ADM*, 5 (2) (1891): 1.
Gold Coast Census Office. *Census Report, 1921, for the Gold Coast Colony, Ashanti, the Northern Territories and the Mandated Area of Togoland*. Accra: Govt. Press, 1923.
Haagsma, Juanita A. et al. 'Assessing Disability Weights Based on the Responses of 30,660 People from Four European Countries', *Population Health Metrics*, 13 (2015): 10–24.
Hammer, Jeffery S. and P. Berman. 'Ends and Means in Public Health Policy in Developing Countries', *Health Policy*, 32 (1995): 29–45.
INDEPTH Network. 'Better Health Information for Better Health Policy', last modified 10 December 2018, http://indepth-network.org/about-us.
INDEPTH Network. 'Better Health Information for Better Health Policy – Dodowa Health Research Centre', last modified 3 May 2020, http://www.indepth-network.org/member-centres/dodowa-hdss.
INDEPTH Network. 'Better Health Information for Better Health Policy – Kintampo Health Research Centre', last modified 3 May 2020, http://www.indepth-network.org/member-centres/kintampo-hdss.
INDEPTH Network. 'Better Health Information for Better Health Policy – Navrongo Health Research Centre', last modified 3 May 2020, http://www.indepth-network.org/member-centres/navrongo-hdss.
INDEPTH Network Secretariat. 'Developing and Validating a Standardized Verbal Autopsy Tool to Elicit Most Probable Cause of Death for Low- and Middle-Income Countries', last modified 10 December 2018, http://www.indepth-network.org/sites/default/files/content/resources/files/SECRETARIAT Developing and validating a standardized Verbal Autopsy final.pdf.
Institute for Health Metrics and Evaluation. 'Director's Statement', last modified 11 December 2018, http://www.healthdata.org/about/director-statement.
Institute for Health Metrics and Evaluation. 'Global Burden of Disease (GBD)', last modified 10 December 2018, http://www.healthdata.org/gbd.
Kushitor, Mawuli K. and Sandra Boatemaa. 'The Double Burden of Disease and the Challenge of Health Access: Evidence from Access, Bottlenecks, Cost and Equity Facility Survey in Ghana', *PloS One*, 13 (2018): e0194677.
Lancet. 'Global Burden of Disease 2016', last modified June 11, 2019, https://www.thelancet.com/journals/lancet/issue/vol390no10100/PIIS0140-6736(17)X0041-X.
Maldonado, Tiago and T. Morira. 'Metrics in Global Health: Situated Differences in the Valuation of Human Life', *Historical Social Research*, 44 (2): 202–24.
Minnesota Population Center. 'Integrated Public Use Microdata Series, International: Version 7.0 [Dataset]', last modified 13 November 2018, https://international.ipums.org/international/citation.shtml.
Murray, Christopher J. L. 'Quantifying the Burden of Disease: The Technical Basis for Disability-Adjusted Life Years', *Bulletin of the World Health Organization*, 72 (1994): 429–45.
Murray, Christopher J. L. and A. D. Lopez. 'Measuring Global Health: Motivation and Evolution of the Global Burden of Disease Study', *Lancet*, 390 (2017): 1460–4.
Ng, Nawi et al. 'Using the INDEPTH HDSS to Build Capacity for Chronic Non-communicable Disease Risk Factor Surveillance in Low and Middle-income Countries', *Global Health Action*, 2 (1) (2009): 1984.
Nord, Erik. 'Uncertain Ties about Disability Weights for the Global Burden', *Lancet Global Health*, 3 (2015): e661–2.
Nyame, Solomon et al. 'Capacity and Readiness for Implementing Evidence-Based Task-Strengthening Strategies for Hypertension Control in Ghana: A Cross-Sectional Study', *Global Heart*, 14 (2) (2019): 129–34.
Oduro, Abraham Rexford et al. 'Profile of the Navrongo Health and Demographic Surveillance System', *International Journal of Epidemiology*, 41 (4) (2012): 968–76.

Parks, R. 'The Rise, Critique and Persistence of the DALY in Global Health', last modified 11 July 2019, http://www.ghjournal.org/the-rise-critique-and-persistence-of-the-daly-in-global-health/#.

Reidpath, Daniel D., Pascale A. Allotey, and Robert A. Cummins. 'Measuring Health in a Vacuum: Examining the Disability Weight of the DALY', *Health Policy Plan*, 18 (2003): 351–6.

Sanuade, Olutobi and Charles Agyemang. 'A Review of Stroke in Ghana'. In *Chronic Non-Communicable Diseases in Ghana: Multidisciplinary Perspectives*, edited by Ama de-Graft Aikins, Samuel Agyei-Mensah, and Charles Agyemang, 29–40. Accra: Sub-Saharan Publishers, 2013.

Sarfo, Fred S. et al. 'Trends in Stroke Admission and Mortality Rates from 1983 to 2013 in Central Ghana', *Journal of the Neurological Sciences*, 357 (2015): 240–5.

Serra, Gerardo. '"Hail the Census Night": Trust and Political Imagination in the 1960 Population Census of Ghana', *Comparative Studies in Society and History*, 60 (3) (2018): 659–87.

Streatfield, Peter Kim et al. 'Adult Non-Communicable Disease Mortality in Africa and Asia: Evidence from INDEPTH Health and Demographic Surveillance System Sites', *Global Health Action*, 7 (1) (2014): 25365.

United Nations. 'Principles and Recommendation for Population and Housing Censuses'. Revision 2, Statistical Papers, Series M. No. 67/Rev. 2, 2008, United Nations, New York.

World Health Organization. 'Verbal Autopsy Standards: the 2012 WHO Verbal Autopsy Instrument', Geneva: WHO, 2012.

Yazoume, Ye et al. 'Health and Demographic Surveillance Systems: A Step Towards Full Civil Registration and Vital Statistics System in Sub-Sahara Africa?', *BMC Public Health*, 12 (2012): 741.

Part 3

8

Dealing with Non-Communicable and Infectious Conditions

Amy Moran-Thomas

Imagine that you felt a little dizzy in the heat and collapsed while making lunch, Salimata told me. Imagine that you wake up in a hospital and feel terrible pain in your leg – but when you look down to where it hurts the most, all you see is an empty space. That was how Salimata described the first time that she was diagnosed with type 2 diabetes. She said it took months to begin absorbing the reality that her leg had been lost due to a chronic condition that no-one had ever suspected she had. Years later, she still woke up feeling its presence sometimes. As we sat talking on the smoothed earth of her family courtyard, in the Savelugu area of Northern Ghana, the flip-flop sandals she wore on her open palms when moving rested on the ground between us. They bore imprints of the body's weight, as cheap rubber sandals often do, only of handprints instead of footprints.

At the time in 2009, I had been observing the Guinea Worm Eradication Program surveillance team going from village to village, meticulously searching for guinea worm ulcers on people's legs or feet. The team could barely find any traces of guinea worm, but people kept approaching with other kinds of ulcers and wounds. There was no system that their specialised team had to count non-guinea-worm ulcers or provide those people with treatment. I had been surprised at the time to hear mention of diabetes, which I had always learned was an 'urban' disease. Yet this constellation of villages in Northern Ghana was the least urban place I had seen in my life – many of the communities unreachable by car, women walking miles daily to carry back home buckets of water, some villages hours from the nearest cell signal.

GUINEA WORM IS A MEDICAL EMERGENCY, the campaign's glossy decal stickers read. But the people I met extruding guinea worms did not seem to think it was nearly as urgent as the foreign photographers taking pictures of them. Meanwhile a diabetes ulcer becoming infected had been categorised as nobody's emergency, even though a resulting amputation could result in searing pains and patterned disability for a lifetime. I wondered what the driving value system was that produced this uneven attention, in which such divergent care priorities could be made of look-alike ulcers on legs? Guinea worms actually produce and secrete morphine to soothe their hosts' legs or feet during the few days they take to emerge. In contrast, many people with diabetes worldwide today end up having limbs amputated in overstrained hospitals without receiving any morphine.

Co-terminus realities

When I brought these observations about people's comments on diabetes to the Ministry of Health physician mentoring my project, he encouraged me to pay attention to all ulcers, not just those caused by guinea worm, and suggested that I visit the local diabetes clinic to talk with his colleagues there.[1] I will never forget the morning that followed, which began by observing the bustling office of the guinea worm eradication programme. Inside the office, several dozen campaign staff, Ghanaian Ministry of Health officials on laptops and Carter Center consultants were debating how best to locate a woman with guinea worm who had run away so as not to receive treatment. Guinea worm hurts for several days but doesn't kill, though it appears grotesque to foreigners who are not accustomed to seeing three-foot-long parasites. These worms have been the target of major US-driven eradication efforts for several decades. Later that same morning, I travelled a few minutes across town to the Tamale public hospital's once-weekly diabetes clinic for the Northern Region. More than 30 patients waited outside for hours for a doctor who never arrived.

I waited awkwardly with those patients for a few hours on the wooden benches of the hospital courtyard until they were finally sent home for the day. The research collaborator I worked with in Tamale, Emmanuel, translated from Dagbani, and I took notes as several people approached me to describe their routines living with diabetes in a region where over half the rural population survives on less than a dollar a day.[2] Some described walking dirt paths by lantern light from their far-flung villages or crossing rivers by canoe in order to reach a road that would lead to the hospital by dawn. As was clinic policy, the first 30 patients who arrived at the Friday diabetes clinic were handed ticket-like numbers, and the rest were sent home until the following week. 'I am number 17,' offered the young woman next to me. She had arrived by *tro-tro* minibus taxi around 4.00 a.m., in order to secure a place.

When I met with the government doctor the next week, he explained he had been called away on another emergency. He spoke about the difficulty of being the only doctor assigned to treat diabetes in a region of 1.8 million people, and only on Friday mornings. 'I am one man,' he said. 'It is just me.' He told me the weekly clinic felt very different from when it first opened: many of his original patients had already died.

Outside his office door, a man with no legs was being carried toward us on the shoulders of two young men in lieu of a wheelchair. 'We used to have dozens of children with type 1 diabetes here,' the physician said, but there were frequent interruptions in the region's insulin supply. The emotional labour of triaging insulin often fell to pharmacists, who had to decide which of the physicians' prescriptions they would actually fill with the very limited supply. Children first. 'They used to come every Friday. But many of them lived in the villages. We lost them; they died, one by one. They are all gone now.'

'What about the Salifu girl?' asked his assistant, an attentive man in a long robe who had worked at the diabetes clinic since it first opened years ago. 'We haven't heard anything since she went back to Kampong.' The doctor nodded and smiled faintly in recognition. 'That's right, we do have one left. Her name was Safia.'

Neglected tropical disease philanthropy and global health aid become a different picture when thinking of these comparative scenes (the same city's gutted public diabetes clinic versus its bustling guinea worm eradication programme office and countless other places like them) as *coterminous realities*, drawing from the same limited pool of healthcare workers and monies spliced into vertical programmes. The institutional 'politics of prioritisation' that many social scientists have described at play in global health funding also impacts on how complex causalities are studied, risks are interpreted and clinical care structures are resourced.

I continued to be struck by this when I wrapped up my research in Northern Ghana and headed for a year of fieldwork in southern Belize, where I had intended (once again) to study a parasitic worm disease intervention.[3] But, once again, people were much more interested in talking about diabetes. An ocean away, thinking across these different encounters helped me to understand that what I was seeing was part of a worldwide problem. Patients, families and other caregivers alike were struggling to achieve diabetes treatment regimens in overstrained health systems where neither type 1 nor type 2 diabetes has historically been considered high priority by the foreign institutions guiding money toward infectious conditions. In nearly all countries, in the wake of structural adjustment policies, health systems have been deeply contoured by an 'alphabet soup' of acronyms belonging to foreign NGOs, where piecemeal funding over the past century has inevitably come with certain priorities and strings attached.[4]

In Belize, diabetes had become the leading cause of death nationwide by 2010. One in four people (and one in three women) in Stann Creek District were living with the condition.[5] The rising blood sugar linked to diabetes involved translations and terms that travelled across languages: *súgara* in Garifuna, *shuga* in Belizean Kriol, *azúcar* in Spanish, *kiha kiik* in Kekchi Mayan, or *ch'uhuk k'iik* (sweet blood) in Mopan and Yukatec.[6] As I tried to make sense of what people described as spreading 'sugar' on both sides of the Atlantic, I was struck by the larger questions being highlighted time and again as people shared their takes on aetiologies of their conditions.

'Catching it'

As rising diabetes levels settled into the social fabric in Belize, rumours kept popping up that certain forms could be contagious. I heard numerous stories about husbands and wives becoming afraid to sleep in the same room, with amputated limbs mentioned as the defining feature of these anxieties. 'Well, here it comes for me,' Laura recalled thinking when she was diagnosed with diabetes in her twenties. 'I knew it was coming for me, because my mother had it, my sister ... we all have it.' The personified pathogens that people kept using to allude to their diabetic injuries came from the language of infection: many said of diabetes sugar that they 'caught it'. More ominously, others said of sugar '*it* caught *me*'. These terms were based on people's first-hand observations of patterns; their mental maps of neighbourhoods and families. The deeper puzzle, I began to think, was not why a fast-spreading fatal disease might be interpreted as somehow infectious, but rather how our terms for framing and addressing public health conditions had come to be so dualistic in the first place.

The old paradigm of environmental miasma located disease agents in contaminated atmospheres and places, repurposing an ancient Greek

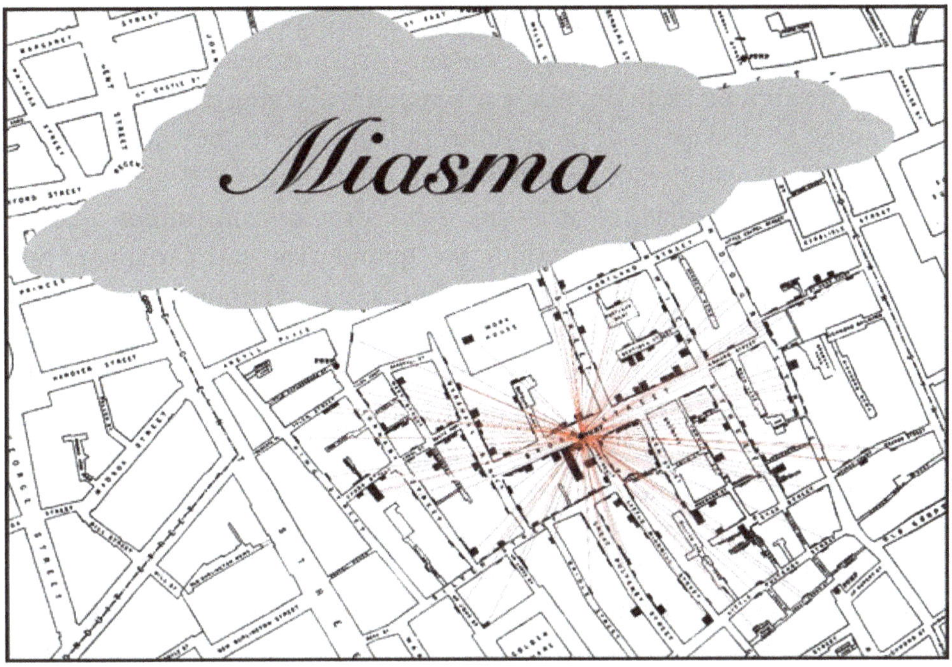

Figure 8.1 Map of 1854 London cholera epidemic by John Snow, with overlaid illustration contrasting miasma and contagion models drawn by James Young.

word for ritual pollution (*míασμα*). In the nineteenth century, germ theory began to replace miasma paradigms with an emergent dichotomy (which, as historians of medicine remind us, held many swerves and nuances that came to be glossed over in the simplified version of this history that got widely taken up into policy).[7] Dominant models today still describe two basic ways to think about diseases: they are either 'communicable' or 'non-communicable'. In this binary schema, infectious diseases need to be addressed in terms of interrupting contagion between people, vectors and environments via targeting specific exposures to disease-specific germs or biological pathogens. Meanwhile, since non-communicable diseases are by definition non-transmissible, they are commonly analysed in biomedicine as a risk assumed to be linked to an individual's own inborn genetic constitution[8] or framed as resulting from personal choices and 'lifestyle' behaviours.[9]

In historical genealogies, the infectious/non-communicable dualism is a relatively recent invention. Even physicians and researchers who dedicate their lives to studying intersections between such dualistic categories can end up positioned by the disciplinary traditions of distinct academic journals and departmental specialities. I wondered what binary models of causation can tend to foreclose, seeing the disjuncture between diabetic injuries and how they often get cast in common public health models. Communicability is not just a matter of seeing and interpreting the causes of disease, as many anthropologists note, but also a factor shaping the plausibility and workability of treatment.[10]

The larger project, which this essay draws from, offers a series of grounded scenes to think about the quandaries that caregivers and families are increasingly facing around such overlooked aspects of diabetes complications. It explores the working idea of *para-communicable conditions* to reflect on the implications of our models of communicability and causality raised by diabetes' patterned injuries. Seen through practices that make another model of problem and response visible, the work that people are facing on the ground shows the material effects of infectious/non-communicable dualisms: how data gets lost when it's assumed in advance that we know what a condition's markers look like, and how those distortions impact real access to the available infrastructures of care.

Viewed in this way, each end-of-the-line injury, such as a diabetes-linked amputation, could be read as another of what Marcel Mauss called a 'total social fact' – at once political, legal, economic, institutional, ecological, alimental, spiritual and social.[11] A total social fact demands a total social response. But only 2 per cent of all global health funding currently goes to all chronic conditions combined – leaving people around the world to negotiate the serious gaps between how these problems' causalities and urgencies get cast in the paperwork of public health models, versus how they are now manifesting in bodies.

I was initially surprised that rumours of contagious diabetes seemed to spread, rather than subside, as time wore on and as people in Belize became more familiar with the illness and observed it more closely in their own communities. Public health authorities often cite education about causality as one of the most important tools to curb diabetes. But in this case, it was not that people had never received diabetes education; it was that the one-size-fits-all biomedical education did not always square with the realities they saw over time. Diabetes moved like an epidemic. It killed like an epidemic. In Belize's southern Stann Creek District, diabetes affected 10 or 20 times more people than HIV/AIDS, and everyone knew that AIDS was an epidemic. Diabetes was spreading quickly in local communities, and a 'non-transmissible' disease is not supposed to spread, let alone spread faster than its contagious comorbidities. So what was happening in the space between local patterns and the biomedical explanations for 'non-communicable' conditions? Many people had learned and considered the classic biomedical account of diabetes as non-transmissible – but at times this account did not align with their lived observations and evident bodily realities.

As historian Allan Brandt notes, 'the problem of causation is critically important because it reflects directly on the fundamental moral issue of responsibility for disease'.[12] This point hit home more concretely for me when I gave a public presentation on an early version of this project's findings one morning to a small crowd in Dangriga. The audience came mostly from local branches of the Belize Diabetes Association and a local organisation providing supportive care for ageing. I began our conversation that day with a cursory slide showing the World Health Organization map of diabetes deaths (see Figure 8.2). I had assumed that was the part everyone would already know, but the global map seemed to be the only image I showed that surprised anybody. People raised eyebrows at each other. *Wait, versions of this are happening across the world?* Some people reflected later that they had become so used to stories attributing the local rise in diabetes to their local 'cultural foods' or their personal responsibility alone, that it shook up their perspectives just to take a step back and think of diabetes *as* an epidemic – a much bigger story, whatever that might mean.

There is a lot on the line in 'explaining epidemics', as historian Charles Rosenberg once put it.[13] Didier Fassin and others have examined the way global funding and resources tend to move according to the moral rationales of humanitarian 'crisis'.[14] This kind of intervention 'has come to define itself through exception', Peter Redfield aptly observes, though that framing quickly 'loses its transcendent magic' when 'diseases prove chronic'.[15] One woman in Belize described to me how a team of US medical students visiting her village had been fascinated by her ankle wound when they believed she had leishmaniasis (a tropical disease caused by sandfly-borne protozoa parasites), but stopped visiting when it turned out to be a diabetic ulcer. As Priscilla Wald notes in *Contagious*, senses of urgency are deeply contoured by 'how both scientists and the lay public understand the nature and consequences of infection, how they imagine the threat, and why they react so fearfully to some disease outbreaks and not others at least as dangerous and pressing'.[16]

A cursory glance into the archives yields more than 50 years of ignored calls for a response to diabetes in the world. 'Diabetes is no longer a rare syndrome in the tropics, and in many parts is being diagnosed with increasing frequency,' Dr Silas Dodu wrote in the *British Medical Journal* in 1967. Returning home to Ghana after medical school in London, Dodu linked the phenomenon he observed to the spread of 'white man's food'.[17] Several years later, the Pan American

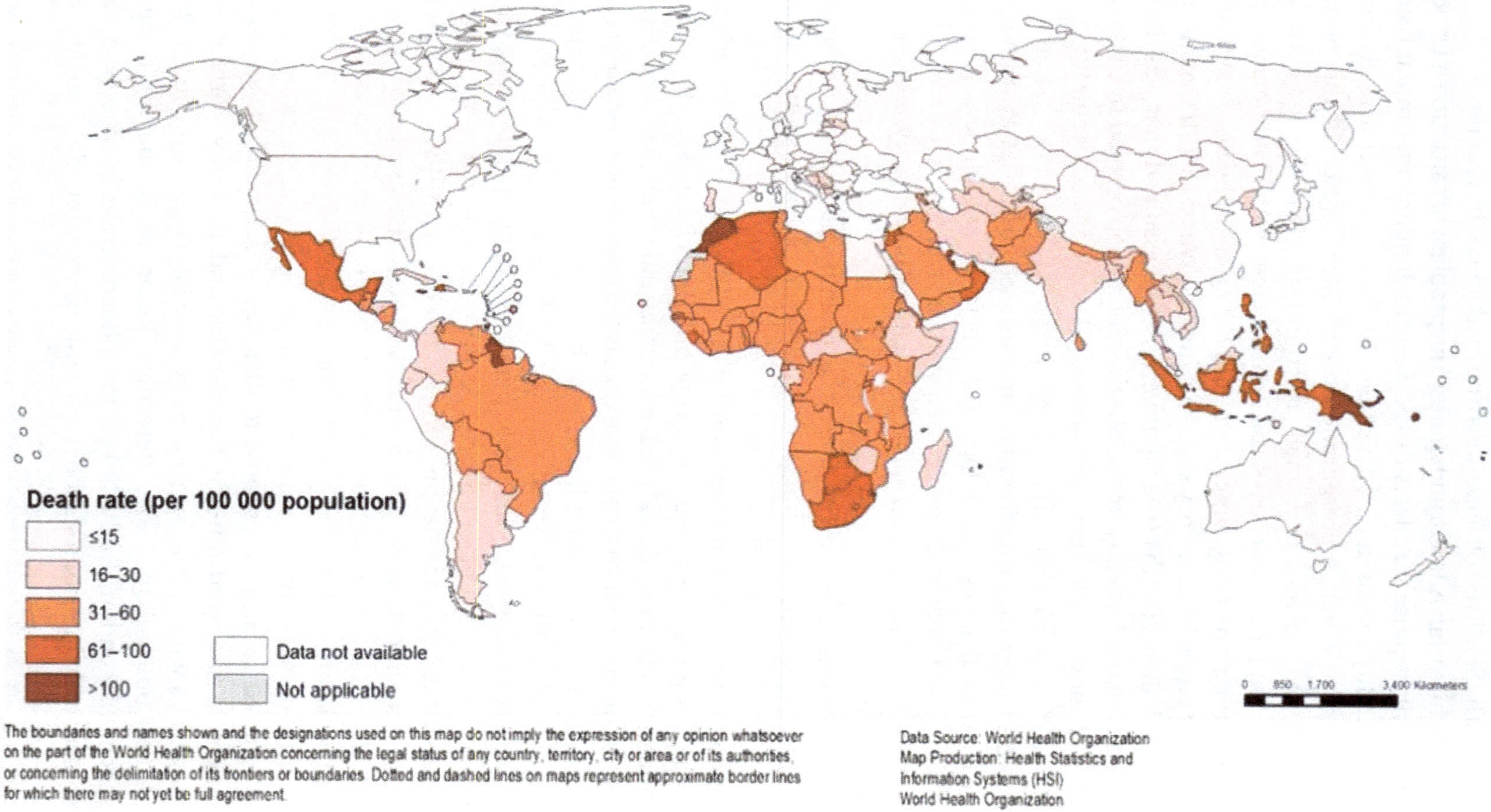

Figure 8.2 'Diabetes Mortality: Age-Standardized Death Rate per 100 000 Population, 2012'. © 2014 World Health Organization.

Health Organization (PAHO) sounded a similar alarm on the other side of the Atlantic. 'Right now the seriousness of the problem is reflected by the large number of diabetics who suffer, die, or become invalids,' reads their 1975 diabetes report, 'fatalities considered largely preventable because effective treatments for these diseases were known'.[18] Their astute and progressive policy recommendations are disturbing to revisit today, because they detail precise knowledge and actionable suggestions for policies to prevent diabetes injuries from spreading further – published before HIV/AIDS ever became legible as an epidemic, and before any of the people I met struggling to live with diabetes across Ghana and Belize had ever been born.

The perceived non-urgency of diabetes also intersects with debates about its contributing causalities.[19] Some molecular pathologists today, for example, see their work within a 'new toxicology paradigm of endocrine and metabolic disruption' that reframes diabetes as a 'hidden cost' to polluted landscapes.[20] Such links were first grasped largely through industrial accidents: for example, diabetes rates in a small town in Italy spiked in the 20 years after its chemical plant exploded.[21] Altered atmospheres also get absorbed: a recent long-term study of 1.7 million US veterans estimated about 14 per cent of diabetes cases could be associated with air pollution alone, regardless of what foods individuals ate.[22]

Reading such studies, I kept thinking about the many places I saw saturated with chemicals and plastics. It takes decades for food containers to photo-degrade into the tiny slivers visible in the ocean, for example. Little pieces get eaten by fish, moving up the food chain and seeping into water, often leaching BPA (an industrial chemical used to make certain plastics) which is also associated with diabetes risk.[23] Another study of 3,080 farmworkers in rural India found that exposure to organophosphate chemicals contributed to diabetes, apparently because the insecticides designed to kill crop pests also interacted with the living microbes crucial to metabolic balance inside people's digestive tracts.[24] This is only one of several mechanisms by which endocrine-disrupting chemicals can contribute to diabetes, a disease of the endocrine system.[25] The metabolic absorptions that connect human bodies and larger environs include a range of biological mechanisms that register daily exposures, what Arline Geronimus and colleagues call bodily 'weathering'.[26] This term refers to stress-related epigenetic traumas linked to social inequity. Other scholars further emphasise that any human's eating also includes the microbes in their bodies and the health of the plants and animals they eat.[27]

Amidst these complex interactions, diseases are not binary either-or conditions, as so many scholars have noted. They emerge from uneven landscapes of exposure with many kinds of transmissions. People I met often narrated these suspicions in great detail, though without having a way to offer the kind of systematic data scientists would recognise. 'They don't talk about it, but I think our diabetes is also caused by all the chemicals,' one woman in Belize told me. Publications supporting her general suspicion about such associations indeed existed in the literature.[28] But proof was not possible to demonstrate causality for *her* case of diabetes in particular, which is of course the point about not being able to tell where sugar begins or ends. The haze of what anthropologist Vanessa Agard-Jones calls 'accreted violence' from agricultural pesticides and the afterlives of plantation practices of depletion[29] remains a legacy throughout much of the world. In this context of limited foods and abundant chemicals, one woman's name for her glucose meter, 'sugar machine', struck me as an apt frame for the way this region – if not much of the agroindustrial world system – is fast becoming a 'diabetes machine'.

What is communicable?

The popularisation of germ theory often gets celebrated in public health memory today as linked to John Snow's team identifying and interrupting patterns of water-borne cholera in London. Or at least, that is the version of epidemiological history that often gets recounted on the first day of a public health policy class. The Broad Street Pump is today the namesake for the John Snow Society's annual 'Pumphandle Lectures' in public medicine. Tiny pictures of the red pump are featured on neckties and curated in museum exhibits. They remain potent icons, although historians like Nancy Krieger and Michael Worboys describe a story infinitely more complicated than the mythological version of this paradigm shift that came to be memorialised. (A complex debate about whether a 'bacteriological revolution' in fact occurred in the history of biology and medicine at all runs parallel to these changes in public health practice, full of many more grey areas and disagreements than would later be recalled.[30]) During slow shifts in nineteenth-century medical knowledge – as today – there was a huge gap between the nuance about causal debates in scientific research labs, versus the narratives driving public health policy.

Even *within* the parable of Snow and the pumphandle, in fact, there is a flipside to public health's founding story that could be read as an equally suggestive symbolic scene: the moment that germ theory became the *only* dominant way disease-causing exposures were taken seriously, this was used by companies as a shield to avoid responsibility for industrial harms. As early as 1855, John Snow was called in a legal case about de-regulating industrial pollution from factories. He testified that chemicals could 'not cause disease; those poisons do not reproduce themselves in the constitution'.[31] When prodded further about reported symptoms of toxic exposure amongst workers, Snow responded: 'Persons are often very much influenced by the imagination.'

To approach escalating chronic disease patterns, we need ways to recognise and publicise potential exposures of processed diets, industrial toxins, and cumulative wears on the body caused by systemic inequalities and stressors, as well as biological germs – an epidemiology of what Adia Benton has called 'connectors', rather than vectors alone.[32] This nexus requires attention, as anthropologists have emphasised, on 'the bioecologies at play' between porous boundaries and reactive membranes, human and environmental health and the historical forces and social systems of disregard that shape them both.[33]

For this task, either-or labelling of 'contagious' versus 'non-communicable' disease is insufficient to describe the prevalence of human-made diseases now becoming so visible around the world.[34] Diabetes is not an exception to, but *iconic* of, growing chronic epidemics – such as cancer clusters,[35] or the soaring prevalence of asthma and other autoimmune conditions.[36] Audre Lorde's observations more than 40 years ago continue to resonate: it remains be all too easy for health institutions and doctors to overlook 'the spread of radiation, racism, woman-slaughter, the chemical invasion of our food, pollution of our environment' as aspects of chronic exposure.[37]

Talking to public health practitioners and policy makers about diabetes, I found it helpful to have a different name for this in-between territory of exposures, and came to describe it as *para-communicable* – chronic conditions that may be materially transmitted as bodies and ecologies intimately shape each other over time, with unequal and compounding effects for historically situated groups of people. It is offered in recognition of the work those living with chronic conditions are already doing constantly, in exploring 'a space of thirdness' beyond public health's bifurcated categories, where space between can offer 'triangulation, possibility, and potentiality, an intermediate area'.[38] This interstitial term also attempts to span the gaps between different kinds of knowledge making – such as academic conferences where keywords to describe the 'biosocial' dimensions of exposure have become extremely plentiful[39] – and the arenas of clinical practice and triage where they were often illegible or simply fell out of the frame.

Chronic exposures to stressful climates and the chemical contamination of food, air and water only compound more commonly recognised issues related to limited access to healthy foods. And of course, industrialised food products can also cause harmfully high blood sugar levels through their depleted nutritional content. The divides of 'food apartheid' unfold with vast historical inequalities, including internally within countries considered affluent.[40] Compounding these divides, through recent international trade policy changes, it is more difficult for healthy foods to circulate across national borders.[41] In different ways, such global food geographies frequently reflect larger forces of racialised blame and disregard, leaving individuals to navigate constraints on their own. 'How am I going to make a diet? There is only one kind of food here,' I often heard patients tell the visiting Cuban physician, who would laugh kindly but never really had an answer. In neighbouring Guatemala, Emily Yates-Doerr observed that nutrition experts intentionally avoided describing problems of macro-infrastructure that neither they nor their patients could change, when that advice could have registered as cold or uncaring.[42] Caregivers tried to avoid depressing conversations, in hopes of generating a healthy sense of optimistic possibility – focusing on the scale within their grasp. This usually meant trying to equip patients to negotiate existing foodways. But who will rework larger food *systems*?

These questions only multiply in the face of changing climates: rising levels of carbon dioxide in the atmosphere can leave crops with less protein and nutrient content, as grain plants adapt to try to survive in changed atmospheres.[43] Fossil fuels at the point of extraction can also drive more people to rely on cheap store-bought foods, as in the case Abosede Babatunde documents surrounding oil spills in Nigeria.[44] The packaged sustenance that people often turn to, trying to escape toxins, is familiar across global markets – sodas like Coca-Cola are only the most iconic[45] of many processed foods containing sugar, white flour and white rice that today are cheaply available worldwide.

In contrast, every local diet that has been dismantled by these industrial diets is unique – meaning that any advice about eating requires hard work and local texture in order to be meaningful for people.[46] One morning, I joined a group in Dangriga that gathered to share cooking ideas to modify Belizean and Garifuna dishes for those with diabetes. They wondered if local labs could be capacitated to investigate nutritional content of certain dishes, or to monitor their fish and water for traces of toxic chemicals.

Some described a fog-like feeling to living with a sense of ambient risk. Yet at the same time, cloudiness can be strategically used by industries to confuse accountability.[47] Such corporate strategies require clarity from social scientists also grappling with uncertainty. For instance, key theorists of 'syndemic' models – describing how multiple epidemics interact – recently expressed concern that the term can take on a miasma-like cloudy quality if it is taken up imprecisely, or without follow-up steps to trace specific pathways and signatures of responsibility.[48] Anthropologists like Elizabeth Hoover and Liz Roberts follow the work of collectives seeking ways to build a counter-science, through sustained collaborations and a grassroots-guided 'science of the in-between'.[49]

I initially thought it would be fairly easy to apply for a grant to support the kind of local projects that people in Belize suggested. But it turns out that certain prominent diabetes grants explicitly decline to fund research that generates locally relevant dietary and care translations; they reason that such outcomes would not be globally 'generalisable'. Yet diabetes prevention relies on locally specific texture in order to gain traction and uptake. If only approaches imagined as 'generalisable' receive policy funding, then most well-resourced interventions end up framing what is happening with individuals as the problem.

Not only did the infectious/non-communicable dualism often appear ill suited to capture a full picture of diabetes causation, but there seemed to be a looping effect of these attributions – certain diseases' 'geography of blame' can in turn shape institutional funding and access to medical technologies that already exist.[50] I came to see *para-communicability* as the partially connected set of ways in which aetiology, treatment, morbidity and mortality are imagined and enacted.

Different material histories and policy interventions (or their absence) may actually produce biologically different versions of diabetes, on the population level as well as for individual bodies. Diseases overlap. Epidemics intersect. What an epidemic *is* becomes different – not just in scale, but potentially in its transmissibility. The two first cases of drug-resistant bacteria documented in the United States both occurred in diabetic ulcers – apparently from separate instances of horizontal gene transfer, by which bacteria can nearly instantaneously swap genes with other living or dead bacteria.[51] One study culturing 150 diabetic ulcers found that '91 per cent of the bacteria were resistant to three or more antibiotics', with high percentages of widely feared bacteria like vancomycin-resistant *Enterococcus* and methicillin-resistant *Staphylococcus aureus* (MRSA).[52] In cases where people live for months or years walking in sandals with open diabetic wounds on their feet, it is also possible that horizontal gene transfer occurred directly between the bacteria infecting lower limb ulcers and the bacteria living in local soils.

This tendency for unchecked diabetes injuries to foster drug-resistant bacteria may have implications for future antibiotic efficacy and diseases of all kinds. Yet if drug-resistant bacteria sound like an urgent global issue in a way the foot ulcers fostering them do not, then that is another example of why the diabetes epidemic will continue to grow.

Notes

1 This acute awareness I encountered among Ghanaian physicians in Tamale at that time often stood in contrast to the uneven 'vertical' streams of international funding that they were navigating. Such national experts' concern has shaped an important literature on diabetes issues in Ghana, particularly over the past decade, where recent studies have revealed diabetes to be more prevalent among the poorest tiers of patients in a number of contexts, and a growing public health issue almost everywhere. See de-Graft Aikins, Agyei-Mensah, and Agyemang (eds.), *Chronic Non-Communicable Diseases in Ghana*; Danquah et al., 'Diabetes Mellitus Type 2 in Urban Ghana'; Bukhman et al., 'Endemic Diabetes'; Mbanya et al., 'Diabetes in Sub-Saharan Africa'.

2 World Bank, 'Republic of Ghana'.

3 I am extremely grateful to all of those who took time to speak with me and who contributed to mentoring this research over the years. These ethnographic descriptions spanning Ghana and Belize are offered here in the spirit of mutual care and critical inquiry, with respect for policymakers' dedication and difficult work. I gratefully acknowledge the support of the Wenner-Gren Foundation, the West African Research Association, Princeton Center for Health & Wellbeing, a Mellon-ACLS Writing Fellowship, the Princeton Health and Development Grand Challenges Initiatives, a writing fellowship at the Rachel Carson Center for Environment and Society, and support from the MIT School of Humanities, Arts, and Social Sciences. This research was approved by the Belize Ministry of Health, the Belize Institute for Social and Cultural Research, Ghana Health Services Ethical Review Committee and the Princeton University Institutional Review Board. Warm thanks to my wonderful colleagues in the MIT History, Anthropology, and STS programme for their support, and for the insights shared on an early version of this paper by Megan Vaughan and participants of the UCL workshop on the Epidemiological Imagination. Deep thanks to Kafui Adjaye-Gbewonyo and Marissa Mika for sustaining our collective conversation.

4 See Pfeiffer and Chapman, 'Anthropological Perspectives'; and Crane, *Scrambling for Africa*.

5 Gough et al., 'Survey of Diabetes, Hypertension and Chronic Disease Risk Factors'.

6 *Sugar* is also a common name for diabetes on both sides of the Atlantic and around the world; see de-Graft Aikins, *Sugar Disease, Bitter Medicine*; Moran-Thomas, *Traveling with Sugar*.

7 For a much more complex version of this history of competing paradigms, see Krieger, *Epidemiology and the People's Health*, 100.

8 Paradies, Montoya, and Fullerton, 'Racialized Genetics and the Study of Complex Diseases'; Montoya, *Making the Mexican Diabetic*.

9 See important critiques, for example, in Hatch, *Blood Sugar*.

10 See, for example, Briggs, 'Towards Communicative Justice in Health'.

11 Mauss, *The Gift*, 76–8.

12 Brandt, 'Behavior, Disease, and Health in the Twentieth Century United States', 56.

13 Rosenberg, *Explaining Epidemics*.

14 Fassin, *Humanitarian Reason*.

15 Redfield, *Life in Crisis*, 72.

16 Wald, *Contagious*, 3.

17 Dodu, 'Diabetes in the Tropics'; Ghana Medical Association, 'A Tribute to Professor Silas R. A. Dodu'.

18 Litvak, 'Diabetes Mellitus'.

19 Hamdy, 'When the State and Your Kidneys Fail'; Murphy, 'Alterlife and Decolonial Chemical Relations'; Nading, 'Local Biologies, Leaky Things, and the Chemical Infrastructure of Global Health'; Shapiro, 'Attuning to the Chemosphere'.
20 Neel and Sargis, 'The Paradox of Progress'.
21 Bertazzi et al., 'Health Effects of Dioxin Exposure'.
22 Bowe et al., 'The 2016 Global and National Burden of Diabetes Mellitus'.
23 Vogel, 'The Politics of Plastics'.
24 Velmurugan et al., 'Gut Microbial Degradation'.
25 Colborn, Dumanoski, and Myers, *Our Stolen Future*.
26 Geronimus et al., '"Weathering" and Age Patterns of Allostatic Load Scores'.
27 Landecker, 'Post-Industrial Metabolism'; Solomon, *Metabolic Living;* Lamoreaux, 'What if the Environment is a Person?'.
28 Mesnage et al., 'Multiomics Reveal Non-Alcoholic Fatty Liver Disease in Rats'.
29 Agard-Jones, 'Chlordécone'.
30 Historians of science recount a much more nuanced and complicated version of this paradigm shift; see Worboys, 'Was There a Bacteriological Revolution'.
31 Lilienfeld, 'John Snow'.
32 For a key ethnography of the implications of such focus on infectious conditions alone, see Benton, *HIV Exceptionalism*. See also framing works such as Reynolds Whyte, 'The Publics of the New Public Health'; Biehl and Petryna, *When People Come First*.
33 See Fischer, 'The Peopling of Technologies'; Niewöhner and Lock, *Situating Local Biologies*; Todd, 'Fish, Kin and Hope'; Whitmarsh, 'Troubling Environments'.
34 This essay aims to give primacy to the ethnographic realities that its observations first grew out of – namely, the lived effects of this infectious/NCD dualism within global health funding flows as observed in 2008–10. The working third term of 'para-communicable' disease began as an exploratory name for those disjunctures at that time; see Moran-Thomas, 'The Paradox of Non-Communicable Epidemic'. It has been exciting to see some resonant thinking, in the years since then, independently arise elsewhere, exploring different names for similar questions; see especially Seeberg and Meinert, 'Can Epidemics Be Noncommunicable?'.
35 Jain, *Malignant*.
36 Fortun and Fortun, 'Scientific Imaginaries and Ethical Plateaus'; Kenner, *Breathtaking*; Vaughan, 'Conceptualising Metabolic Disorder in Southern Africa'.
37 Lorde, *The Cancer Journals*, 77.
38 Eng and Han, *Racial Melancholia, Racial Dissociation*.
39 This often-repeated observation resonates, of course, with the huge existing literature on biosocial dimensions of health and disease causality in anthropology and allied social sciences; see, for instance, Daniel, Moore, and Kestens, 'Framing the Biosocial Pathways'; and Gravlee, 'How Race Becomes Biology', 57.
40 For more on the long tradition of struggles for food justice within the US context, see, for example, Reese, *Black Food Geographies*.
41 Gálvez, *Eating NAFTA*.
42 Yates-Doerr, *The Weight of Obesity*.
43 Plumer, 'How More Carbon Dioxide Can Make Food Less Nutritious'; see also Zhu et al., 'Carbon Dioxide (CO2) Levels this Century'.
44 Babatunde, 'The Curse of Oil'.
45 Elmore, *Citizen Coke*.
46 For more on the history of this issue in Belize, see Palacio, 'Food and Social Relations in a Garifuna Village'; Palacio, *The Garifuna*; and Wilk, *Home Cooking in the Global Village*.
47 Langston, *Toxic*; Nash, *Inescapable Ecologies*; Nestle, 'Coca-Cola Says its Drinks Don't Cause Obesity'.
48 Mendenhall and Singer, 'The Global Syndemic of Obesity'.
49 Roberts, 'What Gets Inside'; Hoover, *The River Is in Us*.
50 Farmer, *Infections and Inequalities*.
51 Quammen, *The Tangled Tree*.
52 Jain and Barman, 'Bacteriological Profile of Diabetic Foot Ulcer'.

Bibliography

Agard-Jones, Vanessa. 'Chlordécone'. Manufacturing of Rights: Beirut, 14 May 2015, last modified 26 May 2015, https://www.youtube.com/watch?v=yvqVkR4Iuqs.

Babatunde, Abosede. 'The Curse of Oil: Unpacking the Challenges of Food Security in Nigeria's Delta'. New York: Social Science Research Council Grant, 2017.

Benton, Adia. *HIV Exceptionalism: Development through Disease in Sierra Leone*. Minneapolis, MN: University of Minnesota Press, 2015.

Bertazzi, Pier et al. 'Health Effects of Dioxin Exposure: A 20-Year Mortality Study', *American Journal of Epidemiology*, 153 (11) (2001): 1031–44.

Biehl, João. *The Will to Live: AIDS Therapies and the Politics of Survival*. Princeton, NJ: Princeton University Press, 2007.

Biehl, João and Adriana Petryna. *When People Come First: Critical Studies in Global Health*. Princeton, NJ: Princeton University Press, 2013.

Bowe, Benjamin et al. 'The 2016 Global and National Burden of Diabetes Mellitus Attributable to PM2-5 Air Pollution', *Lancet Planetary Health*, 2 (7) (2018): e301–12.

Brandt, Allan M. 'Behavior, Disease, and Health in the Twentieth Century United States: The Moral Valance of Individual Risk'. In *Morality and Health*, edited by Allan Brandt and Paul Rozin, 53–78. New York: Routledge, 1997.

Briggs, Charles L. 'Towards Communicative Justice in Health', *Medical Anthropology: Cross-Cultural Studies in Health and Illness*, 36 (4) (2017): 287–304.

Briggs, Charles L. and Clara Mantini-Briggs. *Tell Me Why My Children Died*. Durham, NC: Duke University Press, 2016.

Bukhman, G. et al. 'Endemic Diabetes in the World's Poorest People', *Lancet Diabetes and Endocrinology*, 3 (6) (2015): 402–3.

Colborn, Theo, Dianne Dumanoski, and John Peterson Myers. *Our Stolen Future*. New York: Plume, 1997.

Crane, Johanna T. *Scrambling for Africa: AIDS, Expertise, and the Rise of American Global Health Science*. Ithaca, NY: Cornell University Press, 2013.

Daniel, Mark, Spencer Moore, and Yan Kestens. 'Framing the Biosocial Pathways Underlying Associations Between Place and Cardiometabolic Disease', *Health and Place*, 14 (2) (2008): 117–32.

Danquah, I. G. et al. 'Diabetes Mellitus Type 2 in Urban Ghana: Characteristics and Associated Factors', *BMC Public Health*, 12 (2012): 210.

de-Graft Aikins, Ama. *Sugar Disease, Bitter Medicine: Living with Diabetes in Ghana*. Cambridge: International African Institute, forthcoming.

de-Graft Aikins, Ama, Samuel Agyei-Mensah, and Charles Agyemang (eds.). *Chronic Non-Communicable Diseases in Ghana: Multidisciplinary Perspectives*. Accra: University of Ghana, 2014.

Dodu, Silas. 'Diabetes in the Tropics', *British Medical Journal*, 2 (5554) (1967): 747–50.

Elmore, Bartow. *Citizen Coke: The Making of Coca-Cola Capitalism*. New York: W.W. Norton, 2016.

Eng, David and Shinhee Han. *Racial Melancholia, Racial Dissociation*. Durham, NC: Duke University Press, 2019.

Farmer, Paul. *Infections and Inequalities*. Berkeley, CA: University of California Press, 1999.

Fassin, Didier. *Humanitarian Reason*. Berkeley, CA: University of California Press, 2011.

Fischer, Michael. 'The Peopling of Technologies'. In *When People Come First*, edited by João Biehl and Adriana Petryna, 347–74. Princeton, NJ: Princeton University Press, 2013.

Fortun, Kim and Mike Fortun. 'Scientific Imaginaries and Ethical Plateaus in Contemporary U.S. Toxicology', *American Anthropologist*, 107 (1) (2005): 43–54.

Gálvez, Alyshia. *Eating NAFTA: Trade, Food Policies, and the Destruction of Mexico*. Oakland, CA: University of California Press, 2018.

Geary, James. *I Is an Other*. New York: Harper, 2011.

Geronimus, Arline T. et al. '"Weathering" and Age Patterns of Allostatic Load Scores among Blacks and Whites in the United States', *American Journal of Public Health*, 96 (5) (2006): 826–33.

Ghana Medical Association. 'A Tribute to Professor Silas R.A. Dodu', *Ghana Medical Journal*, 41 (3) (2007): 151–3.
Gough, Ethan et al. 'Survey of Diabetes, Hypertension and Chronic Disease Risk Factors'. Belize City: Pan American Health Organization and Belize Ministry of Health, 2008.
Gravlee, Clarence. 'How Race Becomes Biology: Embodiment of Social Inequality', *American Journal of Physical Anthropology*, 139 (1) (2009): 47–57.
Haagsma, J. A. et al. 'The Global Burden of Injury: Incidence, Mortality, Disability-Adjusted Life Years and Time Trends from the Global Burden of Disease Study, 2013', *Injury Prevention*, 22 (1) (2016): 3–18.
Hamdy, Sherine. 'When the State and Your Kidneys Fail: Political Ecologies in an Egyptian Dialysis Ward', *American Ethnologist*, 35 (4) (2008): 553–69.
Hatch, Anthony Ryan. *Blood Sugar: Racial Pharmacology and Food Justice in Black America*. Minneapolis, MN: University of Minnesota Press, 2016.
Hoover, Elizabeth. *The River Is in Us: Fighting Toxics in a Mohawk Community*. Minneapolis, MN: University of Minnesota Press, 2017.
International Diabetes Federation. 'Diabetes Atlas', last modified 2019, http://www.diabetesatlas.org/.
Jain, Lochlann. *Malignant: How Cancer Becomes Us*. Berkeley, CA: University of California Press, 2013.
Jain, Sudhir K. and Rashmisnata Barman. 'Bacteriological Profile of Diabetic Foot Ulcer with Special Reference to Drug-Resistant Strains in a Tertiary Care Center in North-East India', *Indian Journal of Endocrinology and Metabolism*, 21 (5) (2017): 688–94.
Kaiser, Kristine. 'Preliminary Study of Pesticide Drift into the Maya Mountain Protected Areas of Belize'. *Bulletin of Environmental Contamination and Toxicology*, 86 (1) (2011): 56–9.
Kenner, Ali. *Breathtaking: Asthma Care in a Time of Climate Change*. Minneapolis, MN: University of Minnesota Press, 2018.
Kistenberg, Rob. 'Amputation Prevention Strategies in Developing Nations: A Study of Belize'. MPH thesis, Houston, University of Texas, 2005.
Krieger, Nancy. *Epidemiology and the People's Health*. Oxford: Oxford University Press, 2013.
Lamoreaux, Janelle. 'What if the Environment is a Person? Lineages of Epigenetic Science in a Toxic China', *Cultural Anthropology*, 31 (2) (2016): 188–214.
Landecker, Hannah. 'Post-Industrial Metabolism: Fat Knowledge', *Public Culture*, 25 (3) (2013): 495–522.
Langston, Nancy. *Toxic Bodies*. New Haven, CT: Yale University Press, 2011.
Lilienfeld, D. E. 'John Snow: The First Hired Gun?', *American Journal of Epidemiology*, 152 (1) (2000): 4–9.
Litvak, Jorge. 'Diabetes Mellitus: A Challenge for the Countries of the Region', *PAHO Bulletin*, 9 (4) (1975): 317–24.
Livingston, Julie. *Improvising Medicine*. Durham, NC: Duke University Press, 2012.
Lorde, Audre. *The Cancer Journals*. San Francisco, CA: Aunt Lute Books, 1980.
Mauss, Marcel. *The Gift*. London: Cohen and West, 1966.
Mbanya, J. C. et al. 'Diabetes in Sub-Saharan Africa', *Lancet*, 375 (9733) (2010): 2254–66.
Mendenhall, Emily and Merrill Singer. 'The Global Syndemic of Obesity, Undernutrition, and Climate Change', *Lancet*, 393 (10173) (2019): 741.
Mesnage, Robin et al. 'Multiomics Reveal Non-Alcoholic Fatty Liver Disease in Rats following Chronic Exposure to an Ultra-Low Dose of Roundup herbicide', *Scientific Reports*, 7 (39328) (2017): doi:10.1038/srep39328.
Montoya, Michael. *Making the Mexican Diabetic*. Berkeley, CA: University of California Press, 2010.
Moran-Thomas, Amy. 'The Paradox of Non-Communicable Epidemic', *West African Research Association*, Spring (2010): 8.
Moran-Thomas, Amy. 'Metabola: Chronic Life in Belize'. PhD dissertation, Princeton University, 2012.
Moran-Thomas, Amy. *Traveling with Sugar: Chronicles of a Global Epidemic*. Berkeley, CA: University of California Press, 2019. Open access at https://dspace.mit.edu/handle/1721.1/125712.
Murphy, Michelle. 'Alterlife and Decolonial Chemical Relations', *Cultural Anthropology*, 32 (4) (2017): 494–503.

Nading, Alex. 'Local Biologies, Leaky Things, and the Chemical Infrastructure of Global Health', *Medical Anthropology*, 36 (2) (2016): 141–56.

Nash, Linda. *Inescapable Ecologies*. Berkeley, CA: University of California Press, 2007.

Neel, Brian A. and Robert M. Sargis. 'The Paradox of Progress: Environmental Disruption of Metabolism and the Diabetes Epidemic', *Diabetes*, 60 (7) (2011): 1838–48.

Neil, M. J. E. 'Pain After Amputation', *British Journal of Anaesthesia Education*, 16 (3) (2015): 107–12.

Nelson, Alondra. *The Social Life of DNA*. Boston, MA: Beacon Press, 2016.

Nestle, Marion. 'Coca-Cola Says its Drinks Don't Cause Obesity. Science Says Otherwise', *Guardian*, 11 August 2015.

Niewöhner, Jorg and Margaret Lock. *Situating Local Biologies: Anthropological Perspectives on Environment/Human Entanglement*. New York: Springer, 2018.

Palacio, Joseph. 'Food and Social Relations in a Garifuna Village.' PhD dissertation, University of California, Berkeley, 1982.

Palacio, Joseph. *The Garifuna: A Nation across Borders – Essays in Social Anthropology*. Benque Viejo del Carmen, Belize: Cubola Books, 2005.

Paradies, Y.C., J. M. Montoya, and S. M. Fullerton. 'Racialized Genetics and the Study of Complex Diseases: The Thrifty Genotype Revisited', *Perspectives in Biology and Medicine*, 50 (2) (2007): 203–27.

Pecoraro, Roger, Gayle Reiber, and Ernest Burgess. 'Pathways to Diabetic Limb Amputation: Basis for Prevention', *Diabetes Care*, 13 (5) (1990): 513–21.

Pfeiffer, James and Rachel Chapman. 'Anthropological Perspectives on Structural Adjustment and Public Health', *Annual Review of Anthropology*, 39 (2010): 149–65.

Plumer, Brad. 'How More Carbon Dioxide Can Make Food Less Nutritious', *New York Times*, 23 May 2018.

Quammen, David. *The Tangled Tree: A Radical New History of Life*. New York: Simon & Schuster, 2018.

Ralph, Laurence. 'What Wounds Enable: The Politics of Disability and Violence in Chicago', *Disability Studies Quarterly*, 32 (3) (2012): http://dx.doi.org/10.18061/dsq.v32i3.3270.

Redfield, Peter. *Life in Crisis*. Berkeley, CA: University of California Press, 2013.

Reese, Ashanté. *Black Food Geographies: Race, Self-Reliance, and Food Access in Washington, D.C.* Chapel Hill, NC: University of North Carolina Press, 2019.

Reynolds Whyte, Susan. 'The Publics of the New Public Health: Life Conditions and "Lifestyle Diseases" in Uganda'. In *Making and Unmaking Public Health in Africa*, edited by Ruth Prince and Rebecca Marsland, 187–207. Athens, OH: Ohio University Press, 2014.

Roberts, Elizabeth. 'What Gets Inside: Violent Entanglements and Toxic Boundaries in Mexico City', *Cultural Anthropology*, 32 (4) (2017): 592–619.

Rosenberg, Charles. *Explaining Epidemics and Other Studies in the History of Medicine*. Cambridge: Cambridge University Press, 1992.

Seeberg, Jens and Lotte Meinert. 'Can Epidemics Be Noncommunicable?', *Medicine Anthropology Theory*, 2 (2015): 54–71.

Shapiro, Nicholas. 'Attuning to the Chemosphere', *Cultural Anthropology*, 30 (3) (2015): 368–93.

Solomon, Harris. *Metabolic Living: Food, Fat, and the Absorption of Illness into India*. Durham, NC: Duke University Press, 2016.

Sontag, Susan. *Illness as Metaphor and Aids and Its Metaphors*. New York: Picador, 1988.

Sweeny, Robert. 'Para-Sights: Multiplied Perspectives on Surveillance Research in Art Educational Spaces', *Surveillance & Society*, 3 (2/3) (2005): 240–50.

Todd, Zoe. 'Fish, Kin and Hope: Tending to Water Violations in *amiskwaciwâskahikan* and Treaty Six Territory', *Afterall*, 43 (2017): 102–7.

Vaughan, Megan. 'Conceptualising Metabolic Disorder in Southern Africa: Biology, History and Global Health', *BioSocieties* (2018): 1–20.

Velmurugan, G. et al. 'Gut Microbial Degradation of Organophosphate Insecticides Induces Glucose Intolerance via Gluconeogenesis', *Genome Biology*, 18 (1) (2017): 8.

Vogel, Sarah. 'The Politics of Plastics: The Making and Unmaking of Bisphenol A "Safety"', *American Journal of Public Health*, 99 (S3) (2009): S559–66.

Wald, Priscilla. *Contagious*. Durham, NC: Duke University Press, 2008.

Whitmarsh, Ian. '"Troubling Environments": Postgenomics, Bajan Wheezing, and Lévi-Strauss', *Medical Anthropology Quarterly*, 27 (4) (2013): 489–509.
Wilk, Richard. *Home Cooking in the Global Village*. Oxford: Berg, 2005.
Worboys, Michael. 'Was There a Bacteriological Revolution in Late Nineteenth- Century Medicine?', *Studies in History and Philosophy of Science*, 38 (1) (1007): 20–42.
World Bank, 'Republic of Ghana: Tackling Poverty in Northern Ghana.' PREM 4 / AFTAR, Report No. 53991-GH (2011).
Yates-Doerr, Emily. *The Weight of Obesity: Hunger and Global Health in Postwar Guatemala*. Berkeley, CA: University of California Press, 2015.
Zhu, Chunwu et al. 'Carbon Dioxide (CO2) Levels this Century Will Alter the Protein, Micronutrients, and Vitamin Content of Rice Grains with Potential Health Consequences for the Poorest Rice-Dependent Countries', *Science Advances*, 4 (5) (2018): 1012.

9

Epidemiological Transition Theories, Health and Illness: First 1000 Day Approach

Michelle Pentecost

Introduction

In March 2013, the South African Department of Health released its *Roadmap to Nutrition in South Africa 2013–2017*. Central to its strategy to improve nutrition was a focus on a window of opportunity: the first 1000 days. Shaped by new knowledge in the field of the Developmental Origins of Health and Disease (DOHaD), the 1000 days between conception and a child's second birthday has been presented in contemporary epidemiology as a critical period that will determine future health and potential. 'The first 1000 days of life' has transformed from a neat catchphrase into an important part of primary care policy in South Africa, such that today 'first 1000 days interventions' are a standard part of epidemiological and policy terminology to refer to a host of public health interests in early life.

In this chapter, I use the lens of the 'first 1000 days' to consider the application of epidemiological transition theories to knowledge of health and illness in African contexts, using a case study from South Africa. I take the 'first 1000 days' concept as one point within a long history of scientific and policy approaches to nutrition and health in South Africa. This allows for three discussions that elucidate changing understandings and applications of transition theories in South Africa. First, I consider the historical context of theories of nutrition, health and disease. I trace the emergence of a concern about what today are labelled 'non-communicable' diseases or NCDs in South Africa and the 'nutrition transition' theories that underpin this. Second, I consider what the first 1000 days framework, now well established in public health and policy language in South Africa, can tell us about how notions of transition have shifted. Specifically I am interested in how established epidemiological approaches to the temporal relationship between exposure and outcome are disrupted, the effect this has on the long-standing dichotomy of communicable and non-communicable disease and what kinds of new evidence and new interventions emerge as a result. Third, I discuss how 'the first 1000 days' project is expanding in South Africa to include a strong focus on early childhood development and consider the concomitant shifts underway in how 'transition' is understood and how this makes visible new potential burdens of disease in Africa, especially related to mental health. I conclude with some considerations of the political and conceptual work that 'transition' performs, such that it persists as a defining foundational concept for understanding patterns of health and disease, even as explanatory frameworks change.

As an entry point to these discussions, I will start with an ethnographic portrait of Ndileka, a young woman who I first met while conducting fieldwork in Cape Town in 2014. My ethnographic research, spanning 2013–15, focused on the rollout of the South African *Roadmap to Nutrition in South Africa 2013–2017*. In particular I was concerned to understand what it means to focus nutrition interventions in the 'first 1000 days of life' and, during this fieldwork period, I surveyed 60 women who attended ante-natal clinics in Khayelitsha, a large sub-district of the Cape Metropole that includes both formal housing and informal settlements. I spent 15 months conducting participant observation with 15 of these women and their families. Ndileka gave birth to her second child shortly after our first meeting. The experiences of Ndileka and her infant allow me to introduce in more detail the South African context in which the 'first 1000 days' policy has been rolled out.

'The children of this century are not eating that'

> It is late 2014 and a dry and dusty day in Khayelitsha, Cape Town, South Africa. I am here to visit Ndileka, who has recently given birth to her second daughter. It is a slow morning of tidying her small home – a zinc dwelling in the backyard of her landlord. She is breastfeeding the baby and we are catching up while I play with her first born, two-year-old Aviwe. Ndileka needs bread and milk, and invites me to walk to the spaza (kiosk) with her. We peer through

> the metal grate at the small window for exchanging goods and cash. A half loaf of bread costs five rand and fifty cents; a full loaf ten rand. Amagwinya (fried buns) cost two rand each. Ndileka deliberates out loud – if she buys amagwinya she doesn't have to add anything to it: it can be eaten plain. She decides on the half-loaf of bread instead – a 'healthier' option. Apart from bread and milk, Ndileka doesn't buy anything else at this spaza. She says that most things are more expensive than they are at the supermarket. 'A two litre Coke is seventeen rand here', she says, 'and only fifteen rand at the supermarket. At home it is the same.' For Ndileka, 'home' is a remote rural village close to Mount Frere in the Eastern Cape Province. She describes her village as a 'real' rural area, because the tar road starts a very long way from the homestead. I ask her a bit more about what is available in the village and where people buy food. She explains that there are spaza shops in the village that sell bread and milk, 'but no sugar, no fish oil, no important things'. For other items, they must buy them at the supermarket in the closest town. I ask if there are any crops in the village. She says that 2012 was good for potatoes and cabbages, but there haven't been any vegetables in the last year. There is no electricity in the village, although there is always talk about when it might arrive. There is no lack of wood, because the village is in a forest. 'Certain things work better on the fire, like samp and beans, or baked bread,' Ndileka tells me. Ndileka misses the ground maize meal and pumpkin she would eat as a child. 'The children of this century are not eating that – they only eat noodles and pasta.' Once at home, Ndileka sets about making black chicory coffee and uses the half-loaf to make four apricot jam sandwiches. She gives one sandwich to Aviwe. She will eat the remaining three for lunch.
>
> Field note excerpt, November 2014

Ndileka's nostalgia for ground maize, her frequent comparisons with what was available in the homestead versus the township and her concern about the ubiquitous instant noodles that have become a staple of urban diets[1] exemplified the experiences of the young women that I came to know in Khayelitsha. Nearly all had a strong connection to another home in the Eastern Cape Province. A number of women spoke, as Ndileka did, about the food that they only consumed when in the village, how 'back home' meat was reserved for important occasions, unlike in the township where shisa nyama (grilled meat) is sold on every corner. Many could recall when large supermarkets had arrived in the towns of the Eastern Cape, making life there more and more like life in the city.

Ndileka's story encapsulates the concerns that this chapter will address. Her migrations back and forth between an Eastern Cape village and the Cape Town Metropole are the migrations of hundreds of thousands of people, part of a mass urbanisation that has taken place in South Africa since the advent of democracy. Her reflections on changing patterns of consumption point to the supermarketisation, intensified food marketing practices, increased foreign direct investment in food production and distribution, and incorporation into global markets that now characterise the South African food system.[2] The sugar and flour that made up her lunch that day – three jam sandwiches – are the staples for many low-income urban residents, for whom there is frequently low dietary diversity and tenuous food security.[3]

While Ndileka and others like her would be categorised as food insecure, she was also categorised during her ante-natal visits as 'overweight' according to Body Mass Index criteria. Her household exemplifies the dual burden of adult obesity and child undernutrition that has been called the 'nutrition transition paradox'.[4] The notion that nutrition interventions in early life can mitigate against the persistence of this cycle of under- and overnutrition is the basis of the first 1000 days campaign.

The first 1000 days in South Africa: a brief history

Since it was first proposed in a 2008 *Lancet* 'Series on Maternal and Child Undernutrition',[5] the first 1000 days concept has become a rallying point for international efforts against malnutrition and the first 1000 days slogan has been taken up across different platforms that include the World Health Organization (WHO), the United Nations' (UN) Scaling Up Nutrition programme (SUN) and its country members, as well as 80 non-governmental (NGO), donor and private sector partners.

The 2008 *Lancet* series highlighted the persistent burden of under-nutrition in 36 countries and recommended the integrated delivery of nutrition interventions with maternal and child health packages.[6] The series presented review data from five cohort studies in India, Guatemala, the Philippines, Brazil and South Africa (the COHORTS Consortium), which suggested that height for age at two years (roughly 1000 days after conception) could best predict future human capital – defined by adult height, educational achievement, income and offspring's birth weight.[7] In the same year, the UN Secretary-General established the High-Level Task Force on Food and Nutrition Security and the 2008 Copenhagen Consensus concluded that nutrition was one of the most cost-effective investments for development.[8] These events and recommendations later formed the basis for the SUN programme and the '1000 Days: Change a Life, Change the Future' campaign. Using the new evidence base for action, and in line with the World Bank's shift to reposition nutrition as central to development,[9] SUN aimed to scale up nutrition interventions and re-centre nutrition as a key concern for all sectors.[10] 'Change a Life, Change the Future' was launched on 21 September 2010 by the then United States Secretary of State Hillary Clinton and Irish minister Micheal Martin at the UN General Assembly, where a group of countries pledged to invest in nutrition and in the first 1000 days.[11]

The *Lancet*'s 2013 follow up series 'Maternal and Child Nutrition' recommended that interventions in the first 1000 days would also mitigate against potential future burdens of overnutrition and non-communicable disease (NCDs) – a term introduced by the World Health Organization in the early 2000s to include chronic respiratory conditions, cancer, diabetes and cardiovascular disease.[12] The 2013 *Lancet* series highlighted that interventions in early life may also mitigate against this disease burden.[13]

In South Africa, the focus of the first 1000 days has been taken up explicitly within nutrition policy since 2013. While South Africa is not a formal member country of the SUN network, the *Roadmap to Nutrition in South Africa 2013–2017* was rolled out in partnership with the WHO, UNICEF and the Global Alliance in Nutrition (GAIN) and is based on the SUN framework.[14] The Roadmap states:

> There is now a need to focus on priority target groups and interventions that can have the biggest impact, namely in the life-cycle stages before and during pregnancy and in the first two years of life. Optimal nutrition during this period lays the foundation for a long and healthy life and reduces the risk of developing diet-related chronic diseases. The first 1000 days is therefore internationally recognized as the 'window of opportunity' for direct nutrition interventions.[15]

In the Western Cape Province, where I have conducted fieldwork since 2013, the nutrition policy and the first 1000 days approach forms part of the province's *Healthcare 2030: The Road to Wellness* policy mandate.[16]

The first 1000 days focus translates into the majority of the policy's recommended interventions targeting infants, children and pregnant and lactating women. The package of interventions that Ndileka and her child received includes: a therapeutic feeding scheme for the treatment of moderate to severe child undernutrition, a micronutrient and deworming programme and six behaviour change interventions, including the promotion of exclusive breastfeeding, education on complementary feeding, and dietary education for weight management during pregnancy and lactation. The package also includes a therapeutic intervention for malnutrition in pregnancy based on mid-upper-arm circumference (MUAC) measurement. An important outcome of this policy document is the integration of nutrition interventions into maternal and child health services, including the Basic Antenatal Care (BANC) and Prevention of Mother to Child Transmission of HIV infection (PMTCT) programmes. In practice, this translates into the inclusion of MUAC and body mass index (BMI) measurements at the first ante-natal visit. If a woman's MUAC and BMI measurements indicate undernutrition according to protocol criteria then she is referred to a therapeutic nutrition programme; if she is 'normal' weight or overweight, as was the case with Ndileka, she receives nutrition and lifestyle modification counselling.

Current integrative approaches to nutrition intervention in South Africa stand in contrast to preceding nutrition policy that focused on 'disease-specific nutrition support', nutrition education and advocacy and the (controversial) role of nutrition in the management of HIV and AIDS.[17] This is one shift in a long history of changing conceptions of nutrition and best practice in South Africa. I turn now to this history and the notions of transition that have characterised it.

Theories of population and nutrition transition in South Africa

In the South African context the concept of transition has particular salience, as a framework for understanding political processes as well as changes in demography and population health. The history of nutrition interventions in South Africa is distinctly shaped by histories of colonialism and apartheid. Dutch (1652–1800) and then British (1800–1910) colonialism established public health legislation and biomedical hospital care in South Africa, with missionaries playing a significant role in the delivery of healthcare.[18] 1910 to 1948 saw progressive advocacy for a unified national health service based on a primary healthcare (PHC) model and South Africa is thus often credited as the birthplace of social medicine.[19] The PHC approach has one of its origins in the Pholela Health Centre, established in rural Natal (now KwaZulu-Natal) in 1940 by Sidney and Emily Kark. The comprehensive Pholela model integrated curative and preventive care, provided health education and health promotion and placed health in a family, community and social determinants framework that was profoundly progressive for the time.[20] The Pholela model was influential in the 1942 National Health Services Commission, which resulted in the 1944 Gluckman Report. The report recommended a national health system not dissimilar to the system that would develop in the United Kingdom. However, the planned innovative healthcare and nutrition policies were decisively abandoned after the institution of apartheid policies in 1948.[21]

In his historical account of scientific racism in modern South Africa, Saul Dubow describes the close relationship between the formalisation of apartheid and the shifting notions of heredity and race in the post-war era.[22] While Afrikaner nationalist sentiment in the 1930s drew on Nazi ideologies of racial purity and white racial supremacy, such ideas were no longer acceptable in the post-war period, nor did they account for the heterogeneity of white society in South Africa and the phenomenon of 'poor whites'.[23] The development thesis that characterised international post-war modernisation theories was used to justify apartheid ideology, with apartheid's architects arguing that racial segregation acknowledged 'different stages of development' and allowed people to develop to their own potential.[24] The Population Registration Act of 1950 decreed that each citizen's race would be recorded as either 'white', 'coloured' or 'native'; this was later modified to divide the population into four groups: 'African', 'Indian', 'Coloured' and 'White'.[25] As James Scott describes it, the apartheid project was premised on an 'authoritarian high modernism' that justified 'separate development' policies based on racial classification.[26] While decolonisation projects unfolded elsewhere in Africa in the 1950s, in the South African context the rhetoric of decolonisation was used to rationalise the creation of independent 'homelands' by the apartheid government, which devolved state responsibility for the welfare of homeland residents. Opposition forces to apartheid rejected the term 'homeland', which obscured the exclusionary nature of these divisions, using the word 'Bantustan' to signal the arbitrariness of drawing geographical borders around supposed tribal lines.[27] This historical preface is important for delineating the central importance of the concept of 'transition' to the apartheid project, justifying systematic segregation and discrimination on the basis that different groups, classified according to a state-determined programme of racial characteristics, were at different stages of their transition to civilisation.

Until the late 1950s, the apartheid state's approach to health and nutrition rested on state paternalism and what Diana Wylie refers to as the trope of 'African cultural ignorance'.[28] She traces the halting of state-sponsored health and nutrition services in the homelands in 1959, while South African nutrition science simultaneously presented an alternative image to the international community, contributed to international research on kwashiorkor (severe protein malnutrition) and instituted milk distribution programmes in the 1960s in line with UNICEF recommendations. These schemes and the recording of kwashiorkor statistics were abandoned in 1968. In the 1970s, the state adopted the language of PHC but, as eminent South African paediatrician Hoosen Coovadia noted, this was merely an appropriation of the terms with no meaningful outcomes.[29] A fragmented, grass-roots movement delivered selective primary healthcare in South Africa in the 1980s.[30] While scientists cast the problem of malnutrition in Southern Africa as a multi-sectoral concern, mothers nevertheless emerged as central figures in prevention strategies. A review published in 1990 in the *South African Journal of Family Practice* is emphatic: 'Go for the mother – she is the most important health care worker!'[31] This focus was also evident in training textbooks for health care workers in the early 1990s. For example, the *Manual of Community Nursing and Communicable Diseases: A Textbook for South African Students* includes the statement that 'unenlightened mothers do not comprehend the need for prevention'.[32] The textbook advocates a primary healthcare approach with a strong focus on the health education of the mother, for example in 'housecrafts and the cooking of nutritious meals for the family'.[33]

While undernutrition has long been a target of concern, before the transition to democracy obesity in black Africans attracted little interest, partly because of a theory that Africans developed 'healthy or benign obesity',[34] a concept that lingered in the literature until at least the early 2000s[35] despite extensive work that refutes it.[36] While the 'benign obesity' hypothesis gained little currency in the mid-1990s, there was significant interest in the 'ethnic' differences in the manifestation of obesity and metabolic disease. Research comparing the anthropometry and metabolic responses of different racial groups (using South African census categories) suggested differences in parameters such as insulin resistance,[37] hormone levels[38] and visceral fat,[39] among others.[40] South African biomedicine and nutrition science in the early years of democracy thus appears to have perpetuated conflations of race and genetics, citing 'ethnic variability' as a common explanation for differences in racial health outcomes.[41]

The genetic explanation for rising obesity rates in South Africa has, however, been much less prominent than epidemiological explanations that have cited urbanisation and concomitant dietary and lifestyle change as key drivers of obesity in the urban population.[42] Differences in the health outcomes of racial groups in South Africa in the apartheid period were described as a reflection of separate epidemiological transitions, with whites experiencing a 'First World' pattern, and Blacks a 'Third World' transition that was expected to shift to a 'First World' picture as urbanisation unfolded.[43] Since the advent of democracy, theories of nutrition transition[44] have dominated epidemiological framings of obesity, diabetes and cardiovascular disease in South Africa.[45] Social epidemiologists stress that it is the systematised, structural racism of apartheid that is to blame for the huge variation in health outcomes in South Africa, but also argue that the country displays a 'bipolar' epidemiological transition, modulated by the effects of urbanisation, with an increased incidence of chronic disease and a persistence of infectious diseases, all compounded by the HIV/AIDS epidemic.[46]

There is particular interest in the differences between rural and urban settings in how the epidemiological transition is unfolding. As argued in a recent publication on a rural South African cohort in Agincourt, 'there is on-going need to quantify and characterise [epidemiological transition] and its implications in different sub-populations. This will reveal the history of the burden of disease affecting different ethnic and social groups and help identify and prioritise the interventions with potential for the greatest effect now and in the near future.'[47] The Agincourt study shows how the HIV epidemic is 'reversing' the transition and highlighting gender disparities in health transition and describes this cohort as an exemplar of the national picture of a 'protracted, complex health transition'.[48] It would seem that, since the advent of democracy, the framework of a 'complex health transition' has thus been one way for epidemiologists to capture the heterogeneous and varied population health outcomes of South Africa.

South Africa's national nutrition profile also exemplifies the 'protracted-polarised' model of epidemiological transition,[49] characterised by a dual burden of obesity and undernutrition at the national, community and even household level.[50] The first nationally representative nutrition study on children below six years of age, conducted in 1994, showed that one in four South African children was stunted and that micronutrient deficiencies were prevalent.[51] Obesity rates in black South Africans were first noted as a matter of concern in a 1998 national survey, in which 25.4 per cent of African men and 58.5 per cent of African women were overweight or obese.[52] Women in particular had significantly higher BMIs and rates of abdominal obesity compared to other demographic groups and in contrast to previous studies.[53] Subsequent surveys in 2003, 2009 and 2013 showed an upward trend and a persistently increased risk of obesity in African women compared to other groups.[54] These rates occur in conjunction with high levels of food insecurity, reported by just over half of households surveyed in the 2013 National Survey.

A wealth of research has focused on the challenges of making healthy dietary and lifestyle choices in urban environments,[55] and of the confounding relationships between diet, physical activity and obesity in South Africa. For some urban cohorts, research reports a weak association between dietary intake and BMI,[56] or between BMI and physical activity.[57] Where traditional models of energy balance have been found inadequate to explain the surge in obesity and 'chronic diseases of lifestyle' in South Africa, theories of foetal programming and the Developmental Origins of Health and Disease (DOHaD) have proved a neat fit and have been met with much enthusiasm.[58]

DOHaD and transition theory

Developmental Origins of Health and Disease (DOHaD) research provides a convincing explanation for the nutrition transition paradox, conceptualised as intergenerational metabolic disease. David Barker and Clive Osmond's 1986 article documenting the association between childhood nutrition and adult ischaemic heart disease in England and Wales[59] is often credited as a turning point in chronic disease epidemiology and the basis of the developmental programming hypothesis. In 1992, Hales and Barker introduced the 'thrifty phenotype hypothesis' to explain similar associations between poor nutrition in early life with later susceptibility to type 2 diabetes, noting that 'rapid transition from subsistence to good or overnutrition' seemed to be an important reason for this outcome.[60] The theory that the thrifty phenotype hypothesis is most relevant to 'transitioning societies' was consolidated in a special issue of the *British Medical Bulletin* in 2001, which noted that populations undergoing a transition from undernutrition to adequate nutrition experience a combination of undernutrition in early life and overnutrition in adulthood,[61] and that this observation is particularly important to 'non-industrialised countries' undergoing 'rapid economic development and modernisation'.[62]

Association studies across different regions supported the hypothesis and, following a number of World Congresses, the field of the Developmental Origins of Health and Disease had formalised, with its own society, membership and journal: the *Journal of Developmental Origins of Health and Disease*. DOHaD correlates adverse conditions in early life with an increased propensity for disease in adulthood, places these phenomena within the context of developmental plasticity and, linking with expanding knowledge on epigenetics, understands adult morbidity as the outcome of programming effects during critical developmental periods.[63] In the case of nutrition, undernutrition in early life invokes a predisposition to store energy. In the nutrition transition model, the food-scarce environment of childhood in a developing setting transitions to an industrialised environment of cheap, calorific foods in adulthood. DOHaD scientists describe this as environmental mismatch.[64] DOHaD has thus offered one explanation for a long-standing conundrum for nutritional scientists stymied by rising obesity rates in regions of relative food insecurity.[65] The rapidly expanding DOHaD research base has thus laid the foundation for a renewed interest in understandings of transition and in the early life period as a time of critical intervention. In the South African context, a better understanding of the developmental origins of under- and overnutrition is framed as a way in which the nutrition transition might be 'steered in a more positive direction'.[66]

Birth cohort studies provide a useful epidemiological model for testing out DOHaD hypotheses. For example, the Consortium of Health-Orientated Research in Transitioning Societies (COHORTS) has been a key site of knowledge production in this area. The consortium comprises five birth cohorts including the 1982 Pelotas (Brazil) Birth Cohort Study, the Institute of Nutrition of Central America and Panama Nutrition Trial Cohort (Guatemala), the New Delhi Birth Cohort (India), the Cebu Longitudinal Health and Nutrition Survey cohort (Philippines) and the Birth-to-Twenty Plus (South Africa) cohort.[67] Since its inception in 1990, Birth-to-Twenty has provided a range of data on child and adolescent health in South Africa.[68] Most importantly for the story of the first 1000 days, this cohort has provided the first longitudinal picture of child health in the country and the COHORTS Consortium provided the data on which the *Lancet* nutrition series of recommendations is based. As the consortium's title suggests, an important commonality across the five sites is that they are thought to be undergoing demographic, epidemiological and nutrition transitions. For DOHaD research then, it is clear that 'transition' is a central concept.

Importantly, however, DOHaD models of disease causation depart from prevailing models in their conceptualisation of risk, exposure, environment and communicability. First, DOHaD research has effected a fundamental change in how chronic disease epidemiology conceives of exposures and outcomes. Life-course epidemiology as a discipline has expanded and formalised with DOHaD knowledge as an important stimulus.[69] Unlike traditional epidemiological models for chronic disease, life-course models 'explicitly require the temporal ordering of exposures and their inter-relationships',[70] which occur across the life course and across generations.[71] These new configurations of exposure and outcome alter the ways in which science and policy conceive of and articulate risk.

Second, in these frameworks the binary gene/environment framework that characterised approaches to disease aetiology in the late twentieth century is superseded by great variation in how epidemiologists now conceptualise the environment.[72] In many cases the mother/infant dyad or the consumption of food becomes a proxy for 'environment' so that experiments or interventions can be effectively designed and executed.[73]

Finally, and most importantly for transition theories, DOHaD theory converges interventions for communicable and non-communicable diseases on one early life window. For epidemiological transition theory, this category of 'chronic' or 'degenerative' diseases has traditionally characterised the last stage of transition, the Age of Receding Pandemics.[74] 'Transitioning societies' that have dual burdens of undernutrition and infectious disease, and overnutrition and chronic disease, confound this model. Non-communicable diseases in this framework become entities that are communicable by virtue of the potential for transgenerational transmission of disease risk. DOHaD theory thus has important implications for notions of 'communicable' and 'non-communicable' disease.[75] As Seeberg and Meinert have argued, the framework of non-communicable disease overlooks the 'biosocial communicability of disease'.[76] While DOHaD mechanisms may offer an important opportunity in this sense for building nuanced understandings of the social and political contexts of the intergenerational transmission of disease risk,[77] the persistent attachment to 'transition', as a commonality across regions labelled as 'developing', or 'of the global south', elides this opportunity for more sophisticated understandings of situated biologies.

The COHORTS consortium is illustrative. The cohorts commenced at different times: Guatemala's cohort is the oldest, followed by New

Delhi, Brazil, Philippines and finally South Africa's, which started in 1990, four years before apartheid's official end. A 'transitioning society' in the COHORTS and DOHaD framework has defining characteristics that include: low-middle-income status; high rates of maternal and/or child undernutrition, and 'undergoing rapid demographic, nutritional and epidemiological transitions'.[78] Despite the huge inter-country variation for experiences of the latter, the term 'transition' denotes a commonality between the Brazilian, Guatemalan, Philippine, Indian and South African sites. This term acts as a common placeholder for history, culture and social change: the factors that shape local or situated biologies. Needless to say, these locations have all experienced important socio-political changes during the lives of these cohorts. The cohorts have very different histories, starting at different points in time and with very different socio-political landscapes and trajectories. Under the umbrella term of 'transitioning societies', however, the coordinates for how biology is situated in each of these sites recede from view and the means by which scientific knowledge is rendering comparable across sites is foregrounded.

At a regional scale, there is a similar problem with nutrition transition models that focus singularly on rural to urban flows of people and discount the significant circulation of peoples between rural and urban sites. Like Ndileka, urban dwellers who have migrated from rural homesteads often move cyclically and seasonally between the cities and the countryside. At an individual level, as Ndileka's case also illustrates, the cycles of food deficit and food abundance on which DOHaD logic is premised are also punctuated by seasonality, rural–urban circulations and the extent to which one can draw on networks of social capital in leaner times. All of this presents problems for how DOHaD science continues to *define boundaries* in ways that social theorists have long refuted.[79]

The DOHaD focus on transitioning societies might simply be a function of DOHaD's perceived explanatory power for describing disease burdens in these regions. Yet what I have elsewhere called 'DOHaD geographies' demonstrate remarkable continuities with past logics of intervention in those parts of the world marked as 'third-world', 'low-middle-income', 'developing' or 'Southern'.[80] Campaigns like the first 1000 days contribute to 'boundary-making' in defining the who, what and how of intervention, focusing on women and children in 'developing' contexts. In the same way that humanitarian imagery designed to elicit empathy and compassion is so often racialised,[81] so too does DOHaD imagery re-enact a particular imagination of the other in need. In sum, DOHaD justifies a continued epidemiological appetite for transition theories, reproduces geographies of past interventions and reimagines a long-standing focus on the mother/child dyad to target critical periods in early life.

Moving towards mental health in Africa: articulating new transitions

At the same time as DOHaD research and interventions in Africa and elsewhere figure 'transitioning societies' as a key target for nutrition interventions, DOHaD research and the discourse of transition also offers mechanisms and frameworks by which other disease burdens are made visible and opens up new avenues for intervention, particularly related to early childhood development and mental health. As a recent global health policy white paper on child mental health argues, achievements in reducing infant mortality and increasing child survival have allowed for a shift in focus for the global child health field, to focus on hitherto understudied priorities, such as mental health.[82] The authors cite 'simultaneous epidemiologic and social transitions' as the impetus for broadening the scope of global health intervention in early life. With progress in infant mortality and infectious disease rates in Africa, there is a new motivation to focus on mental health, particularly in the global mental health movement, whose proponents argue that global health programmes have overlooked mental health in low- and middle-income countries.[83] The early life period is a focus here again as a key window for intervention, with the first 1000 days cited as an important opportunity for improving infant mental health in Africa.[84] Since 2016, the Western Cape first 1000 days campaign focuses on love and stimulation in addition to nutrition. Ndileka, her second child then two years old, would receive advice about reading, playing music and singing, developing gross and fine motor coordination, playing with toys and colours and giving the child love and attention. The first 1000 days campaign in South Africa thus exemplifies a seeming convergence of interventions for non-communicable disease, cognitive and emotional development and mental health, focusing as it does on 'growing', 'loving' and 'playing'.[85]

As global mental health practitioners call for an expanded approach to child development that encompasses child mental health as a response to 'simultaneous epidemiological and social transitions',[86] it is important to note the other transitions taking place, particularly in the framing of childhood. The 'quantified child' already circulates in South

African public discourse[87] as a panacea for the country's social ills, a notion that resonates with older concerns about the implications of childhood conditions for future adult health and economic productivity in transition theories.[88] The shift to focus on metrics exemplifies what Wahlberg and Rose have described as a key shift in descriptions of the world's health, from mapping disease burdens to mapping disease patterns. They consider the expansion of population assessments beyond mortality and morbidity rates to include measures of life quality (such as years of potential life lost [YPLL] and quality-adjusted life years [QALY]), as part of an 'on-going governmentalisation of living'.[89] Importantly, these new metrics make visible new patterns and burdens of disease with impacts on life's quality, such as neuropsychiatric and mental health conditions.

Discussion

The notion of a 'transitioning society' is central to DOHaD theory. Demographic, epidemiological and nutrition transition theories have been a standard part of the epidemiological lexicon for explaining changing patterns of fertility, morbidity and mortality since the mid-twentieth century. Social scientists have long questioned whether these models are indeed as robust as they are perceived to be for explaining changing patterns of health and disease across different historical and social contexts.[90] Others have cautioned that transition models reify a teleological logic of linear progress that flattens out complexity,[91] or indeed furthers an imperial narrative of 'modern' versus 'traditional' societies that still require periods of transition and development.[92] For global health, transition narratives of nutrition and non-communicable disease resurface old developmental and modernising logics,[93] and in African contexts these map onto well-worn racialised theories of the dangers of urbanisation for rural Africans.[94] Despite these substantive critiques and the problems posed to transition models by local histories of HIV/AIDS,[95] the transformation of HIV from an infectious to a chronic illness with the rollout of antiretrovirals,[96] the concurrent burdens of infectious and non-communicable disease and the new syndemics that blur these categories,[97] transition theories persist as a powerful explanatory framework on the African continent and in 'developing' contexts more broadly.

The notion that societies are transitioning persists as a defining foundational concept for understanding patterns of health and disease, even as explanatory frameworks for these patterns change. The tenacity of transition theories speaks to their enduring usefulness as a means of understanding large-scale demographic and population changes. Yet social scientists' attention to the heterogeneity of experiences of these broader changes and the over-reliance on modernisation theories in understanding them[98] is a continual reminder that models are not neutral. As Stanley Ulijaszek has argued for understanding obesity, models are often useful, but they are always conditional.[99] Transition theories are useful for their broad explanatory power, in this case as an explicit background to DOHaD frameworks of health and disease and the specific distributions of over- and undernutrition that these models predict in 'transitioning' contexts. DOHaD theory does offer a powerful explanation for South Africa's nutritional profile and, in the case of Ndileka, a useful framework for understanding her health outcomes and those of her children.

At the same time a cautious approach in extrapolating from one context to another is a necessary counterbalance to grand narratives that tend back towards transition narratives that centre on capitalism, development and modernisation.[100] For example, the powerful discourse of urbanisation as the driving force behind significant changes in the South African population's health profile is worth closer scrutiny, particularly in its conception of the urban and the city. As Ruth Toulson has argued:

> there is a fine line to be drawn between urban determinism – the suggestion that the city is *the* pivotal force in shaping individual lives, a perspective that ignores both human agencies and the complexities of causality – and anthropology that relegates the city to mere context, ethnographies that, almost by chance, take place in urban contexts but say little about the realities of city life.[101]

In addition, epidemiological research and social theory alike must also take into account that conflict, migration and instability are potentially more salient descriptors for the life experiences of a large number of the global population in the twenty-first century. Like Ndileka and her family, many people move between rural and urban homes based on access to employment, education or healthcare and on care and kinship obligations. These movements are themselves structured by a long history of segregation, gendered migrant labour and forced removals.[102] It is clear that labour migration has shaped patterns of disease in South Africa, through both the occupational exposures and tuberculosis so evident in mining communities since the 1880s, and the spread of HIV.[103] Transition theories need to take into account these forms of 'temporary' or 'circular' migration, including that people may often choose to return to a rural home when they are dying.[104] Other 'transitional contexts', such as refugee camps and forced displacements, will also require novel approaches and interventions.[105]

We cannot rely on a singular grand transition narrative to understand change in polities as diverse as South Africa, India, the Philippines, Brazil and Guatemala; nor is it useful to discard all models or comparisons. As Ulijaszek and colleagues have argued, for transition theories to remain useful they need to better account for the effects of imperialist expansion, colonialism, early and late globalisation and socio-economic inequality.[106] Their expanded model incorporates historical and political-economic factors and provides a better framework for understanding health outcomes in contexts such as South Africa, where on-going transitions – political, economic, nutritional and cycles between rural and urban – are linked by colonial history and apartheid legacy. To understand why Ndileka is overweight yet food insecure requires 'radical contextualisation',[107] spanning histories, lifetimes and critical periods. We must pay attention to both large-scale transitions and the smaller-scale transitions between generations and between individuals. As critics of efforts towards global mental health have similarly cautioned, 'blithe universalism' risks replicating imperial or colonial dynamics.[108] As the first 1000 days movement expands to encompass nutrition, health and now mental health, it will be important to remain mindful of tendencies towards oversimplifications that reinvigorate old tropes of 'Africa' and interventions in the lives of Africans.

Notes

1 Igumbor et al., 'Big Food'; Errington et al., 'Instant Noodles as an Antifriction Device'.
2 Greenberg, 'Corporate Power in the Agro-Food System'.
3 Shisana et al., *South African National Health and Nutrition Examination Survey*.
4 Doak et al., 'The Dual Burden Household'.
5 Bryce et al., 'Maternal and Child Undernutrition'.
6 Bryce et al., 'Maternal and Child Undernutrition'.
7 Victora et al., 'Maternal and Child Undernutrition: Consequences'.
8 Copenhagen Consensus Center, 'Copenhagen Consensus 2008'.
9 World Bank, 'Repositioning Nutrition As Central to Development'.
10 United Nations, 'Scaling Up Nutrition'.
11 Thurow, *The First 1000 Days*.
12 World Health Organization, '2008–2013 Action Plan'.
13 Black et al., 'Maternal and Child Undernutrition and Overweight'.

14 Department of Health: Republic of South Africa, *Roadmap for Nutrition*.
15 Department of Health: Republic of South Africa, *Roadmap for Nutrition*, 15.
16 Western Cape Government, 'Healthcare 2030'.
17 Labadarios et al., 'Review of the South African Nutrition Policy'; Cousins, 'HIV and the Remaking of Hunger and Nutrition'.
18 Coovadia et al., 'The Health and Health System of South Africa'.
19 Trostle, *Epidemiology and Culture*; Kautzky and Tollman, 'A Perspective on Primary Health Care in South Africa'.
20 Kautzky and Tollman, 'A Perspective on Primary Health Care in South Africa'.
21 Marks and Andersson, 'Industrialisation, Rural Health and the 1944 National Health Services Commission'.
22 Dubow, *Scientific Racism in Modern South Africa*.
23 Dubow, *Scientific Racism in Modern South Africa*, 166.
24 Dubow, *Scientific Racism in Modern South Africa*, 277.
25 Posel, 'Race as Common Sense'.
26 Scott, *Seeing like a State*, 89.
27 Beinart and Dubow (eds.), *Segregation and Apartheid*, 16.
28 Wylie, *Starving on a Full Stomach*.
29 Coovadia, 'What Is Progressive about PPHC?'.
30 Kuhn et al., 'Village Health Workers and GOBI-FFF'; den Besten et al., 'Changes in the Anthropometric Status of Rural African Under-Fives; Kautzky and Tollman, 'A Perspective on Primary Health Care in South Africa'.
31 Bac and Glatthaar, 'Protein-Energy Malnutrition Intervention Strategies'.
32 Vlok, *Manual of Community Nursing and Communicable Diseases*, 402.
33 Vlok, *Manual of Community Nursing and Communicable Diseases*, 35.
34 Walker et al., 'Low Frequency of Adverse Sequelae of Obesity'.
35 Walker, Adam, and Walker, 'World Pandemic in Obesity'.
36 Levitt et al., 'The Prevalence and Identification of Risk Factors for NIDDM'; Kruger, Venter, and Vorster, 'Obesity in African Women', 733.
37 Van der Merwe et al., 'Evidence for Insulin Resistance'.
38 Buthelezi et al., 'Ethnic Differences'.
39 Punyadeera et al., 'Weight-Related Differences'.
40 Kruger et al., 'Obesity in South Africa', 491; Van Der Merwe, Terésa, and Pepper, 'Obesity in South Africa', 315.
41 Van Der Merwe, Terésa, and Pepper, 'Obesity in South Africa', 319.
42 Kruger et al., 'Obesity in South Africa'.
43 Myer, Ehrlich, and Susser, 'Social Epidemiology in South Africa', 112.
44 Popkin, 'Nutritional Patterns and Transitions', 138.
45 Bourne et al., 'Nutritional Status of 3–6 Year-Old African Children'; Vorster et al., 'Contribution of Nutrition to the Health Transition'; Steyn et al., 'Anthropometric Profile'; Shisana et al., *South African National Health and Nutrition Examination Survey*.
46 Myer, 'Social Epidemiology in South Africa'.
47 Kabudula et al., 'Progression of the Epidemiological Transition'.
48 Kautzky and Tollman, 'A Perspective on Primary Health Care'.
49 Frenk et al., 'Health Transition in Middle-Income Countries'.
50 Popkin, Adair, and Ng, 'Global Nutrition Transition'.
51 South African Vitamin A Consultative Group (SAVACG), *Children Aged 6–71 Months in South Africa, 1994*.
52 Puoane et al., 'Obesity in South Africa'.
53 Steyn et al., 'Risk Factors for Coronary Heart Disease'.
54 Dept. of Health, 'South African Demographic and Health Survey', 2007; Ardington and Case, 'Health'; Shisana et al., *South African National Health and Nutrition Examination Survey*.
55 Puoane, Bradley, and Hughes, 'Obesity among Black South African Women'; Puoane and Tsolekile, 'Challenges Faced by the Urban Black South Africans'.
56 Bourne et al., 'Nutrient Intake', 238; Kruger et al., 'Physical Inactivity'.
57 Kruger, Venter, and Vorster, 'Obesity in African Women'; Malhotra et al., 'Determinants of Obesity'.
58 Reddy and Mbewu, 'The Implications of the Developmental Origins of Health and Disease'.
59 Barker and Osmond, 'Infant Mortality, Childhood Nutrition, and Ischaemic Heart Disease'.

60 Hales and Barker, 'Type 2 (Non-insulin-dependent) Diabetes Mellitus'.
61 Hales and Barker, 'The Thrifty Phenotype Hypothesis', 8.
62 Fall, 'Non-Industrialised Countries and Affluence'.
63 Godfrey, Gluckman, and Hanson, 'Developmental Origins of Metabolic Disease', 199.
64 Godfrey et al., 'Epigenetic Mechanisms'.
65 Himmelgreen, 'Using a Life Course Approach'.
66 Vorster, Kruger, and Margetts, 'The Nutrition Transition in Africa'.
67 Richter et al., 'Cohort Profile: The Consortium'.
68 Richter et al., 'Cohort Profile: Mandela's Children'.
69 Ben-Shlomo, Cooper, and Kuh, 'The Last Two Decades of Life Course Epidemiology'.
70 Kuh et al., 'Life Course Epidemiology'.
71 Ben-Shlomo, Yoav, and Kuh., 'A Life Course Approach to Chronic Disease Epidemiology'; Hochberg, et al., 'Child Health, Developmental Plasticity, and Epigenetic Programming'.
72 Whitmarsh, 'Troubling "Environments"'; Shostak and Moinester, 'The Missing Piece of the Puzzle?'.
73 Landecker, 'Food as Exposure'; Lock and Palsson, *Can Science Resolve the Nature / Nurture Debate?*.
74 Omran, 'The Epidemiologic Transition'.
75 Pentecost, 'The First Thousand Days: Epigenetics'.
76 Seeberg and Meinert, 'Can Epidemics Be Noncommunicable?'.
77 Lock, 'Comprehending the Body in the Era of the Epigenome'.
78 Richter et al., 'Cohort Profile: The Consortium'.
79 Mol and Law, 'Boundary Variations'.
80 Pentecost, 'The First Thousand Days: Epigenetics'.
81 Benton, 'Risky Business'.
82 Belkin et al., 'Converging on Child Mental Health'.
83 Patel and Prince, 'Global Mental Health'.
84 Tomlinson and Morgan, 'Infant Mental Health Research'.
85 Pentecost and Ross, 'The First Thousand Days: Motherhood'.
86 Belkin et al., 'Converging on Child Mental Health'.
87 Phala, 'Pitching a Super-Ministry for Child Governance'.
88 Mosley and Gray, 'Childhood Precursors'.
89 Wahlberg and Rose, 'The Governmentalization of Living', 62.
90 Frenk et al., 'Health Transition in Middle-Income Countries'; Chen, Kleinman, and Ware (eds.), *Health and Social Change*; Ginsburg and Rapp, 'The Politics of Reproduction'; Nichter and Kendall, 'Beyond Child Survival'; Ulijaszek, Elton, and Mann, *Evolving Human Nutrition*.
91 Carolina and Gustavo, 'Epidemiological Transition'; Johnson-Hanks, 'Demographic Transitions and Modernity'.
92 Brown and Bell, 'Imperial or Postcolonial Governance?'.
93 Yates-Doerr, *The Weight of Obesity*; Solomon, *Metabolic Living*; Pentecost, 'The First Thousand Days: Epigenetics'.
94 Vaughan,'Conceptualising Metabolic Disorder'.
95 Vaughan, 'Conceptualising Metabolic Disorder'.
96 Livingston, 'AIDS as Chronic Illness'.
97 Mendenhall and Norris, 'When HIV Is Ordinary and Diabetes New'.
98 Kreager et al., *Population in the Human Sciences*.
99 Ulijaszek, *Models of Obesity*.
100 Chakrabarty, 'Postcoloniality and the Artifice of History'.
101 Toulson, 'Theorizing the City', 29.
102 Lurie and Williams, 'Migration and Health in Southern Africa'.
103 Myer, 'Social Epidemiology in South Africa'.
104 Lurie and Williams, 'Migration and Health'; Clark et al., 'Returning Home to Die'.
105 Richter, Lye, and Proulx, 'Nurturing Care for Young Children'.
106 Ulijaszek, Elton, and Mann, *Evolving Human Nutrition*.
107 Chapman and Berggren, 'Radical Contextualization'.
108 Summerfield, 'Global Mental Health'.

Bibliography

Ardington, Cally and Anne Case. 'Health: Analysis of the NIDS Wave 1 Dataset Discussion Paper No. 2', Cape Town: National Income Dynamics Study, 2009.

Bac, Martin and Ingrid I. Glatthaar. 'Protein-Energy Malnutrition Intervention Strategies'. *South African Family Practice*, 11 (1990): 284–91.

Barker, David J. and Clive Osmond. 'Infant Mortality, Childhood Nutrition, and Ischaemic Heart Disease in England and Wales', *Lancet*, 1 (8489) (1986): 1077–81, doi.org/10.1016/S0140-6736(86)91340-1.

Beinart, William and Saul Dubow (eds.). *Segregation and Apartheid in Twentieth Century South Africa*. London: Routledge, 1995.

Belkin, G. et al. 'Converging on Child Mental Health – toward Shared Global Action for Child Development', *Global Mental Health*, 4 (2017): e20, doi.org/10.1017/gmh.2017.13.

Ben-Shlomo, Yoav, Rachel Cooper, and Diana Kuh. 'The Last Two Decades of Life Course Epidemiology, and Its Relevance for Research on Ageing', *International Journal of Epidemiology*, 45 (4) (2016): 973–88, doi.org/10.1093/IJE/DYW096.

Ben-Shlomo, Yoav and Diana Kuh. 'A Life Course Approach to Chronic Disease Epidemiology: Conceptual Models, Empirical Challenges and Interdisciplinary Perspectives', *International Journal of Epidemiology*, 31 (2002): 285–93.

Benton, Adia. 'Risky Business: Race, Nonequivalence and the Humanitarian Politics of Life', *Visual Anthropology*, 29 (2) (2016): 187–203, doi.org/10.1080/08949468.2016.1131523.

den Besten, L. et al. 'Changes in the Anthropometric Status of Rural African Under-Fives during a Decade of Primary Health Care', *American Journal of Tropical Medicine and Hygiene*, 98 (6) (1995): 361–6.

Black, Robert E. et al. 'Maternal and Child Undernutrition and Overweight in Low-Income and Middle-Income Countries', *Lancet*, 6736 (13) (2013): 427–51, doi.org/10.1016/S0140-6736 (13)60937-X.

Bourne, Lesley et al. 'Nutrient Intake in the Urban African Population of the Cape Peninsula, South Africa. The BRISK Study', *The Central African Journal of Medicine*, 39 (1994).

Bourne, Lesley et al. 'Nutritional Status of 3–6 Year-Old African Children in the Cape Peninsula', *East African Medical Journal*, 71 (11) (1994): 695–702.

Brown, Tim and Morag Bell. 'Imperial or Postcolonial Governance? Dissecting the Genealogy of a Global Public Health Strategy', *Social Science & Medicine*, 67 (10) (2008): 1571–9, doi.org/10.1016/j.socscimed.2008.07.027.

Bryce, Jennifer et al. 'Maternal and Child Undernutrition: Effective Action at National Level', *Lancet*, 371 (9611) (2008): 510–26, doi.org/10.1016/S0140-6736(07)61694-8.

Buthelezi, Ernest P. et al. 'Ethnic Differences in the Responsiveness of Adipocyte Lipolytic Activity to Insulin', *Obesity Research*, 8 (2) (2000): 171–8, doi.org/10.1038/oby.2000.18.

Carolina Martínez, S. and Leal F. Gustavo. 'Epidemiological Transition: Model or Illusion? A Look at the Problem of Health in Mexico', *Social Science & Medicine*, 57 (3) (2003): 539–50, doi.org/10.1016/S0277-9536(02)00379-9.

Chakrabarty, Dipesh. 'Postcoloniality and the Artifice of History: Who Speaks for "Indian" Pasts?', *Representations*, (37) (1992): 1–26, http://www.jstor.org/stable/2928652.

Chapman, Rachel R. and Jean R. Berggren. 'Radical Contextualization: Contributions to an Anthropology of Racial/Ethnic Health Disparities', *Health*, 9 (2) (2005): 145–67, https://doi.org/10.1177/1363459305050583.

Chen, Lincoln C., Arthur Kleinman, and Norma C. Ware (eds.). *Health and Social Change in International Perspective*. Cambridge, MA: Harvard University Press, 1993.

Clark, Samuel J. et al. 'Returning Home to Die: Circular Labour Migration and Mortality in South Africa', *Scandinavian Journal of Public Health*, 69 (2007): 35–44, doi.org/10.1080/14034950701355619.

Coovadia, Hoosen et al. 'The Health and Health System of South Africa: Historical Roots of Current Public Health Challenges', *Lancet*, 374 (9692) (2009): 817–34, doi.org/10.1016/S0140-6736(09)60951-X.

Coovadia, Hoosen M. 'What Is Progressive about PPHC?' In *Women's Health and Apartheid: The Health of Women and Children and the Future of Progressive Primary Health Care in Southern Africa: Proceedings of the Third Workshop of the Project on Poverty, Health, and the State in*

Southern Africa, edited by Marcia Wright, Z. Stein, and J. Scandlyn. New York: Columbia University, 1988.

Copenhagen Consensus Center. 'Copenhagen Consensus 2008 – Results'. Copenhagen, 2008.

Cousins, Thomas. 'HIV and the Remaking of Hunger and Nutrition in South Africa: Biopolitical Specification after Apartheid', *BioSocieties*, 10 (2) (2015): 143–61, doi.org/10.1057/biosoc.2015.8.

Department of Health, Medical Research Council, OrcMacro. 2007. *South Africa Demographic and Health Survey 2003*. Pretoria: Department of Health.

Department of Health: Republic of South Africa. *Roadmap for Nutrition in South Africa 2013–2017*. Pretoria: Department of Health, 2013.

Doak, Colleen M. et al. 'The Dual Burden Household and the Nutrition Transition Paradox'. *International Journal of Obesity*, 29 (1) (2005): 129–36, doi.org/10.1038/sj.ijo.0802824.

Dubow, Saul. *Scientific Racism in Modern South Africa*. Cambridge: Cambridge University Press, 1995.

Errington, Frederick, Tatsuro Fujikura, and Deborah Gewertz. 'Instant Noodles as an Antifriction Device: Making the BOP with PPP in PNG', *American Anthropologist*, 114 (1) (2012): 19–31, doi.org/10.1111/j.1548-1433.2011.01394.x.

Fall, Caroline H. D. 'Non-Industrialised Countries and Affluence', *British Medical Bulletin*, 60 (2001): 33–50, doi.org/10.1093/bmb/60.1.33.

Frenk, Julio et al. 'Health Transition in Middle-Income Countries: New Challenges for Health Care', *Health and Policy Planning*, 4 (1) (1989): 29–39.

Ginsburg, Faye and Rayna Rapp. 'The Politics of Reproduction', *Annual Review of Anthropology*, 20 (1991): 311–43, http://www.popline.org/node/386510.

Godfrey, Keith M., Peter D. Gluckman, and Mark Hanson. 'Developmental Origins of Metabolic Disease: Life Course and Intergenerational Perspectives', *Trends in Endocrinology and Metabolism: TEM*, 21 (4) (2010): 199–205, doi.org/10.1016/j.tem.2009.12.008.

Godfrey, Keith M. et al. 'Epigenetic Mechanisms and the Mismatch Concept of the Developmental Origins of Health and Disease', *Pediatric Research*, 61 (5) Pt 2 (2007): 5R–10R, doi.org/10.1203/pdr.0b013e318045bedb.

Greenberg, Stephen. 'Corporate Power in the Agro-Food System and the Consumer Food Environment in South Africa', *Journal of Peasant Studies*, 44 (2) (2017): 467–96, doi.org/10.1080/03066150.2016.1259223.

Hales, C. Nicholas and David J. P. Barker. 'The Thrifty Phenotype Hypothesis', *British Medical Bulletin*, 60 (2001): 5–20, www.ncbi.nlm.nih.gov/pubmed/11809615.

Hales, C. Nicholas and David J. P. Barker. 'Type 2 (Non-Insulin-Dependent) Diabetes Mellitus: The Thrifty Phenotype Hypothesis', *Diabetologia*, 35 (1992): 595–601.

Himmelgreen, David A. 'Using a Life Course Approach and a Bio-Cultural Perspective to Understand the Food Insecurity and Obesity Paradox', *Cadernos de Saude Publica*, 29 (2) (2013): 230–1, www.ncbi.nlm.nih.gov/pubmed/23459805.

Hochberg, Z. et al. 'Child Health, Developmental Plasticity and Epigenetic Programming', *Endocrine Reviews*, 32 (2) (2011): 159–224, doi.org/10.1210/er.2009-0039.

Igumbor, Ehimario U. et al. '"Big Food," the Consumer Food Environment, Health, and the Policy Response in South Africa', *PLoS Medicine*, 9 (7) (2012): e1001253, doi.org/10.1371/journal.pmed.1001253.

Johnson-Hanks, Jennifer. 'Demographic Transitions and Modernity', *Annual Review of Anthropology*, 37 (1) (2008): 301–15, doi.org/10.1146/annurev.anthro.37.081407.085138.

Kabudula, Chodziwadziwa W. et al. 'Progression of the Epidemiological Transition in a Rural South African Setting: Findings from Population Surveillance in Agincourt, 1993–2013', *BMC Public Health*, 17 (1) (2017): 1–15, doi.org/10.1186/s12889-017-4312-x.

Kautzky, Keegan and Stephen M. Tollman. 'A Perspective on Primary Health Care in South Africa'. In *South African Health Review 2008*, edited by P. Barron and J. Roma-Reardon, 17–30. Durban: Health Systems Trust, 2008.

Kreager, Philip et al. *Population in the Human Sciences: Concepts, Models, Evidence: An Introduction*. Oxford: Oxford University Press, 2015.

Kruger, H. Salome., Christina S. Venter, and Hester H. Vorster. 'Obesity in African Women in the North West Province, South Africa Is Associated with an Increased Risk of Non-Communicable Diseases: The THUSA Study', *British Journal of Nutrition*, 86 (6) (2001): 733, doi.org/10.1079/BJN2001469.

Kruger, H. Salome et al. 'Physical Inactivity Is the Major Determinant of Obesity in Black Women in the North West Province, South Africa: The THUSA Study', *Nutrition*, 18 (5) (2002): 422–7, doi.org/10.1016/S0899-9007(01)00751-1.

Kruger, H. Salome et al. 'Obesity in South Africa: Challenges for Government and Health Professionals', *Public Health Nutrition*, 8 (5) (2007), doi.org/10.1079/PHN2005785.

Kuh, Diana et al. 'Life Course Epidemiology', *Journal of Epidemiology and Community Health*, 57 (2003): 778–83.

Kuhn, L. et al. 'Village Health Workers and GOBI-FFF: An Evaluation of a Rural Programme', *South African Medical Journal*, 77 (5) (1990): 471–5.

Labadarios, D. et al. 'Review of the South African Nutrition Policy 1994–2002 and Targets for 2007: Achievements and Challenges', *Nutrition*, 21 (2005): 100–8, doi.org/10.1016/j.nut.2004.09.014.

Landecker, Hannah. 'Food as Exposure: Nutritional Epigenetics and the New Metabolism', *BioSocieties*, 6 (2) (2011): 167–94, doi.org/10.1057/biosoc.2011.1.

Levitt, Naomi S. et al. 'The Prevalence and Identification of Risk Factors for NIDDM in Urban Africans in Cape Town, South Africa', *Diabetes Care*, 16 (1993): 601–7.

Livingston, Julie. 'AIDS as Chronic Illness: Epidemiological Transition and Health Care in South-Eastern Botswana', *African Journal of AIDS Research*, 3 (1) (2004): 15–22, doi.org/10.2989/16085900409490314.

Lock, Margaret. 'Comprehending the Body in the Era of the Epigenome', *Current Anthropology*, 56 (2) (2015): 151–77, doi.org/10.1086/680350.

Lock, Margaret and Gisli Palsson. *Can Science Resolve the Nature/Nurture Debate?* Cambridge: Polity Press, 2016.

Lurie, Mark N. and Brian G. Williams. 'Migration and Health in Southern Africa: 100 Years and Still Circulating', *Health Psychology and Behavioral Medicine*, 2 (1) (2014): 34–40, doi.org/10.1080/21642850.2013.866898.

Malhotra, R. et al. 'Determinants of Obesity in an Urban Township of South Africa', *South African Journal of Clinical Nutrition*, 21 (4) (2014): 315–20.

Marks, Shula and Neil Andersson. 'Industrialisation, Rural Health and the 1944 National Health Services Commission in South Africa'. In *The Social Basis of Health and Healing in Africa*, edited by Steven Feierman and John M. Janzen. Berkeley, CA: University of California Press, 1992.

Mendenhall, Emily and Shane A. Norris. 'When HIV Is Ordinary and Diabetes New: Remaking Suffering in a South African Township', *Global Public Health*, 10 (4) (2015): 37–41, doi.org/10.1080/17441692.2014.998698.

Mol, Annemarie and John Law. 'Boundary Variations: An Introduction', *Environment and Planning D: Society and Space*, 23 (5) (2005): 637–42, doi.org/10.1068/d350t.

Mosley, W. Henry and Ronald Gray. 'Childhood Precursors of Adult Morbidity and Mortality in Developing Countries: Implications for Health Programs'. In *The Epidemiological Transition: Policy and Planning Implications for Developing Countries*, edited by James N. Gribble and Samuel H. Preston, 83–114. Washington, DC: National Academies Press, 1993.

Myer, Landon, Rodney I. Ehrlich, and Ezra S. Susser. 'Social Epidemiology in South Africa', *Epidemiologic Reviews*, 26 (2004): 112–23, doi.org/10.1093/epirev/mxh004.

Nichter, Mark and Carl Kendall. 'Beyond Child Survival: Anthropology and International Health in the 1990s'. *Medical Anthropology Quarterly*, 5 (3) (1991): 195–203.

Omran, Abdel R. 'The Epidemiologic Transition: A Theory of the Epidemiology of Population Change', *Milbank Memorial Fund Quarterly*, 49 (1971): 509–38.

Patel, Vikram and Martin Prince. 'Global Mental Health: A New Global Health Field Comes of Age', *Journal of American Medical Association*, 303 (19) (2012): 1976–77, doi.org/10.1001/jama.2010.616.

Pentecost, Michelle. 'The First Thousand Days: Epigenetics in the Age of Global Health'. In *The Palgrave Handbook of Biology and Society*, edited by Maurizio Meloni, John Cromby, Des Fitzgerald, and Stephanie Lloyd, 269–94. London: Palgrave Macmillan, 2018.

Pentecost, Michelle and Fiona C. Ross. 'The First Thousand Days: Motherhood, Scientific Knowledge, and Local Histories', *Medical Anthropology* (2019), doi.org/10.1080/01459740.2019.1590825.

Phala, Ronnie. 'Pitching a Super-Ministry for Child Governance: A Wish List for the Future'. *Daily Maverick*, 12 July 2018, www.dailymaverick.co.za/opinionista/2018-07-12-pitching-a-super-ministry-for-child-governance-a-wish-list-for-the-future/.

Popkin, Barry M. 'Nutritional Patterns and Transitions', *Population and Development Review* 19 (1) (1993): 138–57.

Popkin, Barry M., Linda S. Adair, and Shu Wen Ng. 'Global Nutrition Transition and the Pandemic of Obesity in Developing Countries', *Nutrition Review*, 70 (1) (2011): 3–21, doi.org/10.1111/j.1753-4887.2011.00456.x.

Posel, Deborah. 'Race as Common Sense: Racial Classification in Twentieth-Century South Africa', *Africa Studies Review*, 44 (2) (2001): 87–113, doi.org/10.2307/525576.

Punyadeera, C. et al. 'Weight-Related Differences in Glucose Metabolism and Free Fatty Acid Production in Two South African Population Groups', *International Journal of Obesity and Related Metabolic Disorders*, 25 (2001): 1196–205.

Puoane, Thandi, Hazel Bradley, and Gail D. Hughes. 'Obesity among Black South African Women', *Human Ecology*, (13) (2005): 91–5.

Puoane, Thandi and Lungiswa Tsolekile. 'Challenges Faced by the Urban Black South Africans in the Prevention of Non-Communicable Diseases', *Tribes and Tribals*, 2 (2008): 9–14.

Puoane, Thandi et al. 'Obesity in South Africa: The South African Demographic and Health Survey', *Obesity Research*, 10 (10) (2002): 1038–48, doi.org/10.1038/oby.2002.141.

Reddy, Sasiragha and Anthony Mbewu. 'The Implications of the Developmental Origins of Health and Disease on Public Health Policy and Health Promotion in South Africa', *Healthcare*, 4 (4) (2016): 83, doi.org/10.3390/healthcare4040083.

Richter, Linda M., Stephen J. Lye, and Kerrie Proulx. 'Nurturing Care for Young Children under Conditions of Fragility and Conflict', *New Directions for Child and Adolescent Development*, 159 (2018): 13–26, doi.org/10.1002/cad.20232.

Richter, Linda et al. 'Cohort Profile: Mandela's Children: The 1990 Birth to Twenty Study in South Africa', *International Journal of Epidemiology*, 36 (3) (2007): 504–11, doi.org/10.1093/ije/dym016.

Richter, Linda M. et al. 'Cohort Profile: The Consortium of Health-Orientated Research in Transitioning Societies', *International Journal of Epidemiology*, 41 (3) (2012): 621–6, doi.org/10.1093/ije/dyq251.

Scott, James. *Seeing like a State: How Certain Schemes to Improve the Human Condition Have Failed*. New Haven, CT: Yale University Press, 1998.

Seeberg, Jens and Lotte Meinert. 'Can Epidemics Be Noncommunicable?', *Medicine Anthropology Theory*, 2 (2) (2015): 54–71.

Shisana, O. et al. *South African National Health and Nutrition Examination Survey (SANHANES-1)*. Cape Town: HSRC Press, 2013.

Shostak, Sara and Margot Moinester. 'The Missing Piece of the Puzzle? Measuring the Environment in the Postgenomic Moment'. In *Postgenomics: Perspectives on Biology and the Genome*, edited by S. Richardson and H. Stevens, 192–209. Durham, NC: Duke University Press, 2015.

Solomon, Harris. *Metabolic Living: Food, Fat, and the Absorption of Illness in India*. Durham, NC: Duke University Press, 2016.

South African Vitamin A Consultative Group (SAVACG). *Children Aged 6–71 Months in South Africa, 1994: Their Anthropometric, Vitamin A, Iron and Immunisation Coverage Status*. Johannesburg: SAVACG, 1995.

Steyn, K. et al. 'Anthropometric Profile of a Black Population of the Cape Peninsula in South Africa', *East African Medical Journal*, 75 (1) (1998): 35–40.

Steyn, K. et al. 'Risk Factors for Coronary Heart Disease in the Black Population of the Cape Peninsula: The BRISK Study', *South African Medical Journal = Suid-Afrikaanse Tydskrif Vir Geneeskunde*, 79 (8) (1991): 480–5, www.ncbi.nlm.nih.gov/pubmed/2020891.

Summerfield, Derek. '"Global Mental Health" Is an Oxymoron and Medical Imperialism', *BMJ*, 346 (2013): 1–2, doi.org/10.1136/bmj.f3509.

Thurow, Roger. *The First 1000 Days: A Crucial Time for Mothers and Children – and the World*. New York: Perseus Books, 2016.

Tomlinson, Mark and Barak Morgan. 'Infant Mental Health Research in Africa: A Call for Action for Research in the Next 10 Years', *Global Mental Health*, 2 (2015): e7, doi.org/10.1017/gmh.2015.4.

Toulson, Ruth E. 'Theorizing the City: Recent Research in Urban Anthropology', *Reviews in Anthropology*, 44 (1) (2015): 28–42, doi.org/10.1080/00938157.2015.1001646.

Trostle, James. *Epidemiology and Culture*. Cambridge: Cambridge University Press, 2004.

Ulijaszek, Stanley J. *Models of Obesity: From Ecology to Complexity in Science and Policy*. Cambridge: Cambridge University Press, 2017.

Ulijaszek, Stanley J., Sarah Elton, and Neil Mann. *Evolving Human Nutrition: Implications for Public Health*. Cambridge: Cambridge University Press, 2012.
United Nations. 'Scaling Up Nutrition: A Framework for Action', *Food and Nutrition Bulletin*, 31 (1) (2010): 178–86.
Van der Merwe, Maria Terésa, and M. S. Pepper. 'Obesity in South Africa', *Obesity Reviews*, 7 (4) (2006): 315–22, doi.org/10.1111/j.1467-789X.2006.00237.x.
Van der Merwe et al. 'Evidence for Insulin Resistance in Black Women from South Africa', *International Journal of Obesity and Related Metabolic Disorders*, 24 (2000): 1340–6.
Vaughan, Megan. 'Conceptualising Metabolic Disorder in Southern Africa: Biology, History and Global Health', *BioSocieties*, 14 (1) (2019): 123–42, doi.org/10.1057/s41292-018-0122-3.
Victora, Cesar G. et al. 'Maternal and Child Undernutrition: Consequences for Adult Health and Human Capital', *Lancet*, 371 (9609) (2008): 340–57, doi.org/10.1016/S0140-6736(07)61692-4.
Vlok, M. E. *Manual of Community Nursing and Communicable Diseases: A Textbook for South African Students*. Lansdowne: Juta, 1991.
Vorster, Hester H. et al. 'Contribution of Nutrition to the Health Transition in Developing Countries: A Framework for Research and Intervention', *Nutrition Reviews*, 57 (11) (1999): 341–9.
Vorster, Hester H., Annamarie Kruger, and Barrie M. Margetts. 'The Nutrition Transition in Africa: Can It Be Steered into a More Positive Direction?', *Nutrients*, 3 (4) (2011): 429–41, doi.org/10.3390/nu3040429.
Wahlberg, Ayo and Nikolas Rose. 'The Governmentalization of Living: Calculating Global Health', *Economy and Society*, 44 (1) (2015): 60–90, doi.org/10.1080/03085147.2014.983830.
Walker, Alexander Robert, B. F. Adam, and B. F. Walker. 'World Pandemic in Obesity: The Situation in Southern African Populations', *Public Health*, 115 (6) (2001): 368–72.
Walker, Alexander Robert et al. 'Low Frequency of Adverse Sequelae of Obesity in South African Rural Black Women', *International Journal of Vitamin & Nutrirtion Research*, 59 (2) (1989): 224–8.
Western Cape Government. 'Healthcare 2030: The Road to Wellness'. Cape Town, 2014.
Whitmarsh, Ian. 'Troubling Environments', *Medical Anthropology Quarterly*, 27 (4) (2013): 489–509, doi.org/10.1111/maq.12061.
World Bank. *Repositioning Nutrition as Central to Development: A Strategy for Large-Scale Action*. Washington, DC: World Bank, 2006.
World Health Organization. '2008–2013 Action Plan for the Global Strategy for the Prevention and Control of Noncommunicable Diseases.' Geneva: World Health Organization, 2009.
Wylie, Diane. *Starving on a Full Stomach: Hunger and the Triumph of Cultural Racism in South Africa*. Charlottesville, VA: University of Virginia Press, 2001.
Yates-Doerr, Emily. *The Weight of Obesity: Hunger and Global Health in Postwar Guatemala*. Berkeley, CA: University of California Press, 2015.

10

Southern Africa and Discussions on Breastfeeding

Catherine Burns

Introduction

Since the 1930s, breastfeeding discussions have been a conduit for anxiety about women's autonomy, malnutrition, child psychological development, and chronic non-communicable diseases (NCDs) in newborns and children. Recently, work on the long-term adverse health outcomes for intermittently, or never, breastfed adults, born in the developed north as well as countries in the south, has taken on a central place in research on breastfeeding and NCDs.[1] Over the last two decades, a body of published work in leading journals has traced links between NCDs and various forms of inadequate breastfeeding, including research into cancers, diabetes, cardiovascular diseases and respiratory diseases – all of which contribute to a high burden of morbidity and mortality in low- and middle-income countries. Kelishadi and Farajian argue in their exhaustive paper reviewing evidence for the protective effects of breastfeeding on chronic non-communicable diseases, 'that NCDs have a complex etiology resulting from the interaction of genetic factors, gender, age, ethnicity, and the environmental factors ... [because] chronic diseases in adulthood have origins in early life ... [there are] beneficial effects of breastfeeding during infancy on chronic diseases in adulthood, particularly on hypertension, obesity, diabetes, hypercholesterolemia, and cardiovascular diseases.'[2]

A key finding of their review of two decades of published work is that breastfeeding of babies can have long-term beneficial health effects at individual and population levels. The culmination of research into the foetal and early infancy origins of adult disease in the 1980s and 1990s linked up with earlier publications from social medicine and community-oriented healthcare models of health promotion. By 2006 a combined form of 'social and environmental approaches to health and health planning', known as the Developmental Origins of Health and Disease (DOHaD), emerged.[3] The DOHaD approach places breastfeeding at the centre of health planning, and infant health at the epicentre of longitudinal studies of sifting adult mortality and morbidity over the life span of people in aggregated cohort studies since the Second World War.[4] Employing the framing of 'the first 1000 days of life', these studies (captured in two landmark volumes in 2006 and 2016 and edited by Peter Gluckman and others) leave open the key question of what correct, attainable and healthy forms of breastfeeding are, and should be, across the globe. (See also Pentecost in this volume.)

To address this key question, this chapter explores the long history of expert knowledge about breastfeeding practices in different regions of Southern Africa – with a specific focus on African women; women of the Indian diaspora, living in and around the East Coast of Southern Africa; and women classified as 'white'. The discussion covers the 1950s through to the present. These women and their breastfeeding practices and beliefs were, and remain, the objects and subjects of scientific and social analysis. In the wake of the HIV epidemic, Southern Africa is a vital source of breastfeeding science today. At the epicentre of the global efforts to understand the links between HIV infection and transmission, the study of breastfeeding has attracted large investments of time and money since the late 1980s. But there is a second reason to focus on breastfeeding knowledge from this region – and the roots of this lie in the work of a collection of remarkable social medicine researchers in South Africa in the 1950s and 1960s. This cohort of researchers included clinicians, epidemiologists, sociologists and anthropologists – and their findings and research methods remain relevant today. The paper demonstrates their influential contribution to these current debates.

Modern scientific knowledge about breastfeeding precedes by almost four decades the often ahistorical, decontexualised and voluminous publication outputs that emerged after the link with HIV transmission emerged. An older body of knowledge, rooted in the research of clinical researchers in the south, generated a baseline of studies about breastfeeding and NCDs and about the impact of early infant nutrition on adult health. This long pre-dated the rise of commercial infant formula production and marketing in the south, and the concomitant emergence of new transnational networks of humanitarianism and maternal feminism. In the wake of effective antiretroviral treatment of pregnant and post-partum women – by the late 2000s and into the 2010s – the focus of breastfeeding research and policymaking shifted to the advocacy of 'exclusive breastfeeding' by global health bodies. To trace the history of this concept, and this approach to infant feeding, I draw on archival state documents and on medical and scientific papers and reports as well as on the memoirs of key actors who drew attention to nutritional cultures, and their links with chronic disease, 70 years ago.

As many commentators have shown, in South Africa over the last two decades public health has become an arena of many bitter – and academically productive – contests.[5] Within this field, debates about breastfeeding have been relatively unexplored. In the 1990s and 2000s anxiety around breastfeeding focused on HIV transmission but, in the period before this and again over the last decade, the focus has been on non-communicable diseases and infant nutrition, and the links between compromised breastfeeding regimes and long-term chronic disease in adults as well as children. A feature of breastfeeding – seldom attended to in nutritional and NCD studies – is that, unlike other forms of human food, it is produced exclusively by women, not always the biological mothers of suckled infants, and is a complex production that includes its deep links to sexuality, mental health, affect and psychological well-being as well as biological vitality.[6] Public health initiatives concerned, internationally and nationally, with maternal health, lactation, weaning and all aspects of infant nutrition have, since the late 1990s, been beset with coerced decisions, cul-de-sacs and about-turns. The knowledge generated in this highly pressured and presentist context stands in contrast to the claims of older breastfeeding studies on health transition, and on social context of health.

This is especially true when considering the research into breastfeeding conducted since the late 1950s, and widely disseminated since the 1970s: successful breastfeeding by any measure at all (exclusive; predominant; partial; or intermittent – concepts discussed below) depends on a woman's full and engaged participation, and on the support around her. Women who are not the biological parents of born infants can also provide infant lactation to other women's offspring – not only as wet nurses (through familial or commercial/labour arrangements), but also as adoptive mothers – with the help of nipple stimulation (practised for hundreds of years), as well as, more recently, with hormonal and chemical interventions.[7] In many parts of Southern Africa infants are suckled for comfort or nourishment, by relatives and care givers other than their mothers. We know that the instinct to suck and the pleasure and comfort thus afforded are part of our mammalian polymorphous sexual lineage.[8] This has huge implications for research. Yet, in recent times, in scholarly works and breastfeeding guidelines emerging from the WHO and UNICEF, the terminological field is focused on the 'mother and her child' relationship, and on what is termed 'exclusive breastfeeding'. This raises many questions about meaning, practice and efficacy.[9] While the World Health Organization (WHO) and the United Nations Children's Fund (UNICEF) guidelines do stress that, to increase rates of the kinds of breastfeeding sought by health experts, supportive interventions are key (and thus state actors; employers; policymakers and households), these documents do not address breastfeeding as a culture, or its contextual variations, or the many complex pressures shaping the form it takes in everyday life.

In describing what experts today mean by 'optimal breastfeeding' the WHO and UNICEF guidelines point out that only about a third of infants aged 0 to 6 months are currently breastfed in this manner globally. They recommend 'early initiation of breastfeeding within 1 hour of birth; exclusive breastfeeding for the first 6 months of life; and [the] introduction of nutritionally-adequate and safe complementary (solid) foods at 6 months together with continued breastfeeding up to 2 years of age or beyond'. In defining exclusive breastfeeding the WHO argues first that the optimal length of time for this practice is six months. In order to achieve exclusive breastfeeding these recommendations argue for some of the widely known guides to breastfeeding that have been researched for over a century such as: direct contact between mother and baby immediately after birth, and the initiation of breastfeeding within the first hour of life. They also recommend a regime called 'breastfeeding on demand' which, as I show in this paper, was eschewed by global health elites for many decades in the twentieth century. The new injunction in WHO definitions of exclusive breastfeeding over the last decade is this: 'not giving babies additional food or drink, even water, unless medically necessary', for six months.[10] This specific requirement is repeated across key guidelines and articles and training sites. It is highly unlikely that this exclusive form of breastfeeding is achievable in many societies in the world, let alone in places like South Africa, where legal and institutional supports are absent.[11] Sidestepping the obvious difficulties of attaining fuller rates of any form of breastfeeding, the WHO guidelines present compelling reasons:

> Children and adolescents who were breastfed as babies are less likely to be overweight or obese. Additionally, they perform better

> on intelligence tests and have higher school attendance. Breastfeeding is associated with higher income in adult life. Improving child development and reducing health costs results in economic gains for individual families as well as at the national level. Longer durations of breastfeeding also contribute to the health and well-being of mothers: it reduces the risk of ovarian and breast cancer and helps space pregnancies – exclusive breastfeeding of babies under 6 months has a hormonal effect which often induces a lack of menstruation. This is a natural (though not fail-safe) method of birth control known as the Lactation Amenorrhoea Method.[12]

The stakes, here, are very high. What then do we know about the roots of lactation cultures and practices, and how can we draw upon this knowledge as it bears on the present?

South African social medicine and paradoxes of breastfeeding

In the late 1940s and early 1950s South African medical and health professionals began collecting and assembling data on breastfeeding in the wider context of social or community health initiatives. They read the published anthropological literature and took account of earlier commentaries on breastfeeding. One of the most extensive and interesting collections was undertaken in and around Durban – a city on the eastern seaboard of South Africa and the largest port on the continent – and at Pholela, a hamlet 100 kilometres inland. The research was headed by Dr Eva Salber and the team of nurses, doctors, health educators and researchers gathered around the Institute of Family Medicine, which was established in a working-class community south of the city in the port area after the Second World War. These core research sites were linked to a network of Health Centres – part of a wider scheme, set up by Dr Sidney Kark and Dr Emily Kark with the help of Dr H. Gluckman (the war-era Health Minister of the then Union of South Africa); Dr Gale (later a Professor of Family and Social Medicine at Makerere University in Uganda); and Dr H. S. Gear (a key state health official, and later an assistant director general at the WHO), and other leading health officials in Jan Smuts' last Cabinet.[13] Shula Marks argues that the combination of socialist and progressive ideas about health in social context, as well as the crucial support for a small number of years from central state policy makers, allowed the Centres to make significant advances in knowledge of health practices and local health needs. Durban in the 1950s was unique in the country because its population consisted of three large groupings of relatively equal numbers: people of African descent, mainly isiZulu speakers; people of Indian descent; and people of European descent (white); as well as a much smaller group of mixed background categorised as 'Coloured'.[14] Eva Salber's research, published first in the early 1950s, showed that, of children born in a clinic or hospital in Durban and its surrounds:

> … at the beginning of their lives white babies were the heaviest, Indian babies the lightest, and coloured and black babies intermediate between the two. By the end of the year white babies were still the heaviest, but black babies had overtaken the coloured infants. Indian babies grew as fast as whites for about two months, but fell away increasingly thereafter. Black babies overtook white ones at about one month, and maintained their lead until thirty weeks of age after which they dropped below them. In interpreting these results I suggested that white infants were underfed in early life due to strictly regulated by-the-clock schedules of nursing. Paediatricians at that time lectured mothers on the dangers of overfeeding. Babies of the other ethnic groups grew well in early life due to their mothers' accepted practice of nursing on demand. But when the latter's children needed other foods in addition to breast milk, the mothers could neither afford the purchase nor were they sufficiently educated in child nutrition.[15]

Salber, and her later globally famous colleagues, Emily and Sydney Kark, were enthusiastic and wrote positively about many of the practices and meanings associated with breastfeeding amongst isiZulu-speaking and South African Indian women. They appreciated the commitment to the labour and duty of motherhood (as it was, and is still, seen by many) and recognised the confidence and power that management of breastfeeding offered many women in these communities.

In their published work, this research team highlighted the layered sexual experience and meaning in the work of breastfeeding and the cross-gender, socially rooted and generative power of breastfeeding's status, with its interlinking web of taboo, avoidance and control. The Karks and Salber traced the way that breastfeeding practices forestalled disharmony, poisoning and other destructive interventions. The roles grandmothers and kinfolk, notably fathers, played in supporting and policing breastfeeding – from support with food and rest and infant care, through to particular religious, sexual and social observances – were closely analysed, as were the ways in which lactating women and their infants were treated with special regard. Salber showed that 'Hindu breastfeeding practice' was quite different from the practices of isiZulu-speakers. Yet in their many positive associations with status and care for breastfeeding, the women in these two communities shared similarities that separated them from more rapidly changing cultures of breastfeeding amongst white women.

In tandem with anthropologists and sociologists working in this region before them, Eva Salber and the Karks concluded that breastfeeding practice was itself embedded in a bigger basket of beliefs and practices, carrying specific understandings of the porous, vulnerable and virtual 'skins' that separated pregnant women from potential evil doers and the ancestors of these women and their menfolk. In turn these virtual 'skins' (and the real and virtual membranes, fontanelles and actual skins) between 'the world' and the infant life of small children were part of a continuum of health beliefs.[16]

In isiZulu-speaking communities breastfeeding in particular was powerfully associated with these porous, vulnerable 'skins'. For isiZulu speakers, and many others south of the Limpopo, a woman's sexual arousal, her contact with ejaculated sperm, or her dreams could all poison her breast milk. Moving through a contaminated or poisoned space (along a river bank, across a road or path) could also trigger contamination. Women could be fed or sprinkled with poison which would infect their breast milk. Attention was given to protecting infants from evil forces, but breast milk was particularly vulnerable. In Durban and in Pholela, Salber and her co-researchers witnessed the effects of these beliefs and associated practices. The Karks summarised their observations made over several years in their widely read and reviewed summative 1999 text, drawing on Salber's extensive work. They revisited the comparisons Salber made across both her clinical and other health records, where she showed that mortality among infants and babies under one year in Natal was heavily associated with early weaning and the onset of infant mixed and cereal feeding. They observed:

> Most Pholela residents and many in Lamontville believed that diarrhoeal diseases were transmitted through the mother, congenitally and through breast feeding. Mothers were believed to have been infected by an ill-wisher who had directed them, by supernatural means, to walk across a place that had been struck

> by lightening, or by a bird (*inyoni*) that had previously flown over the site they traversed. The traditional practitioners' treatments were focused on the diarrhoea itself, involving the use of grass reed enemas, twirling the reed in the anus to draw blood. Their advice to stop breast feeding was consistent with local traditional concepts of causation. Both the advice and the treatment were considered by us to be harmful. However, with the mother's belief that her breast milk had been rendered detrimental and a cause of the baby's illness, neither she nor her mother-in-law could be expected to comply with the advice to continue breast feeding.[17]

To understand how these earlier researchers addressed this challenge to their practice of community-embedded health services, and to weigh the value of their findings about compliance with breastfeeding advice, it is useful to move away from the specifics of the South African case from the 1950s and through the HIV era, and trace a brief history of breastfeeding internationally.

Expert management of the female breast and its milk

Debates in the current literature on NCDs and the protective benefits of breastfeeding start with the premise that it is pre-eminently a biological or physiological process, and the assumption is implicit that it carries the same meaning and function across time and space. This is demonstrably false. The link between the physiological process (hormonal and chemical and so on) and the psychological process for breastfeeding, from the milk-duct opening 'prompts' in the so called 'let down' reflex, to the actual production of breast milk, is a powerful example of the falsity of the mind/body distinction in human experience.[18] Through the history of formal ethnographic studies, social and biological scientists have been animated by comparisons of the social and cultural histories and forms of human lactation. While expert knowledge on this subject from the past is much easier to glean than the popular and ordinary knowledge, classical scholars of the Middle East, India and western Europe have combed the corpus of medical treatises devoted to 'infant health', much of which was in circulation through elite networks thousands of years before the western scientific renaissance. Combined with ancient Roman and Greek medical writings (from Hippocrates, Soranus and especially Galen), scholars have traced complex and regionally specific forms of breastfeeding. Porter, Fildes, Jelliffe and Jelliffe in particular traced the pathways of breastfeeding beliefs from the ancient world into the Middle Ages, and showed how they were carried by the schools of Arabian and Persian commentators and disseminated by medical writers in the renaissance. Histories of printing and the globalisation of literary texts have shown that these expert and elite ideas reached a wider audience in Europe with the advent of printing and the use of vernacular languages in the fifteenth and sixteenth centuries. As several scholars in the field of lactation histories argue, this era of dissemination may lie behind the notable similarity of many descriptions of 'traditional' beliefs about infant feeding found throughout the world today.[19]

Our human ancestors clearly debated how to manage breastfeeding in the context of agricultural and mercantile lifestyles, as well as slave-based, industrial and plantation economies, over thousands of years. For the last several thousand years experts have recorded debates about when to introduce mixed feeding; when to allow wet nursing and artificial feeding; and when and how to supplement breast milk feeds in the life of an infant. By the nineteenth century breastfeeding over the age of three was increasingly deemed harmful and a *Lancet* paper published in 1842 recorded a physician's views that childhood epilepsy and other conditions could be linked to long durations of breastfeeding.[20] Fildes, Jelliffe and Jeliffe and others have pointed to sources from the second century BC exhorting believers to express and disregard colostrum[21]; methods to speed up the excretion of infant meconium[22]; expert literature about colostrum taboos; and the use of devices and pumps to assist with breast milk production – with preserved objects and related texts dating from the 1500 BC era. These scholars argue that this prevalence of assisting devices proves that the so-called 'let-down' reflex may have been inhibited in many settings through '... fears of bewitchment or guilt over non-observance of taboos, especially of a sexual nature'.[23] The links between infant suckling and production of milk seemed to be well understood by ancient societies. In Fildes' work on the history of wet nursing she makes it clear that both the character of wet nurses as women, and the quality of their breast milk, was the subject of much discussion and checking in all the societies for which she found wet-nursing evidence. The explanations for this are clear: the character of the wet nurse as a person was seen as transmittable through the quality, viscosity and taste of her milk. Yet poorer and less healthy women were often employed despite these beliefs. Clearly the individual wet nurse's moral and milk qualities could supersede her poverty, at times her ethnicity and her 'race', and even her religion. Only in the later nineteenth century, with the rise of eugenic fears about 'race decline' and miscegenation, was 'wet nursing' as a whole the subject for concerted critique by experts working on behalf of the state or church. This history, linking eugenicists to breastfeeding debates, is not acknowledged and is, perhaps, ill understood by proponents today of epigenetic arguments made for evolutionary biology in the context of the first 1000 days of life. This is especially in relation to claims to enduring mental and physical benefits, and higher rates of intelligence, in breastfed children.

It is interesting in terms of global health history that it took until the eve of the First World War before breastfeeding was accorded the status of an international conference, with state and civil society participation. In 1913 in Paris the first international conference was held on bottle feeding and other artificial infant-feeding techniques, considering, at the highest state levels, social and political aspects as well as nutritional issues.[24] One of the salient issues in reviewing this literature, in globalised scientific publications, is the homogenisation of ideas about the moral effects of breastfeeding alongside the commercialisation of artificial infant nutrition. A similarly structured, if exactly opposite, body of advice has emerged from elite medical academies in the West since the late 1980s.

From the 1940s to the early 1970s infant and maternal health experts and western paediatricians, and their counterparts in many sectors of the developing world, argued that to breastfeed an infant 'on demand' was a maternal practice of incivility – children nourished in this way would display tendencies towards savage mentality; laziness; over-sensuality; over-dependence and immaturity; and so on. In this literature, the moral and social consequences of indolent 'demand' feeding were ascribed harms which varied with prevailing psycho-social and intellectual trends in scientific and public health literature. After 1950, an international breastfeeding literature stressed the individual woman's responsibility for four-hourly or 'by-the-clock' feeding and paid scant attention to the any other issue: the role of fathers, friends or kinfolk, let alone wet nursing; shared suckling; work environment demands; psycho-social conflicts; or other contextually crucial issues. Instead the health educator, the nurse, the doctor and the social worker became the mediating experts around a single woman's breastfeeding. The state's health mechanisms and regulating bodies took over a major role in breastfeeding management.[25]

This was true in Southern Africa as in Europe – though in South Africa the particularities of white infant health as a key state goal often muddied the waters of public health policy for far longer than in other contexts.[26] The Second World War and its aftermath produced a challenge to this: communal non-commercial infant milk-banks were established in the same ways that blood banks were set up, and infant feeding was for a time regarded through the lenses of non-interventionist, non-marketable, communitarian social health goals.[27] But this era was short lived.

In the 1960s and 1970s the 'by the clock' view predominated in expert discourses and, around the world, women moved away from breastfeeding towards bottle feeding in greater or lesser numbers. Tragically in places like Botswana and South Africa – where clean water sources and cheap or subsidised infant formula were restricted to small parts of the population – the cost of new infant formula feeding was a dramatic rise in infant and child mortality.[28] By the 1980s, public health expertise, pressed into reconsiderations of prevailing views and practices by non-governmental organisations, many led by women health activists like La Leche League International, began to draw on fringe research into infant nutrition and breastfeeding. They began to turn the behemoth of 'clocked and controlled' breastfeeding around. By the later 1980s the evidence for the long-term ill effects of formula infant feeding was unmistakable. The results of large-scale research on the chemical and hormonal and physiological apparatus of lactation showed that clock feeding would actually reduce overall milk production as well as weaken the content of human breast milk.[29] From 1990 WHO and UNICEF decided that the evidence for breastfeeding as 'best practice' for infant health worldwide, and in every setting, was conclusive. They jointly adopted the 'Innocenti Declaration' (named after the town where they met) titled: 'The Protection, Promotion and Support of Breastfeeding'. After this point all national governments were urged to develop national breastfeeding policies and set appropriate national targets, and states were required to set up national systems for monitoring the attainment of targets. Critical of the role and profiteering of major infant formula production corporations, regulations to restrict and control the commercial sale of infant formulas were adopted. This took place alongside an attack on the practice of commercial formula producers giving out free formula samples at birth clinics, especially in poor and under-resourced regions, and the prevention of the inappropriate use, by state or UNICEF/WHO-sponsored health services, of formula products. These Conventions came into effect as the Soviet Union was breaking up and many other eastern European states were in a process of great upheaval and change. In South Africa, the apartheid regime was finally crumbling. In the same decade in South Africa nationally constituted progressive health organisations and some areas of the state health service began laying out and even implementing some of the best-practice maternal and health policy ideals and goals set out in these infant health Conventions. In recognition of the distortions and injustices of the past and the imbalances in South Africa's health resource management, one of the first acts of the new Mandela government after 1994 was the creation of free public health access for all children under six and pregnant women. Lactation support and a positive approach to breastfeeding was a corner-stone of this plan.[30] A new version of 'breast is best' entered centre stage. By 1992 the mood in public health, paediatric and maternal health discourses and associated recommended practices had swung in the opposite direction of the previous era: the new science of breastfeeding now required what was termed (for the first time) exclusive breastfeeding as best practice. But little research had yet been done on just what 'exclusive' breastfeeding would mean in lived experience for lactating women of the world.[31]

Exclusive breastfeeding: an invention of public health doctrines

These crucial questions frame this final section of the paper: what is exclusive breastfeeding and how long should a woman who is breastfeeding continue in order to prevent the transmission of infectious diseases, protect against the acquisition of communicable diseases, and provide protection for the child as it matures? Answering these questions requires further historical explanation and demands that we draw on the expertise of social and cultural studies conducted in tandem with clinical science.

For most of the twentieth century when scientists, maternal and infant health advocates spoke of exclusive breastfeeding they meant that infants derived *most* of their nourishment from suckling their mother's breast milk. Studies conducted in over a dozen national contexts have convincingly shown that in no place on earth did women breastfeed exclusively.[32] (This is according to the definition of exclusive breastfeeding in which no food or liquid product, other than mere drops for medication, or less than 10 millilitres of water or juice over time, are given until the age of six months of infant life has been reached.) Clara Aarts, working on evidence from a breastfeeding research centre in Uppsala, Sweden, has provided a rubric for determining 'exclusivity', and by this measure most mothers in most parts of the world breastfeed their biological infants exclusively for less than a month. In addition to mixing breast milk with some bottle feeds of milk replacement (an almost ubiquitous practice in the developed world, and widespread in poor countries as well), and in addition to the adding of cereals and other foods to the diets of very young infants – common in many parts of Africa and the Caribbean – some women across the world routinely share suckling of infant young. They do so with non-biological mothers and also offer water, teas and fruit juices instead of human or animal milk. In addition, exclusive breastfeeding may be delayed by a few days at the start of life in some settings. In India, parts of South Africa and many other places, women routinely express their colostrum[33] and replace this with other feeding for two to five days.[34] Already, by the late 1980s, a critique of this form of breast milk and mixed feeding existed. Worldwide public health and maternal and infant health activists and experts questioned the widely taught theory that infants needed to be weaned onto high-protein foods and that bottle feeding with formula feeds was a good way to gradually wean children. A revolution in infant-feeding ideologies and technologies was under way and at the same time a new epidemic forced much of this work against the wall: the discovery that HIV infection could be transmitted by human lactation.

As late as the mid-1980s it was still unclear to the world's virologists whether HIV infection could be transmitted through human lactation. In their survey of the HIV/AIDS transmission literature, 'HIV Infection in Developing Countries', Drs M. Carael and P. Piot, then world experts in the emerging field of HIV/AIDS, wrote:

> As elsewhere, there is no evidence for HIV transmission in the tropics by casual contact, by anthropods, or within household and occupational settings such as the hospital ... The potential for transmission of HIV by breast milk should be elucidated urgently because of its important public health consequences.[35]

Thus by the late 1980s and early 1990s the first papers were being published establishing breast milk as a possible transmission route. Work was underway to protect milk banks at major state hospitals throughout the world and then to measure and analyse viral load in breast milk. Researchers also began to investigate the layers of infection possibilities for HIV-infected infants and to establish the mechanism through which some HIV-free infants born to HIV-infected mothers maintained their negative status. By 1992 the pressure was intense and scientists began proposing the cessation of breastfeeding in all HIV-positive mothers of newborns and infants. Starting in the late 1990s, Coutsoudis, Pillay, Spooner, Khun, Coovadia and their team, working from Durban, published a series of articles on exclusive breastfeeding and HIV status.[36] The work of key individuals on this team received widespread dissemination through the web of medical and health journals. Studies in other countries repeated and some took issue with these findings, and in South Africa, a team in Johannesburg based at Chris Hani Baragwanath Hospital entered into debate with their fellow researchers.[37]

The work of Coutsoudis et al. began building a case for advice that even HIV-positive mothers could breastfeed with little risk if they employed exclusive breastfeeding. Furthermore, even if this method risked some infection, this was a potentially better public health choice than the already established riskier choice of infant formula for women unable to keep up the costs and the correct proportions of mixed formula, and unable to provide 100 per cent sterile water and bottles to prevent other life-threatening infections. The literature on infant ill-health in poor communities with the latter conditions was, as we have mentioned, already well established. The abstract of their 1999 *Lancet* paper is instructive:

> We compared transmission rates in exclusively breastfed, mixed-fed, and formula-fed (never breastfed) infants to assess whether the pattern of breastfeeding is a critical determinant of early mother-to-child transmission of HIV-1 ... Our findings have important implications for prevention of HIV-1 infection and infant-feeding policies in developing countries and further research is essential. In the meantime, breastfeeding policies for HIV-1-infected women require urgent review. If our findings are confirmed, exclusive breastfeeding may offer HIV-1-infected women in developing countries an affordable, culturally acceptable and effective means of reducing mother-to-child transmission of HIV-1 while maintaining the overwhelming benefits of breastfeeding.[38]

The key concluding clause, 'exclusive breastfeeding may offer HIV-1-infected women in developing countries an affordable, culturally acceptable, and effective means of reducing mother-to-child transmission of HIV-1', set experienced South African researchers to deep thinking. Familiar with the complex terrain, after years in local clinical services and in neo-natal and maternity wards of the region's biggest tertiary hospital at that time, King Edward VIII hospital in Durban, these researchers and clinical workers were also familiar with the local contexts of poor households and the complex challenges faced by poor families and mothers caring for infants and their children in impoverished homes. The research emerging out of laboratories and clinical wards and reported on in the *Lancet* piece (and others like it) begged many questions: what were the 'culturally accepted' forms of breastfeeding referred to in the piece? And how had these developed or changed over time in other contexts of pressure or challenge? Could these cultures of breastfeeding be adapted to 'exclusive breastfeeding'? How was this linked to sexual practice and desire, and to couples and their coupling before and during pregnancy and in the post-partum period? And then, how could successes and failures be ethically determined and studied in field work involving such crucial matters of life and death as well as desire?

From 2000 to 2003 a highly trained lactation and public health nurse, Thoko Ndaba, conducted a series of extensive interviewers with women in a region highly affected by HIV in the Durban hinterland.[39] She found no evidence, even after extensive community health education and support, that women were able to exclusively breastfeed: migration, waged employment, shared child rearing practices and local forms of sexual intimacy with partners and babies' fathers mitigated against this. In the years between the completion of her study and the first Cochrane Review of breastfeeding evidence (published in 2005), reviewers found that the evidence for exclusive breastfeeding versus other forms of mixed feeding regimes remained weak. In 2016 the Cochrane Review conducted an update of work from 2005 to 2016, and the authors argued:

> Mothers require information on the frequency and duration of breastfeeds but they receive conflicting advice. Current guidelines encourage baby-led breastfeeding. It is important to systematically review the evidence, to inform women's decisions on the relative effectiveness of each method. This is also important as baby-led breastfeeding is not always followed, as many women and caregivers seem more comfortable with scheduled rather than baby-led feeding patterns … We looked for studies that compared baby-led with scheduled (or mixed) breastfeeding for successful breastfeeding for healthy newborn babies. However, no studies were found that met the inclusion criteria. It is recommended that no changes are made to current practice guidelines without undertaking robust research, to include many patterns of breastfeeding and not limited to baby-led and scheduled breastfeeding. Future exploratory research on baby-led breastfeeding is also needed that takes the mother's perspective into consideration.[40]

As I argued above, the archive of the research collected by the Karks and Salber is instructive. In examining the similarities and differences between South African Indian and isiZulu communities, and their responses to the challenges of malnutrition and sickness in Durban and Pholela in the late 1940s and early 1950s, they explored the widely shared belief that diarrhoeal diseases were transmitted through the mother via breastfeeding. Supernatural forces and infection by ill intent were blamed, and the concomitant community and familial advice was to stop breastfeeding. The solution proffered in this context was a compromise: 'The health centre's advice to use the special skim milk powder preparation diluted with cooled boiled water, using sterilised bottles and rubber teats, was, fortunately, acceptable to them.'[41] Lest readers infer that traditions of breastfeeding were confined to mothers of African descent, their work showed that this was widespread in the region:

> Hindu newborns were also thought to be in need of protective cleansing and treatment. However, non-invasive treatments such as massage of mother and baby with various oils together with prayers and incantations were used ... In the Durban Indian communities of Merebank and Springfield there did not appear to be any conflicts between the concepts of cause and treatment of gastroenteritis or acute respiratory infections with those of the health centre practice. They assigned the cause of illness or misfortune to themselves; some of the vows they made as to future behaviour if the baby survived or got well were very demanding, and were taken in order to expiate their feelings of guilt.[42]

The level of detail and the commitment to breastfeeding advice in these accounts, within contexts both meaningful and efficacious to women, remains powerful when read today. What emerges is a detailed history and aetiology of breastfeeding – assigning the causes of infant illness by community knowledge, and also the location of therapeutics in breastfeeding cessation. This body of ethnographic and historical record offers insights to current debates and understandings of DOHaD approaches, in the light of the burst of new scientific work on NCDs. We have in the South African data the following key themes: the social embeddedness of the practice of breastfeeding occurring in tandem with complex management required to thwart the potential dangers involved in breastfeeding – managed through taboos, avoidance and so on; and then the relationship of these to sexuality and child spacing. In the light of this, a strong disjuncture emerges around current exhortations to exclusively breastfeed, especially when this appears not to have been practised in South Africa, or anywhere else, in human records. And lastly, the tensions over advice versus practice – between generations of women as well as clinicians – that continue to shape current understandings, as noted in the 2016 Cochrane Review cited above.

Thus in Southern Africa, over the last decade and more, initial exhortations to formula feed because of poisoned milk (directed towards HIV-infected women with babies) were followed by WHO and other exhortations to exclusively breastfeed – for all women and also for HIV-positive women with infants. How did these exhortations clash with local understandings, making it impossible either ideologically or materially for many women to successfully take up advice and act upon it?

A suggestive conclusion

Both of these explanations for infant ill-health causation in Hindu and isiZulu Natal families in the 1950s, provided by the Karks in their summary of infant sickness, are worth deep examination: firstly, an externalising explanation for ill-will (but which still places all the onus for cure and altered behaviour on women as mothers); and secondly, an internalising explanation (placing emphasis for sickness on the level of an individual woman's goodness and worth). These explanations for successful and faulty breastfeeding linger as spectres as we consider the implications of NCD work on the centrality of newborn and early infant nutrition on life-long health, at an individual and population level.

As we have seen, the evidence for the link between early lactation experiences of infants and their lifetime burden of chronic non-communicable diseases is persuasive. The stakes are huge. In taking up the challenge of the Cochrane Review experts in 2016, the carefully planned and detailed team-based work of Eva Salber and the Karks provides just such a model for the work ahead today. For all of these reasons the archive of extant work on breastfeeding in South Africa, before and through the era of HIV, provides a rare and valuable resource, supporting the view of breastfeeding as a complex and layered set of practices, including in regions where traditional forms of breastfeeding – as described in the scientific literature – live on.

Notes

1 Kelishadi and Farajian, 'The Protective Effects of Breastfeeding'; Katarzyna et al., 'Family Factors'; Costanian, 'Inadequate Prenatal Care Use and Breastfeeding Practices'; Gowshall and Taylor-Robinson, 'The Increasing Prevalence of Non-Communicable Diseases'.

2 Kelishadi and Farajian, 'The Protective Effects of Breastfeeding', 1.

3 Gluckman and Hanson (eds.), *Developmental Origins of Health and Disease*.
4 Gluckman, Buklijas, and Hanson, 'The Developmental Origins of Health and Disease (DOHaD) Concept'.
5 Cullinan and Thom (eds.), *The Virus, Vitamins and Vegetables*; Baldwin-Ragaven, de Grunchy, and London (eds.), *An Ambulance of the Wrong Colour*; Cameron, *Witness to Aids*; Mbali, 'AIDS Discourses and the South African State'; Mbali, 'TAC in the History of Rights-Based, Patient-Driven AIDS Activism'; McGregor, *Khabzela*; Digby and Phillips, *At the Heart of Healing*.
6 Avery, Duckett, and Frantzich, 'The Experience of Sexuality during Breastfeeding'; Polomeno, 'Sex and Breastfeeding'; Alder and Bancroft, 'The Relationship between Breastfeeding Persistence, Sexuality and Mood'; Sibeko and Dhansay et al., 'Beliefs, Attitudes, and Practices of Breastfeeding Mothers'.
7 Auerbach, 'Induced Lactation'; Szucs et al., 'Induced Lactation and Exclusive Breast Milk Feeding'; Newman and Goldfarb, *The Protocols for Induced Lactation*.
8 Mobbs, 'Human Imprinting and Breastfeeding'; Mobbs et al., 'Imprinting, Attachment and Displacement'.
9 World Health Organization, 'Exclusive Breastfeeding'; Kramer and Kakuma, 'Optimal Duration of Exclusive Breastfeeding'; *Lancet*, 'Breastfeeding'.
10 World Health Organization, 'Infant and Young Child Feeding'.
11 Jaga mentions South Africa's stated commitment to support breastfeeding, its support for the United Nation's Sustainable Development Goals recommendations on breastfeeding, as well as a country-specific Code of Good Practice in the Basic Conditions of Employment Act (which mandates two 30-minute breastfeeding breaks for lactating workers in a day). However, Jaga has also established that human resource departments, employers, as well as the public sector, and all registered unions – including the female-dominated Southern African Clothing and Textile Workers Union (SACTWU) – neither know about nor offer support for breastfeeding.
12 World Health Organization, 'Infant and Young Child Feeding'.
13 Marks, 'South Africa's Early Experiment in Social Medicine'; Marks, 'Doctors and the State'.
14 Kuper, Watts, and Davies, *Durban*, 43; for a recent exploration of race in relation to schooling in Durban, see Hunter, *Race for Education*.
15 Salber, *The Mind is not the Heart*, 116; Kark and Kark, *Promoting Community Health*; Salber, 'Growth of South African Babies'; Salber and Bradshaw, 'Birth Weights of South African Babies'.
16 Hunter, *Reaction to Conquest*; Schapera, *Married Life in an African Tribe*; Junod, *The Life of a South African*; Krige, *The Social System of the Zulus*; Ngubane, *Body and Mind in Zulu Medicine*.
17 Kark and Kark, *Promoting Community Health*, 144.
18 Fildes, *Breasts, Bottles and Babies*; Jelliffe and Jelliffe, *Human Milk in the Modern World*; Wickes, 'A History of Infant Feeding'; Porter (ed.), *The Cambridge Illustrated History of Medicine*; Porter and Bynum, *Companion Encyclopedia of the History of Medicine*.
19 Hymansen, 'A Short Review of the History of Infant Feeding'.
20 Martin traces views about breastfeeding in the *Lancet*. In 1842 it recorded the case of a woman who breastfed her child for over three years and then developed epilepsy. The attending physician wrote: 'The worst symptoms of debility at last attended this monstrous proceeding'. See R. Martin, 'Commentary'.
21 'Colostrum is the earliest breast milk produced, beginning in mid-pregnancy (12–18 weeks) and is continually produced for the first few days after the baby's birth. It is thick, sticky, concentrated milk and is usually yellow, clear or white, although it could be other colours as well. It is made up of immune factors, protein, sugar, and fats.' La Leche League International, 'Colostrum'.
22 'Meconium is the thick, sticky, tarry-appearing foetal stool that is passed in the several days after birth (and sometimes before birth). It is the digested residue of swallowed amniotic fluid.' Hull, 'Meconium'.
23 Jelliffe and Jelliffe, *Human Milk*, 164.
24 Wickes, 'History of Infant Feeding', 416–22.
25 Links between the rise of eugenics and imperial motherhood were demonstrated in one of the most widely cited papers in this field, on infant rearing and campaigns aimed at the European working class. See Davin, 'Imperialism and Motherhood'. The link between motherhood and breastfeeding and eugenics in the 1930s has been traced also by Bock, 'Racism and Sexism in Nazi Germany'. The history of colonial debates about this has been

addressed in Hunt's *A Colonial Lexicon*. The way in which the South African state mobilised these arguments to create and defend 'whites' and white women has been examined by Klausen in *Race, Maternity, and the Politics of Birth Control*. I have traced this in relation to motherhood campaigns aimed at black South African women in Burns, 'Reproductive Labours', and in Burns, 'Sexual and Reproductive Health and Rights'.

26 This is explored in detail in Burns, 'Reproductive Labours'. See Brown, 'Facing the "Black Peril"'; Klugman, 'Population Policy in South Africa'.

27 W. Laubengayer, 'The Evolution of the Art of Infant Feeding in Relation to the Development of the Science of Nutrition' (Unpublished PhD Thesis, Ithaca: Cornell University, 1935).

28 Greiner summarises this in 'Exclusive Breastfeeding'. For a paper weighing the complexity of defining exclusive breastfeeding in practice see Noel-Weiss et al., 'Questioning Current Definitions for Breastfeeding Research'.

29 A useful summary of all nutritional science of breastfeeding literature from the 1950s to 2000 is in Latham, *Nutritional Data on Breastfeeding*; also very helpful is Wolf, 'Low Breastfeeding Rates'; Simonds, 'Watching the Clock'.

30 This is summarised in Coovadia et al., 'The Health and Health System of South Africa' and Chopra et al., 'Saving the Lives of South Africa's Mothers, Babies, and Children'.

31 The Cochrane Review studied the evidence for different forms of breastfeeding globally. This was updated again in 2016. The review found many gaps in research and many inconclusive studies – and set out the many flaws in cited research and the basis on which better research has to proceed in this area. See Balogun et al., 'Interventions for Promoting the Initiation of Breastfeeding'.

32 Couto de Oliveira et al., 'Extending Breastfeeding Duration through Primary Care' and Heinig, 'Development of Effective Strategies to Support Breastfeeding'.

33 La Leche League International, 'Colostrum'.

34 Aarts, 'Exclusive Breastfeeding'; Aarts et al., 'How Exclusive is Exclusive Breastfeeding?'.

35 Carael and Piot, 'HIV Infection in Developing Countries'.

36 Coutsoudis et al., 'Influence of Infant-Feeding Patterns'.

37 McIntyre and Gray, 'What Can We Do to Reduce Mother to Child Transmission of HIV?'.

38 Coutsoudis et al., 'Method of Feeding and Transmission of HIV-1 from Mothers to Children'; Coovadia et al., 'Mother-to-Child Transmission of HIV-1 Infection'.

39 Ndaba, 'Breast Feeding Patterns of HIV Positive Mothers'.

40 Fallon et al., 'Baby-led Compared with Scheduled (or Mixed) Breastfeeding'.

41 Kark and Kark, *Promoting Community Health*, 144.

42 Kark and Kark, *Promoting Community Health*, 144.

Bibliography

Aarts, C. 'Exclusive Breastfeeding – Does It Make a Difference?: A Longitudinal, Prospective Study of Daily Feeding Practices, Health and Growth in a Sample of Swedish Infants'. PhD defended and published by the University of Uppsala, Sweden, 2001.

Aarts, C. et al. 'How Exclusive Is Exclusive Breastfeeding? A Comparison of Data since Birth with Current Status Data', *International Journal of Epidemiology*, 29 (2000): 1041–6.

Alder, E. and J. Bancroft. 'The Relationship between Breastfeeding Persistence, Sexuality And Mood in Postpartum Women', *Psychological Medicine*, 18 (1988): 389–96.

Auerbach, K. G. 'Induced Lactation: A Study of Adoptive Nursing by 240 Women', *American Journal of the Diseases of Children*, 135 (4) (1981): 340–3.

Avery, M. D., L. Duckett, and C. R. Frantzich. 'The Experience of Sexuality during Breastfeeding among Primiparous Women', *Journal of Midwifery & Women's Health*, 45 (2006): 227–37.

Baldwin-Ragaven, L., J. de Grunchy, and L. London (eds.). *An Ambulance of the Wrong Colour: Health Professionals, Human Rights and Ethics in South Africa*. Cape Town: University of Cape Town Press, 1999.

Balogun, Olukunmi O. et al. 'Interventions for Promoting the Initiation of Breastfeeding'. *Cochrane Database of Systematic Reviews*, 1. Art. No.: CD001688 (2016).

Bock, G. 'Racism and Sexism in Nazi Germany: Motherhood, Compulsory Sterilization, and the State', *Signs*, 8 (3) (1983): 4004–21.

Brown, B. 'Facing the "Black Peril": The Politics of Population Control in South Africa', *Journal of Southern African Studies*, 13 (1987): 256–73.

Burns, Catherine. 'Reproductive Labours: The Politics of Women's Health in South Africa, 1900–1960'. Unpublished PhD, Northwestern University, Evanston, 1995.

Burns, Catherine. 'Sexual and Reproductive Health and Rights', *South African Health Review*. Durban: Health Systems Trust, 2010.

Cameron, E. *Witness to Aids*. Cape Town: Tafelberg, 2005.

Carael, Michel and Peter Piot. 'HIV Infection in Developing Countries', *Journal of Biosocial Science*, 10 (1989): 44.

Chopra, M. et al. 'Saving the Lives of South Africa's Mothers, Babies, and Children: Can the Health System Deliver?' *Lancet: Health in South Africa Series*, 374 (9692) (2009): 835–46.

Coovadia, H. et al. 'The Health and Health System of South Africa: Historical Roots of Current Public Health Challenges', *Lancet: Health in South Africa Series*, 374 (9692) (2009): 817–34.

Coovadia, H. et al. 'Mother-to-Child Transmission of HIV-1 Infection during Exclusive Breastfeeding in the First 6 Months of Life: An Intervention Cohort Study', *Lancet*, 369 (9567) (2017): 1107–16.

Costanian, C. 'Inadequate Prenatal Care Use and Breastfeeding Practices in Canada: A National Survey of Women', *BMC Pregnancy and Childbirth*, 16 (2016).

Couto de Oliveira, M. N. et al. 'Extending Breastfeeding Duration through Primary Care: A Systematic Review of Prenatal and Postnatal Interventions', *Journal of Human Lactation*, 17 (4) (2001): 326–43.

Coutsoudis, A. et al. 'Influence of Infant-Feeding Patterns on Early Mother-to-Child Transmission of HIV-1 in Durban, South Africa: A Prospective Cohort Study. South African Vitamin A Study Group', *Lancet*, 354 (9177) (1999): 4716.

Coutsoudis, A. et al. 'Method of Feeding and Transmission of HIV-1 from Mothers to Children by 15 Months of Age: Prospective Cohort Study from Durban, South Africa', *AIDS*, 15 (2001): 379–87.

Cullinan, K. and A. Thom (eds.). *The Virus, Vitamins and Vegetables*. Johannesburg: Jacana, 2009.

Davin, A. 'Imperialism and Motherhood', *History Workshop Journal*, 5 (1) (1978).

Digby, A. and H. Phillips. *At the Heart of Healing: Groote Schuur Hospital 1938 to 2009*. Cape Town: Jacana Press, 2008.

Fallon, A. et al. 'Patterns of Breastfeeding, According to the Baby or According to the Clock', last modified 27 September 2016, www.cochrane.org/CD009067/PREG_patterns-breastfeeding-according-baby-or-according-clock. Accessed 4 August 2019.

Fallon, A. et al. 'Baby-Led Compared with Scheduled (or Mixed) Breastfeeding for Successful Breastfeeding', *Cochrane Database of Systematic Reviews*, 9 (CD009067) (2016).

Fildes, V. *Breasts, Bottles and Babies: A History of Infant Feeding*. Edinburgh: Edinburgh University Press, 1986.

Fokazi, Sipokazi. 'Employers Can Milk Breastfeeding for Their Own Benefit', last modified 16 May 2019,https://select.timeslive.co.za/news/2019-05-16-employers-can-milk-breastfeeding-for-their-own-benefit-says-expert.

Gluckman, P., T. Buklijas, and M. A. Hanson. 'The Developmental Origins of Health and Disease (DOHaD) Concept: Past, Present, and Future'. In *The Epigenome and Developmental Origins of Health and Disease*, edited by C. Rosenfeld. Amsterdam: Elsevier, 2016.

Gluckman, P. and M. Hanson (eds.). *Developmental Origins of Health and Disease*. Cambridge: Cambridge University Press, 2006.

Gowshall, M. and S. D. Taylor-Robinson. 'The Increasing Prevalence of Non-Communicable Diseases in Low-Middle Income Countries: The View from Malawi', *International Journal of General Medicine*, 2811 (2018): 255–64.

Greiner, Ted. 'Exclusive Breastfeeding: Measurement and Indicators', *International Breastfeeding Journal*, 9 (18) (2014), doi.org/10.1186/1746-4358-9-18.

Heinig, M. J. 'Development of Effective Strategies to Support Breastfeeding', *Journal of Human Lactation*, 17 (4) (2001): 293–4.

Hull, Jeffrey W. 'Meconium', last modified 2012, www.drhull.com/EncyMaster/M/meconium.html.

Hunt, N. R. *A Colonial Lexicon of Birth Ritual, Medicalization, and Mobility in the Congo*. Durham, NC: Duke University Press, 1999.

Hunter, Mark. *Race for Education*. Cambridge: Cambridge University Press, 2019.

Hunter, Monica. *Reaction to Conquest: Effects of Contact with Europeans on the Pondo of South Africa*. Oxford: Oxford University Press, 1936.

Hymansen, A. 'A Short Review of the History of Infant Feeding', *Archives of Pediatrics*, (1934): 51.

Jelliffe, B. D. and E. F. P Jelliffe. *Human Milk in the Modern World*. Oxford: Oxford University Press, 1978.

Junod, H. *The Life of a South African Tribe*. Neuchatel: IAF, 1912.

Kark, S. and E. Kark. *Promoting Community Health from Pholela to Jerusalem*. Johannesburg: Witwatersrand University Press, 2001.

Katarzyna, Z. et al. 'Family Factors Associated with Selected Childhood Nutrition Aspects in Central Poland', *International Journal of Environmental Research and Public Health*, 16 (4) (2019): 541.

Kelishadi, R. and S. Farajian. 'The Protective Effects of Breastfeeding on Chronic Non-Communicable Diseases in Adulthood: A Review of Evidence', *Advanced Biomedical Research*, 3 (3) (2014): 1.

Klausen, S. *Race, Maternity, and the Politics of Birth Control in South Africa, 1910–1939*. Basingstoke and New York: Palgrave Macmillan, 2004.

Klugman, B. 'Population Policy in South Africa: A Critical Perspective', *Development Southern Africa*, 8 (14) (1991): 19–31.

Kramer, M. and R. Kakuma. 'Optimal Duration of Exclusive Breastfeeding, Review', *The Cochrane Library*, 4 (2009).

Krige, E. *The Social System of the Zulus*. New York: Longmans, 1936.

Kuper, L., W. H. Watts, and R. Davies. *Durban: A Study in Racial Ecology*. London: Jonathan Cape, 1958.

La Leche League International. 'Colostrum: General', last modified 2020, www.llli.org/breast feeding-info/colostrum-general.

Lancet. 'Breastfeeding', last modified 2019, www.thelancet.com/series/breastfeeding.

Latham, M. C. *Nutritional Data on Breastfeeding: Food and Agriculture Organization of the United Nations*. Rome: UN Publications, 1997.

Laubengayer, W. B. 'The Evolution of the Art of Infant Feeding in Relation to the Development of the Science of Nutrition'. Unpublished PhD Thesis, Ithaca, NY: Cornell University, 1935.

Marks, Shula. 'South Africa's Early Experiment in Social Medicine', *American Journal of Public Health*, 87 (3) (1997): 452–9.

Marks, Shula. 'Doctors and the State: George Gale and South Africa's Experiment in Social Medicine'. In *Science and Society in Southern Africa*, edited by S. Dubow, 188–211. Manchester: Manchester University Press, 2000.

Martin, R. 'Commentary: Does Breastfeeding for Longer Cause Children to Be Shorter?' *International Journal of Epidemiology*, 30, (3) (2001): 481.

Mbali, M. 'AIDS Discourses and the South African State: Government Denialism and Post-Apartheid AIDS Policy-Making', *Transformation*, 54 (2004): 104–22.

Mbali, M. 'TAC in the History of Rights-Based, Patient-Driven AIDS Activism in South Africa'. In *Democratising Development: The Politics of Socio-economic Rights in South Africa*, edited by K. Stokke and P. Jones, 21– 44. Leiden: Martinus Nijhoff, 2005.

McGregor, L. *Khabzela: The Life and Times of a South African*. Johannesburg: Jacana Press, 2007.

McIntyre, J. and G. Gray. 'What Can We Do to Reduce Mother to Child Transmission of HIV?', *BMJ (Clinical Research Ed.)*, 324 (7331) (2002): 218–21.

Mobbs, E. 'Human Imprinting and Breastfeeding – Are the Textbooks Deficient?' *Breastfeeding Review* (1989): 39–41.

Mobbs, E. et al. 'Imprinting, Attachment and Displacement: A Mini Review of Early Instinctual Behaviour in Newborn Infants Influencing Breastfeeding Success', *Acta Paediatrica*, 105 (1) (2016): 24–30.

Ndaba, T. C. 'Breastfeeding Patterns of HIV Positive Mothers in the Context of Mother to Child Transmission in Kwazulu-Natal.' Unpublished Masters Thesis, UKZN, 2003.

Newman, J. and L. Goldfarb. *The Protocols for Induced Lactation: A Guide for Maximizing Breastmilk Production*. New York: Prima Publishing, 2000.

Ngubane, H. *Body and Mind in Zulu Medicine: An Ethnography of Health and Disease in Nyuswa-Zulu Thought and Practice*. London: Academic Press, 1977.

Noel-Weiss, J. et al. 'Questioning Current Definitions for Breastfeeding Research', *International Breastfeeding Journal*, 7 (1) (2012): 9.

Polomeno, V. 'Sex and Breastfeeding: An Educational Perspective', *Journal of Perinatal Education*, 8 (1) (1999): 30–40.

Porter, R. (ed.). *The Cambridge Illustrated History of Medicine*. Cambridge: Cambridge University Press, 1996.

Porter, R. and W. F. Bynum. *Companion Encyclopedia of the History of Medicine*. London: Routledge, 1993.

Salber, E. J. 'Growth of South African Babies in the First Year of Life', *Human Biology*, 24 (12) (1957): 12–39.

Salber, E. J. *The Mind is not the Heart*. Durham, NC: University of North Carolina Press, 1993.

Salber, E. J. and E. Bradshaw. 'Birth Weights of South African Babies', *British Journal of Social Medicine*, 5 (1951): 1139.

Schapera, I. *Married Life in an African Tribe*. Faber: London, 1940.

Sibeko, L. and M. Dhansay et al. 'Beliefs, Attitudes, and Practices of Breastfeeding Mothers from a Periurban Community in South Africa', *Journal of Human Lactation*, 21 (1) (2005): 313–8.

Simonds, W. 'Watching the Clock: Keeping Time During Pregnancy, Birth, and Postpartum Experiences', *Social Science & Medicine*, 55 (4) (2002): 559–70.

Swindler, Helen. 'Why Breastfeeding is a Workplace Issue', last modified 10 May 2019, www.news.uct.ac.za/article/-2019-05-10-why-breastfeeding-is-a-workplace-issue.

Szucs, K. et al. 'Induced Lactation and Exclusive Breast Milk Feeding of Adopted Premature Twins', *Journal of Human Lactation*, 26 (3) (2010): 309–13.

Wickes, I. G. 'A History of Infant Feeding' Part I, II, III and IV, *Archives of Disease in Childhood*, 28 (1953).

Wolf, J. H. 'Low Breastfeeding Rates and Public Health in the United States', *American Journal of Public Health*, 93 (12) (2003): 2000–10.

World Health Organization. 'Infant and Young Child Feeding', last modified 16 February 2018, www.who.int/news-room/fact-sheets/detail/infant-and-young-child-feeding.

World Health Organization. 'Exclusive Breastfeeding for Six Months Best for Babies Everywhere', last modified 15 January 2011, accessed 20 October 2019, www.who.int/mediacentre/news/statements/2011/breastfeeding_20110115/en/.

11

High BP among Adults and Children with HIV

Betsey Behr Brada

Boitumelo and her *nkoko*

After a few weeks of observing at the Superlative Clinic, Botswana's only outpatient paediatric HIV clinic, I had begun to get used to the routine: At 7.30 a.m. the doors opened to the queue of adults and children waiting outside.[1] The queue then moved inside, where they waited to check in at the reception desk with Mma Goitsemang, the Clinic's receptionist, who assigned them a pink numbered card.[2] The nurse assigned to triage began taking the children one by one to a small room behind the reception area, documenting their weight and temperature. The Clinic's paediatricians, many of them young American physicians, passed silently through the waiting area and into the consulting rooms. The other nurses milled around the reception desk, greeting one another and stacking the binders that held the records of the children scheduled to be seen that day. They eventually began to call the names listed on their binders and escorted each child and the accompanying adult to one of the consulting rooms at the back of the building.

I had arranged the day before to shadow Koketso, the Clinic's young social worker, but it took me some time to find her. She beckoned to me to follow and then walked upstairs to the second floor. This perplexed me: there were no consulting rooms on the second floor, only a classroom, the Clinic's administrative offices, and the computer lab. A poised young woman finishing up her social work degree at the University of Botswana, Koketso usually spent her time on the Clinic's first floor, moving serenely from one consulting room to another as needed: helping one woman apply to Botswana's food basket programme on behalf of her orphaned niece, facilitating a referral for another child to the audiology clinic in Ramotswa, 35km to the south and, with the help of the Clinic's formidable and well-respected head nurse, cajoling a third child's aunt and uncle into monitoring his daily antiretroviral medications (ARVs) more closely.[3] On this morning, however, Koketso was distinctly flustered. Shuffling the papers in her arms, she walked into the classroom where, improbably, we found the Clinic director, Dr Buyaga. The director, who tended to involve himself little in the lives of individual patients or the Clinic's day-to-day activities, was sitting with a young child in tears. The child jumped to her feet as Koketso entered the room and addressed her in Setswana too rapid and broken for me to follow. Dr Buyaga, born and raised in East Africa, gently urged the child in English to sit down, a request Koketso repeated in Setswana. Through sobs and false starts and with Koketso's many whispered asides to me, the child's story slowly emerged.

Boitumelo, nine years old, had lived all of her life with her maternal grandmother – first in the company of her mother and then, after her mother passed away a few years earlier, alone. Boitumelo's *nkoko* (granny) was well known to the Clinic staff. In Botswana women have historically provided the lion's share of care to family members in need, and even when Boitumelo's mother had been alive, her grandmother had most frequently brought the young Boitumelo to the Clinic. It was her grandmother who diligently supervised her daily medications and her medical care more generally while Boitumelo's mother had worked cleaning houses to support her mother and child until she herself became too ill. The reason Boitumelo sat before us in tears was that her beloved grandmother had suffered a stroke two days earlier and was presently confined to a bed in the hospital's adult medical ward, her prognosis uncertain. Boitumelo had been taken in temporarily by her mother's unmarried cousin, but the cousin had pleaded that her job, which required frequent travel, was simply too demanding for her to provide long-term care for Boitumelo. Just that morning, Dr Buyaga explained, the cousin had dropped Boitumelo off at the Superlative Clinic but had insisted she was unable to stay for a meeting with Clinic staff. Boitumelo had no contact with her father, Koketso added, and Boitumelo's mother's only sibling, a brother, had predeceased her. Boitumelo's grandmother's surviving sister was rather frail and relied on an adult son in South Africa for financial support.

As Boitumelo slumped in her chair, Koketso and Dr Buyaga kept returning to the question of how best to maintain Boitumelo's adherence to her ARVs. Boitumelo's grandmother had begun to have trouble with hypertension over the past year, Koketso recounted, and the potential for her failing health to affect her care for Boitumelo had surfaced from time to time as Clinic staff had discussed Boitumelo, but no backup plan had been solidified. Clinic staff had seen several cases where the disruption of a child's living situation had interrupted their adherence, leading them to develop resistance to first-line medications and requiring them to take second-line medications instead.[4] Finally, at Dr Buyaga's urging, Koketso pulled out her cell phone and called SOS Children's Village in Tlokweng.[5] Despite a general apprehension in south-eastern Botswana regarding non-kin-based care for children who had lost one or both parents,[6] Koketso and Dr Buyaga agreed that SOS was the solution best suited to keeping Boitumelo on track with her medications, which had to be taken on a strict schedule every 12 hours. As Koketso collected the child and her belongings, Boitumelo tearfully asked when she would see her *nkoko*, a question that hung in the air as she walked from the room.

Adult hypertension and paediatric HIV in Botswana's treatment era

Drawing on ethnographic fieldwork conducted in south-eastern Botswana in 2006–8 and 2012, this chapter analyses the complex relationships between adult hypertension and paediatric HIV. It highlights the narrowing of disease categories that global health programmes address amid the increased pressures on ageing women to manage both children's HIV infections and their own health. On one hand, cases of paediatric HIV brought hypertensive adult women under the clinical gaze. On the other, the narrow focus within global health initiatives on HIV/AIDS and the even narrower focus within the Superlative Clinic on children hindered efforts to treat kin groups as anything other than a set of discrete units whose relationships with one another were incidental or, at best, a secondary consideration. I show how these tensions played out in clinical encounters, prompting the creation of a Family Clinic that attempted to reconcile these contradictions through a more holistic approach to the care of families. Yet Clinic administrators, I show, increasingly restricted enrolment in Family Clinic due to fears that resources were being diverted from both a specific disease and a specific demographic. Taking a cue from the anthropological literature on syndemics, I illustrate, first, how uncontrolled adult hypertension threatened to amplify or exacerbate paediatric HIV infections and, second, why this posed such a conundrum to US-driven transnational health interventions in Botswana. More broadly, by emphasising the patterns through which syndemics span bodies and generations, this paper demonstrates the limitations of global health interventions that conceptualise diseases as bounded entities rather than as always already embedded in relations.

This story is set against the expansion of access to antiretroviral treatment across the African continent and the emergence of public–private partnerships for global health.[7] Through the late 1990s, as death tolls mounted worldwide, pharmaceutical manufacturers, under fire for allegedly contributing to thousands of deaths by pricing ARVs beyond the reach of those who most needed them, responded with high-profile initiatives, providing discounts to some countries through UN-sponsored programmes, engaging in corporate philanthropy and forming public–private partnerships.[8] Botswana's treatment programme emerged from one such partnership. By 2000, despite decades of steady economic growth and political stability, its relatively robust public health system and its small population, Botswana had one of the highest HIV prevalence rates in the world.[9] High diamond prices may have sheltered Botswana from the radical downscaling of public services that accompanied structural adjustment programmes in the region.[10] Nevertheless, few of Botswana's approximately 1.7 million citizens could afford ARVs through the private sector.

That year, the then-president Festus Mogae raised the possibility of Botswana's 'national extinction' at the International AIDS Conference and requested international assistance.[11] The government began co-operating with the African Comprehensive HIV/AIDS Partnership, a collaboration between the Bill and Melinda Gates Foundation and the Merck Corporation Foundation that supported the healthcare training and infrastructural development the treatment programme required.[12] By 2002 the government was distributing ARVs in Gaborone; even so, the number of deaths attributed to the virus continued to rise, peaking at more than 15,000 in 2003 alone.[13] Three years later the programme had enrolled more than 20,000 patients, the highest ratio of HIV-positive citizens enrolled in treatment on the continent at the time.[14] By 2008, an estimated 80,000 Batswana were receiving ARVs.

As the treatment programme expanded so did the number of partnerships, each awkwardly linking public and private institutions. Located in the grounds of a public hospital, the Superlative Clinic was operated by a partnership between Botswana's Ministry of Health and the Children's HIV/AIDS Network (CHAN), an American NGO that received a portion of its funding through transnational pharmaceutical philanthropy. CHAN had been founded in the late 1990s by a paediatric infectious disease specialist and focused exclusively on the treatment of HIV-positive children, supporting several specialised clinics across Africa. The composition of the Clinic's staff reflected this intermingling of affiliations. Most physicians were Americans with specialised training in paediatrics and HIV treatment.[15] All the nurses were Batswana. More broadly, the presence of foreign specialists in the Clinic was shaped by Botswana's historical emphasis on primary healthcare and reliance on nurses and non-specialist physicians. The country did not open a medical school within its borders until 2009 and, apart from nurses, the government has tended to depend on foreigners and on Batswana trained outside the country to fill positions in public hospitals.[16] While qualified Batswana received government support to study medicine abroad, many remained abroad after their training and only a small fraction of those who returned to work in Botswana's public health system received training in specialised fields such as paediatrics and infectious disease.

The Superlative Clinic was the conjunction, then, of a narrow set of clinicians with a narrow set of patients. In 1999, before ARVs were publicly available, clinicians in Botswana had begun enrolling HIV-positive pregnant women into a UNICEF-sponsored programme aimed at the prevention of mother-to-child transmission (PMTCT) of HIV. These programmes offered HIV-positive pregnant women a short course of ARVs that reduced the likelihood that the child they carried would contract the virus. The programme was highly successful in reducing transmission rates between women and the children they bore, and in 2001 Botswana's government incorporated the PMTCT programme into its national health services.[17] The children attending the Clinic, then, were born before PMTCT became available, born to women unable to access the programme, or belonged to the small number of children for whom the intervention was ineffective. The Superlative Clinic was the only institution in the country dedicated specifically to their care.

These children were viewed with some ambivalence. As I have argued elsewhere, while the survival of HIV-positive children marked the treatment programme's success and the state's ability to keep them alive, their survival served both as a reminder of the epidemic and a lingering threat to the project of managing it.[18] Individually, these children required a great deal of care, straining the already limited resources of extended kin. More broadly, HIV-positive children were incompatible with fantasies of an 'AIDS-free generation', a fact reflected in the public censure towards women who become pregnant after receiving a HIV-positive diagnosis.[19] So, while many children in Botswana depended on members of their extended families, and particularly older women, for elements of daily care, such as feeding, bathing and clothing, caring for these HIV-positive children also entailed the demands of their infections, including adherence to their antiretroviral medications and attendance at regular clinic appointments.[20]

But if the survival of Botswana's HIV-positive children has been both a national project, however ambivalent, as well as part of a more transnational concern around African AIDS orphans, the health of the adults, particularly of the women, who care for them has received far less attention.[21] Behind this story of the emergence of HIV in southern Africa, its climax in the early 2000s, and the implementation of targeted treatment and support programmes, is a story of rising hypertension and other non-communicable diseases (NCDs) against a backdrop of broader demographic changes. As Botswana's public services, including public health, expanded through the first decades of independence, infant mortality rates fell sharply from 98/1000 live births in 1971 to 37/1000 in 1994, and life expectancy increased from 48 years in 1966 to 65.3 years in 1991.[22] The population over the age of 60 doubled between 1971 and 1991.[23] The total fertility rate fell from 6.2 children per woman in 1980 to 2.6 children in 2006.[24] But despite these gains, and even as Botswana began launching HIV awareness campaigns in the late 1980s and early 1990s, Ministry of Health reports pointed to cardiovascular disease as the third leading cause of death in the country, and incidence rates of hypertension and other NCDs continued to rise.[25] The picture presented by Botswana's health statistics from the past three and a half decades, then, is one where, as the HIV epidemic gained hold on the country through the 1990s, those adults who survived this epidemic, which doubled or even tripled mortality among individuals aged 25–40 between 1991 and 1998,[26] shouldered increasing demands to care for ill family members and dependent children even as they faced increasing risks to their own health.[27]

These risks and burdens are distinctly gendered. Data from Botswana's Ministry of Health shows a five-fold increase in the prevalence of hypertension through the 1980s and 1990s, with far more women than men dying as a result of the condition over the latter of those two decades.[28] Very generally, these increases follow broader epidemiological trends of non-communicable diseases (NCDs) in sub-Saharan Africa attributed to a combination of economic development, rapid urbanisation and changes in diet alongside other factors such as patterns of alcohol and tobacco consumption.[29] The conjunction of epidemics of infectious diseases with non-communicable ones constitutes what some clinical researchers have called a 'double burden'.[30] The marked gendered disparity of this double burden has continued into the treatment era of Botswana's HIV epidemic. Analysing survey data collected in 2007, Keetile et al. found that, while the risk of conditions like hypertension increased with age for both women and men, hypertension was much more common amongst women than men (18.9 per cent versus 9.9 per cent) and women were nearly twice as likely to have hypertension as their male counterparts when controlling for age, socioeconomic factors and risk factors.[31] A broader set of risk factors for NCDs more generally were also unevenly distributed across gender: more than half of women surveyed were overweight and nearly a quarter were obese, compared to 22.1 per cent and 5.6 per cent of men, respectively.[32] Women surveyed in 2007 drank less and smoked far less than men did, but they shared with men a diet low in vegetables and fruit and they were more likely than men to be physically inactive, twice as likely as men to be overweight and four to five times more likely than men to be obese.[33] These gendered disparities held constant in survey data collected in 2014.[34]

The gendered embodiment of the double burden in Botswana has materialised at the level of the household. Stover et al. estimate that in 2007 some 130,000 children, or 16 per cent of Batswana under the age of 18, had survived the loss of one or both parents, and that three-quarters of these deaths were attributable to HIV/AIDS.[35] Orphaned children, whether HIV-positive or not, relied predominantly upon elderly female kin: one study found that nearly half of Tswana households caring for an orphan (that is, a child who had lost at least one parent or their primary caregiver) were headed by grandmothers.[36] These elderly women faced their own challenges: a small survey of grandmothers and aunts caring for orphaned Tswana children found that most of the grandmothers reported 'chronic and degenerative conditions'.[37] Despite the existence of social supports such as orphan food baskets and old age pensions, for some Tswana grandmothers the confluence of their own poor health and the needs of the orphaned infants and children in their care has hampered their engagement in agricultural activities or other informal work, thereby contributing to their impoverishment.[38]

It is only quite recently, however, that NCDs have attracted policy attention both in Botswana and in sub-Saharan Africa more generally. Tapela et al. observe that prior to 2016 Botswana lacked any national policy or strategy on NCDs per se.[39] In 2007 the Ministry of Health conducted its first STEPWISE (STEPS) Noncommunicable Disease Risk

Factor Survey, part of the World Health Organization's Adult Risk Factor Surveillance project. This survey indicated that NCDs accounted for 31 per cent of all deaths in Botswana and prompted a series of assessments, policy strategies and legislative tools aimed specifically at tobacco and alcohol, including a 30 per cent levy on alcohol in 2008, and the inclusion of NCDs in Botswana's National Health Policy in 2009.[40] In the wake of the first Africa Regional Ministerial Consultation on NCDs and the United Nations high-level meeting on NCD prevention and control in 2011, the government of Botswana began devising national guidelines for primary healthcare, including clinical guidelines for the management of NCDs. In 2015, it began working toward a multi-sectoral strategy aimed at the prevention and control of NCDs, including them in the country's National Development Plan for 2017–2022.[41]

During my fieldwork in the first decade of Botswana's treatment programme, however, this attention to NCDs was markedly absent despite the fact that many HIV-positive children in Botswana were cared for by, and dependent upon, a generation of women most of whom were currently afflicted by hypertension or other NCDs or whose risk for these conditions was increasing over time. Moreover, despite the relationship between an older woman's own health and her ability to care for HIV-positive children in her care, the health of these women was only intermittently visible within the Superlative Clinic. At Clinic appointments, children's health was meticulously assessed and documented through biometric measurements, physical examinations and laboratory tests; the health of the women accompanying them was monitored incidentally and occasionally documented in passing. Clinic accounts of children's social situations and home visits by the Clinic's social workers took the well-being of adults into account primarily as a factor affecting an HIV-positive child's well-being. As Boitumelo's story illustrates, women's hypertension tended to become most visible in the Superlative Clinic in moments of crisis when paediatricians perceived an acute threat to children's adherence.

My point is not to emphasise the short-sightedness of the Clinic staff or to fault a particular set of clinicians, but to focus on how hypertensive adults, and women in particular, slipped in and out of visibility in the Superlative Clinic. Like the Superlative Clinic staff, I, too, was focused on HIV; hypertension was an afterthought, a phenomenon just out of the corner of my eye. On one hand, this limits what I have to say about it. Yet that limit itself is telling: it was out of the corner of many of my informants' eyes too. But it lurked, an unacknowledged constant in my field notes: child with HIV, granny with hypertension; child with HIV, auntie with diabetes; child with HIV, mother with high blood pressure. It was always there in the background. Indeed, most of the key risk factors for chronic NCDs – being female, old and living in an urban village – describe Boitumelo's *nkoko* to a tee.[42] While occlusion of the caregiving or maternal subject has, arguably, been a fairly constant feature in paediatric HIV, it is the local production of these occlusions and their particularly local effects, as Boitumelo's story reveals, that are the focus of this essay.[43]

In what follows, I use anthropological engagements with syndemics and co-morbidity to draw attention to how forms of relatedness figured in the clinical care given to HIV-positive Batswana children, and the shape of paediatricians' ambivalence toward these children's adult kin and its consequences. While concepts such as syndemics and co-morbidity draw our attention to the compounding effects of multiple afflictions in the same individual body, holding paediatric HIV and adult hypertension in the same frame shows us how these compounding effects can manifest *across* different afflictions in multiple bodies. As I try to think about interactive dimensions of what in the clinic are discrete phenomena, I find it useful to think with a Setswana category of diagnosis, *dikgaba*, where relatedness precedes and is the precondition for the illness. What might we see when we consider syndemics as phenomena that encompass multiple bodies and generations, not just multiple conditions or social factors?[44]

Compounding afflictions

Over the past two decades, anthropologists have defined syndemics in terms of three features: 1) the clustering of two or more diseases within a population; 2) the interaction of these diseases on biological, social and psychological levels; and 3) the social forces that give rise to clustering.[45] A key aspect of the term is that the two diseases are not simply co-present, but that they amplify or enhance one another synergistically.[46] Emphasising the social conditions of health disparities, syndemics:

> involve the interaction of diseases or other adverse health conditions (e.g. malnutrition, substance abuse, stress) as a consequence of a set of intertwined and mutually enhancing epidemics involving disease interactions at the biological level that develop and are sustained in a community/population because of harmful social conditions and injurious social connections.[47]

Some behaviour, in other words, 'exacerbates the negative health effect of any or all of the diseases involved'.[48] Classic cases include SAVA (substance abuse, violence and AIDS) and VIDDA (violence, immigration, depression, diabetes, abuse).[49] While analyses of syndemics, as a biocultural approach, tend to focus on the 'specific pathways by which diseases interact in the body to exacerbate health defects', they explicitly encompass social, economic and environmental factors in these interactions.[50] Syndemics, in short, are more than a sum of an individual's morbidities and more than a sum of the risk factors attributable to the individuals within a population.[51] Social scientists have also turned to the concept of co-morbidity, a concept that has, until recently, gained more traction in biomedicine than in anthropology.[52] Chronic diseases, point out the authors of a recent review, are frequently co-morbid with other infectious diseases, or even other chronic disorders.[53] These scholars emphasise the additive or compounding aspect of co-morbidity: like a syndemic, co-morbidity is more than simply the sum of two diseases. 'Co-morbidity' has more traction in biomedical discourse than does 'syndemic', but the former term has the potential to draw together conversations that might otherwise be split by biomedical frameworks or subdisciplines, paving the ground for broader recognition of the synergistic aspect of co-morbidities, particularly their social aspects.[54]

The strengths of these approaches are many. A syndemics approach pushes against biomedicine's tendency to orient itself toward the identification and isolation of single causes.[55] As Emily Mendenhall demonstrates in her work with Mexican women who have migrated to the United States, feelings as well as structural and symbolic forces promote the clustering and interaction of diabetes and depression, complicating their designation as discretely 'physical' or 'mental' health.[56] Co-morbidity emphasises the compounding effects of multiple afflictions on an individual, including the ways that an individual's ill health can put pressure on their kin, resulting in something of a negative feedback loop as ill individuals, in attempting to compensate for the burnout they perceive amongst their caregivers, exacerbate their own afflictions.[57]

That HIV treatment may take place alongside, in spite of, or encompass other forms of violence and suffering has been well documented.[58] For my purposes, syndemics and co-morbidity are useful in drawing attention to the interactions of simultaneous epidemics of HIV and hypertension as they are distributed across individual biologies *within* families and how those epidemics can amplify one another at the biological level *across* social relationships. In other words, while classic examples of syndemics and co-morbidities illustrate amplification within one individual's body, what happens when we take this analysis to a kin group? Due to the dependence of both HIV-positive children and Clinic staff on adult caregivers to manage children's ongoing adherence, paediatric HIV care offers a compelling, if not unique, point of view into these dynamics. As Clinic staff intermittently noted, the sudden illness or hospitalisation of an adult caregiver could put an HIV-positive child's adherence at risk, possibly amplifying the infection as the child's virus became resistance to treatment. Conversely, the careful management of an adult's hypertension might contribute to a child's ongoing adherence.[59] What might we see when we consider syndemics as phenomena that encompass multiple bodies and generations, not just multiple conditions or social factors?

Thinking with *dikgaba*: Relation as the site of affliction

At this juncture I want to take a slight detour into a rather different epidemiological imagination, one informed by Tswana diagnostic categories that offer a useful shift in perspective. *Dikgaba* is an illness whose features are well documented in ethnographic accounts of Tswana peoples: an illness befalls a child, often a very young, vulnerable or even unborn child. A healer divines that the cause of the child's illness is anger and sorrow on the part of one of the child's elders. It is key that the child herself has done nothing to cause this anger or sorrow. Instead, the child's illness is a consequence of the simultaneously sentimental and somatic bonds that enable kin to 'build up' one another's bodies through a love (*lerato*) which is, as Fred Klaits has argued, necessarily performative, necessarily in action; failures of this love-in-action, conversely, break bodies down.[60] Also key is that the elder may be entirely unaware of the anger or sorrow; instead, *dikgaba* was 'sent by the ancestral spirits as the punishment for the breach of respect to one's elder'.[61] The cure lies in the appeasement of the offended elder, carried out through verbal pronunciations of forgiveness and a ritual washing of the afflicted junior by the offended elder.[62]

Dikgaba diagnoses offer a useful counterpoint to concepts of co-morbidity and syndemic insofar as they *begin* from a group of related kin and trace the problem to its manifestations in individuals. In contrast to the individual afflicted body that tends to populate accounts of co-morbidity and even syndemics, relatedness precedes and is the precondition for *dikgaba*. It is, in a sense, the opposite of contact tracing, which begins with one affected (or infected) individual and traces outwards. You cannot diagnose *dikgaba* in just one person, but neither is it a population-level assessment of risk or a map of transmission. *Dikgaba* can only be understood in terms of a specific group of people whose bodily well-being is contingent on the ongoing dynamics of their interrelatedness – that is, a family, *losika* in Setswana, a term that connotes the interconnectedness of blood vessels.

Dikgaba was not a category for which Batswana reached in clinical settings; using it as a lens through which to view overlapping and intertwining patterns of HIV and NCDs is my move. And yet Batswana, confronted with affliction in clinical settings, sometimes reached beyond individual bodies in an attempt to diagnose affliction at the level of kin groups. Tswana aetiologies of illness and misfortune seeped into ostensibly biomedical spaces, and even into the accounts of biomedical practitioners: Dr Chilube, a Motswana intern, assessing an older woman who had collapsed and been admitted to the hospital unconscious, observed that the children of the family had been involved in a car accident just before the woman collapsed. He was reluctant to discount the explanatory power of the somatic and sentimental relations among kin even if it had no part in shaping his plan of treatment. In the Superlative Clinic 'Tswana medicine' was a more contentious topic: American practitioners, who regarded prayer with approbation, feared herbs would have pharmacological effects and regarded them as incompatible with ARVs. But 'Tswana medicine' was nonetheless sought by some families less as a supplement or substitute for ARVs than for its capacity to address a family's affliction *as* a family.[63]

Thinking with *dikgaba*, in contrast to a more biomedically informed epidemiological imagination, requires that we begin from the premise that one person's illness affects their intimates regardless of whether the condition is transmissible or not, and it pushes us beyond syndemics by demanding that we look at patterns of disease amplified *across* social relations.[64] It helps us understand why Tswana families make healthcare decisions as a collective even when, from a biomedical standpoint, the well-being of more than one body is not at stake.[65] A granny's debilitating stroke threatens to render her grandchild's HIV infection resistant to treatment, but not because the two conditions are present in the same body or because one individual transmits her condition to the other. It is exactly this entanglement, this dependence of individual well-being on collective well-being even when, or especially when, transmission is not the issue that remains so elusive.

Family clinic: The ambivalent position of adults in paediatric HIV treatment

The people in the room during a paediatric consultation at the Clinic commonly consisted of a doctor, a nurse, the child-patient and the child's caregiver. The nurses served as translators in the vast majority of situations as few of the paediatricians spoke more than a smattering of Setswana. A small number were able to conduct the rudiments of a physical examination, such as asking children to open their mouths or remove items of clothing, but anything beyond these requests and greetings, or the most basic questions pertaining to a patient's condition and medical history, was beyond their capabilities. This made it necessary to assign a Setswana-speaking nurse to each consulting room. Consultations sometimes ground to a halt in the circumstance that the adult accompanying the child spoke little English and no nurse was available. The consultation itself consisted of three activities: 1) an assessment of the child's adherence; 2) an assessment of the child's current state of health; and 3) counselling to reinforce a set of messages regarding adherence to the prescribed treatment and proper disclosure of a child's HIV status.[66]

In addition to assessing a child's physical health, the Clinic's paediatricians and nurses were under intense pressure to document the child's 'social situation', as a child's adherence and her well-being more generally were understood to be predicated upon her caregivers' actions. In other words, part of the clinical evaluation was an assessment and documentation of the child's relatives' ability to follow the instructions of Clinic staff. That said, Clinic staff, faced with time constraints, expressed frustration with these tasks and performed them somewhat unevenly. The result was that some patients and their families, as in the case of Boitumelo and her *nkoko*, became quite well known to the Clinic's paediatricians and nurses as well as Koketso and the Clinic's other support staff. Their files contained extensive notes about the child, her family, her caregivers' occupations and health status and other details. In other circumstances, however, paediatricians might know no more about the child in front of them than what was given in a short paragraph in the child's file. In other words, an auntie's hypertension or a granny's diabetes might be well known to Clinic staff, or it might be more or less invisible until a crisis resulted in the child arriving at the Clinic with an adult unfamiliar with the child's condition, her regimen and Clinic procedures or, worse, a child not arriving at the Clinic for her scheduled appointment at all.

These intra-familial co-morbidities, then, were only haphazardly and partially visible for myriad reasons, some of which reflected the ways that transnational health interventions have organised and prioritised healthcare as well as biomedicine's tendency to address seemingly discrete entities in seemingly discrete individuals. The hospital within which the Superlative Clinic was located had a weekly 'Comorbidity Clinic' that focused on hypertension, type 2 diabetes and deep vein thrombosis among HIV-positive adults. Adults, particularly women, who attended the Comorbidity Clinic were asked about their living situations, and clinicians made notes regarding for whom they were caring at home and what source of support they had, if any. But the Comorbidity Clinic and the Superlative Clinic were run by separate partnerships between the hospital and two different private American medical institutions, and the two partnerships' agendas rarely intersected in everyday practice.[67] A paediatrician in the Superlative Clinic might inquire after an auntie's health and, if the auntie replied she had 'high blood" (*madi amatona*), the paediatrician might ask whether the auntie was taking medication and whether she went regularly to her own check-ups.[68] But this information was inconsistently solicited and inconsistently documented and, at the end of the day, was not the paediatrician's priority.

This broader ambivalence toward the heath of adult caregivers and the dependence of the Clinic's child-patients on the actions of these adults is reflected in the Family Clinic. In 2006, Dr Aaron, an American physician trained in adult medicine as well as paediatrics, began seeing some of the HIV-positive adults accompanying children to the Clinic. At first, this Family Clinic gained wide approval. By treating adults and children together, it offered a singularly convenient and inexpensive form of HIV care. Local and expatriate staff praised it for approaching HIV as a condition affecting whole families rather than discrete individuals. HIV-positive adults whose children attended the Clinic appreciated the expedience of 'one-stop shopping'. These adults would otherwise have had to book appointments at the hospital's adult HIV clinic, known as the Infectious Disease Care Clinic (IDCC), and hope that their own appointments coincided with their children's in order to avoid the expense of travelling to the hospital twice. They also valued the Clinic's relative privacy, its discretion and convenience, compared to the IDCC. The care available in the Family Clinic also extended far beyond HIV. While observing in the Family Clinic I witnessed adults receive treatment for everything from hypertension to haemorrhoids to wound care in addition to HIV.

Treatment that strayed too far from HIV care, however, or that involved adults whom Clinic paediatricians suspected were not directly involved in the care of an HIV-positive child (especially men), could cause murmurs among the paediatricians that the Clinic was drifting too far from its mission. The Clinic's American staff resented the expectation that they would work shifts on the hospital's inpatient paediatric ward, but this was a job that could be rotated evenly among them. The Family Clinic, on the other hand, monopolised the time of the one or two Americans trained to treat both adults and children, an arrangement that multiplied feelings of resentment among the Clinic's American staff. Perhaps unsurprisingly, then, despite the ubiquitous praise it garnered, enrolment in the Family Clinic became increasingly restricted over time. Dr Aaron left Botswana seven months after he had arrived and, of the other American physicians, only one or two were trained to treat adults as well as children. As the number of children enrolled in the Clinic increased, Dr Amy, an American paediatrician who served as the Clinic's Associate Director, insisted the Clinic focus on paediatric care and resented the time, space and manpower diverted to adults in the Family Clinic.

By the time I began fieldwork in early 2007, Dr Amy was actively reducing the number of adults enrolled in the Family Clinic and limiting patient participation to those whom, the Clinic's American staff had concluded, needed most to be offered the incentive of adult care in order to bring their children to regular appointments. Many adults who had been treated by Dr Aaron, Dr Amy told me, did not require specialised services and should have sought care at an IDCC or another public clinic. At stake in her strategy was not only the Clinic's and CHAN's commitment to HIV-positive children as a uniquely vulnerable population, but also their ability to demonstrate to their funders (and their competitors) that they offered something unique in the broader landscape of transnational global health interventions. The Family Clinic ran the risk of seeming too general, too duplicative of services already available. To put it bluntly, the Family Clinic was only indirectly in the business of saving children. The fact that so many HIV-positive children, like Boitumelo, depended on the ability of their older female relatives to manage extraordinary threats to their own health was simply not enough to make the NCDs that afflicted those women more than intermittently legible as a priority in the context of US-driven transnational HIV/AIDS interventions in sub-Saharan Africa.

Conclusion

If it is true that multi-scalar histories and political economies are written into our biologies,[69] then it is also true that this fact slips in and out of view even in, or perhaps especially in, clinical settings. The dependence, throughout the twentieth century, of many Tswana families on remittances from men working in South Africa's mines became starkly visible to me in the raspy breathing of Rra Modise, a middle-aged man who came to the hospital to collect his ARVs but whose doctor suspected silicosis. The historical trajectory of Botswana's AIDS epidemic jumped into view when Mma Pitso, whose two children, nine-year-old Neo and seven-year-old Masego, were receiving treatment at the Superlative Clinic, explained to me that her fourteen-year-old son was HIV-negative, as was her youngest child, two-year-old Boinelo. Her eldest child had been born before Mma Pitso contracted HIV; Boinelo had been born after PMTCT became widely available in Botswana. The two middle children were born near the peak of the epidemic but before their mother had access to the ARVs that prevent perinatal transmission. Epidemiological facts themselves have histories, but their visibility at any given moment is a product of social and historical context. As I have shown, the Superlative Clinic staff did attempt, however briefly, to take a broader, family-based approach to children's health that explicitly recognised the impact family members' health had on one another. But it is the failure of any of these initiatives to adequately grasp, let alone address, the interdependency of adults' and children's health that is most telling with regard to the epidemiological imagination in Botswana's HIV treatment era.

This interdependency will continue but its shape is necessarily in motion. Matlho et al. observe that Botswana's epidemic is 'ushering in a diverse cohort of older people living with HIV', both 'those aging with the disease and those who acquired the infections in older age'.[70] While the number of children who have lost one or both parents to the virus appears to be slowly decreasing as infected adults survive longer on ARVs, the adults who do care for orphaned children are increasingly likely to be HIV-positive themselves and to have increasingly complex health needs.[71] Nor can we expect Boitumelo's own needs and desires, her role vis-à-vis her family, or even her status as 'orphan' to remain unchanged.[72] *Dikgaba*, however, cautions us against trying to reconcile statistical views of individuals, however dynamic, without considering relatedness itself as a key epidemiological factor in Africa.

Notes

1 My greatest debts are to the adults and children of the Superlative Clinic. Thanks to Patrick Monnaesi, Noah Christen and Paul Molamphy for their invaluable research assistance, to Megan Vaughan and Marissa Mika for their constructive comments on the paper, and to

my fellow workshop participants for their useful feedback and encouragement. The study protocol was approved by the University of Chicago's Social and Behavioral Sciences Institutional Review Board. My research and writing were supported by the Fulbright-Hays DDRA fellowship program, the Wenner Gren Foundation, the University of Chicago Department of Anthropology and Social Sciences Collegiate Division, the Princeton Center for Health and Wellbeing, and the Reed College Anthropology Department. 'Superlative Clinic' and the names of its staff and patients are pseudonyms.

2 Throughout this essay the uppercase 'Clinic' refers specifically to the Superlative Clinic. Many Batswana use teknonyms, that is, names derived from their children; women are commonly addressed as *mma*, men as *rra*.

3 Antiretroviral medications (ARVs) disrupt the replication of HIV and are used in combination, sometimes known as highly active antiretroviral therapy (HAART). Inconsistent dosing promotes the replication of HIV strains least affected by the medications, leading to treatment failure as the medications become less effective and the child's HIV infection grows more acute. For one account of the history and politics of HAART, see Nguyen, *The Republic of Therapy*, Ch.4.

4 Brada, 'How to Do Things to Children with Words'; Brada, 'Between Discipline and Empowerment'. Second-line medications are given when a patient's initial ARV regimen can no longer control her HIV infection. Given the limited number of ARVs available through Botswana's public health system, children on second-line medication are at risk of developing an infection that cannot be adequately controlled with medication.

5 Founded in Austria in the aftermath of the Second World War, SOS Children's Villages is an international organisation that provides care for children in houses: groups of children, including siblings, live together with an adult rather than in, for example, a dormitory. The Botswana association was formed in 1980.

6 Dahl, 'The "Failures of Culture"'; Dahl, 'Too Fat to Be an Orphan'.

7 Brada, 'Not Here'; Brada, 'The Contingency of Humanitarianism'; Brown, 'Global Health Partnerships, Governance, and Sovereign Responsibility'; Crane, *Scrambling for Africa*; Decoteau, *Ancestors and Antiretrovirals*; Sullivan, 'Mediating Abundance and Scarcity'; Sullivan, 'Enacting Spaces of Inequality'.

8 Biehl, *Will to Live*; Nguyen, *The Republic of Therapy*.

9 In 2000 the adult prevalence rate exceeded 37 per cent. In 2004 UNAIDS estimated the adult prevalence rate to have been above 37 per cent from 2001 to 2003; see Joint United Nations Programme on HIV/AIDS (UNAIDS), 'Epidemiological Fact Sheet and Sexually Transmitted Diseases', 2004. Ten years later UNAIDS revised these figures, estimating the adult prevalence rate in 2005 to have been closer to 25 per cent; see Joint United Nations Programme on HIV/AIDS (UNAIDS), 'The Gap Report'. The severity of Botswana's epidemic is typical of the region: according to one report, in 2007 southern Africa accounted for nearly one-third of all new HIV infections and AIDS deaths worldwide; see Joint United Nations Programme on HIV/AIDS (UNAIDS), 'AIDS Epidemic Update'.

10 Maganu, 'Access to Health Services', 291–301; Pfeiffer and Chapman, 'Anthropological Perspectives'; Poku, *AIDS in Africa*; Schoepf, 'International Aids Research in Anthropology'.

11 Farley, 'At AIDS Disaster's Epicenter'.

12 Ramiah and Reich, 'Public-Private Partnerships'. Each foundation initially contributed $50 million over five years. Merck donated two antiretroviral medications.

13 Joint United Nations Programme on HIV/AIDS (UNAIDS), '2013 Epidemiological Fact Sheet on HIV/AIDS and Sexually Transmitted Diseases', 2013.

14 Darkoh, 'Fighting HIV/AIDS in Africa'.

15 I follow my informants in referring to citizens of the US as 'Americans'.

16 Botswana's Ministry of Health recruited practitioners, including physicians and pharmacists, from other African countries and South Asia.

17 In 2004 HIV testing became a standard component of ante-natal care; by 2006 the proportion of women participating in PMTCT had risen dramatically while the number of perinatally infected children had begun to decline. See Tracy L. Creek et al., 'Successful Introduction of Routine Opt-Out HIV Testing'. Incidence rates among children declined from 4600 in 1999 to approximately 900 in 2008, and Botswana's PMTCT programme is estimated to have averted 10,000 child infections between 2002 and 2007; see Stover et al., 'Estimated HIV Trends and Program Effects in Botswana'.

18 Brada, 'Between Discipline and Empowerment'; see Dahl, 'Beyond the Blame Paradigm'.

19 'AIDS Organizations Grill Tlou for "'Disturbing" Remarks'.

20 On bathing as a site wherein the intersubjective constitution of moral personhood is at stake for Batswana, see Durham, 'Did You Bathe This Morning?'; Livingston, 'Disgust, Bodily Aesthetics and the Ethic of Being Human'.

21 On orphaned children as objects of HIV-related humanitarianism, see Dahl, 'Too Fat to Be an Orphan'; Fassin, 'Children as Victims'; Malkki, *The Need to Help*; Reynolds, 'Low-Hanging Fruit'. While Botswana's HIV/AIDS epidemic has arguably increased children's dependence on extended kin, sending a child to reside with an elderly or infertile female family member is a practice that predates the epidemic; see Ingstad, 'The Value of Grandchildren'; Ingstad et al., 'Care for the Elderly, Care by the Elderly'; Upton, 'Women Have No Tribe'. A child whose parents are living may reside most of the year in a village cared for by an aunt or granny while her parents work elsewhere in Botswana or abroad. Ideally, these arrangements are mutually beneficial and based in reciprocity; in the context of the epidemic, however, existing anxieties and ambivalences regarding obligations to kin have intensified; see Dahl, 'The "Failures of Culture"'; Livingston, *Debility and the Moral Imagination in Botswana*; Reece, 'An Ordinary Crisis?'. In the Superlative Clinic, American paediatricians tended to regard a child's residence with extended kin and particularly movement among multiple residences as threatening to the child's adherence and indicative of a 'bad social situation'; see Brada, 'Between Discipline and Empowerment'.

22 The first statistic is drawn from Tlou, 'Indicators of Health', 306; the second is drawn from Festus Mogae, 'Opening Speech', 12.

23 Botswana Government Selected Demographic Statistics, 2000, cited in Livingston, *Debility and the Moral Imagination*, 278, n9. Livingston cautions that the *total* population grew, not the *proportion* of older people, but that 'popular experiences of an aging population through a rise in the total numbers of elderly in any given family or community contribute to the perceptions that there are many more elderly people now than there were long ago'.

24 The World Bank, 'Forever Young?'; Velkoff and Kowal, 'Population Aging in Sub-Saharan Africa', 14.

25 Tlou, 'Indicators of Health', 308. On the failure of early HIV awareness campaigns in Botswana see Heald, 'It's Never as Easy as ABC'; Ingstad, 'The Cultural Construction of AIDS'.

26 United Nations Development Programme, *Botswana Human Development Report 2000*.

27 Ingstad et al., 'Care for the Elderly, Care by the Elderly'; Livingston, 'Reconfiguring Old Age'; Livingston, 'Pregnant Children and Half-Dead Adults'. These transformations, of course, have much deeper roots: see Livingston, *Debility and the Moral Imagination in Botswana*; Upton, 'Women Have No Tribe'.

28 Ministry of Health, Republic of Botswana, 'Collaboration Report on Developing an Integrated Response'.

29 Cappuccio and Miller, 'Cardiovascular Disease and Hypertension'; Echouffo-Tcheugui et al., 'High Blood Pressure in Sub-Saharan Africa'; Seedat, 'Recommendations for Hypertension in Sub-Saharan Africa'.

30 Boutayeb, 'The Double Burden of Communicable and Non-Communicable Diseases'; Bygbjerg, 'Double Burden of Noncommunicable and Infectious Diseases'; Maher, Smeeth, and Sekajugo, 'Health Transition in Africa'.

31 Keetile, Navaneetham, and Letamo, 'Patterns and Determinants of Hypertension'.

32 Ministry of Health, Republic of Botswana, 'Botswana STEPS Survey 2007 Fact Sheet'.

33 Keetile, Navaneetham, and Letamo, 'Patterns and Determinants of Hypertension'.

34 Ministry of Health, Republic of Botswana, 'Botswana STEPS Survey Report on Non-Communicable Disease Risk Factors'.

35 Stover et al., 'Estimated HIV Trends'.

36 Republic of Botswana, 'National Situation Analysis on Orphans and Vulnerable Children'.

37 Malinga-Musamba, 'The Nature of Relationships', 262.

38 Shaibu, 'Experiences of Grandmothers Caring for Orphan Grandchildren'.

39 Tapela et al., 'Integrating Noncommunicable Disease Services', 143.

40 Ministry of Health, Republic of Botswana, 'MOH/WHO Collaboration Report on Developing an Integrated Response of Health Care Systems to Rapid Population Ageing using Hypertension and Stroke as Tracers to the Health Needs of the Elderly'; cf. Silva et al. 2015; on policy and legislation, see: World Health Organization Regional Office for Africa, 'WHO Country Cooperation Strategy'.

41 Tapela et al., 'Integrating Noncommunicable Disease Services', 143; Ministry of Health and Wellness, Republic of Botswana, 'Botswana National Multisectoral Strategy for the Prevention and Control of Non-Communicable Diseases 2017–2022'.

42 Letamo et al. include being rich among these key risk factors.
43 Bassett, 'Keeping the M in MTCT'; Rosenfield and Figdor, 'Where Is the M in MTCT?'.
44 This is not to say that relatedness precedes or gives shape to diagnosis only in Botswana; indeed, there is a rich anthropological literature to suggest otherwise, for example, Casper, *The Making of the Unborn Patient*; Haraway, 'The Virtual Speculum in the New World Order'; Rouse, 'If She's a Vegetable, We'll Be Her Garden'. Nor does relatedness necessarily precede Tswana diagnoses, though Tswana conceptualisations of health and illness emphasise the entanglement of somatic and sentimental phenomena; see Comaroff and Comaroff, 'On Personhood'; Klaits, *Death in a Church of Life*; Livingston, *Debility and the Moral Imagination in Botswana*. Rather than insist that anthropology's objects epitomise a fundamental relatedness 'we' do not share, I want to highlight the more or less tense process of delimiting a field of intervention in the face of affliction that both biomedical categories and *dikgaba* share. Thanks to Emily Yates-Doerr for pushing me to think carefully about this.
45 Baer, Singer, and Susser, *Medical Anthropology and the World System*; Mendenhall, *Syndemic Suffering*; Mendenhall, 'Syndemics'; Singer, 'A Dose of Drugs'; Singer, *Introduction to Syndemics*; Merrill Singer et al., 'Syndemics and the Biosocial Conception of Health'.
46 Singer and Clair, 'Syndemics and Public Health'.
47 Singer and Clair, 'Syndemics and Public Health', 428–9.
48 Singer et al., 'Syndemics and the Biosocial Conception of Health', 941.
49 Singer, 'A Dose of Drugs'; Mendenhall, *Syndemic Suffering*.
50 Singer et al., 'Syndemics and the Biosocial Conception of Health', 943.
51 Singer, *Introduction to Syndemics*.
52 Mendenhall, 'Beyond Comorbidity'; Nichter, 'Comorbidity'; Weaver, Barrett, and Nichter, 'Special Section on Comorbidity'.
53 Weaver, Barrett, and Nichter, 'Special Section on Comorbidity', 438.
54 Weaver, Barrett, and Nichter, 'Special Section on Comorbidity', 436–8.
55 Singer and Clair, 'Syndemics and Public Health'; Mendenhall, *Syndemic Suffering*; see Good, *Medicine, Rationality and Experience*; Kleinman, *Writing at the Margin*.
56 Mendenhall, *Syndemic Suffering*, 24.
57 Weaver, 'Transactions in Suffering'.
58 Biehl, *Will to Live*; Kalofonos, 'All I Eat Is ARVs'; Nguyen, 'Government-by-Exception'; Rhine, *The Unseen Things*.
59 Could the reverse not also be true? As scholars of Botswana have been careful to point out (for example, Ingstad, 'The Value of Grandchildren'; Ingstad et al., 'Care for the Elderly, Care by the Elderly'), children are not always only recipients of care. A child might offer comfort, perform household chores and give and receive the love that, for Batswana, also builds up bodies: Comaroff and Comaroff, 'On Personhood'; Klaits, *Death in a Church of Life*; Livingston, 'Disgust, Bodily Aesthetics and the Ethic of Being Human in Botswana'; cf. Hunleth, *Children as Caregivers*.
60 Klaits, *Death in a Church of Life*; see Comaroff and Comaroff, 'On Personhood'; Livingston, 'Disgust, Bodily Aesthetics and the Ethic of Being Human in Botswana.'
61 Schapera, *Married Life in an African Tribe*; see Lambek and Solway, 'Just Anger'.
62 Livingston, *Debility and the Moral Imagination in Botswana*; Klaits, *Death in a Church of Life*.
63 Cf. Livingston, 'AIDS as Chronic Illness'.
64 This phenomenon is hardly limited to southern Africa; see work on familial aggregation in mental illness and substance abuse. Another example close to home might be rates of PTSD among American parents of medically fragile children; see Savoie, 'PTSD Helps Parents Keep Their Medically Fragile Children Alive'. These examples, however, emphasise the uniqueness of my case in illustrating this phenomena with regard to infectious diseases and non-communicable diseases rather than mental health.
65 See Livingston's discussion of families who refuse amputation on their children's behalf in *Improvising Medicine*, 85–92.
66 Brada, 'How to Do Things to Children with Words'.
67 On enclaves in global health see Crane, *Scrambling for Africa*; Geissler, 'Public Secrets in Public Health'; Nguyen, *The Republic of Therapy*; Sullivan, 'Mediating Abundance and Scarcity'; Sullivan, 'Enacting Spaces of Inequality'. As I have argued elsewhere, discerning the boundaries between Botswana's 'public' and 'private' or 'global' and 'local' clinical spaces at any given moment was an ongoing problem for all involved; see Brada, 'Not Here'; Brada, 'The Contingency of Humanitarianism'.

68 It should be noted that *madi amatona* is not, or not necessarily, the same thing as 'high blood' or high blood pressure; see Livingston, 'Pregnant Children and Half-Dead Adults'; Livingston, 'Productive Misunderstandings and the Dynamism of Plural Medicine'.
69 Hamdy, *Our Bodies Belong to God*; Lock, *Encounters with Aging*; Nading, 'Local Biologies, Leaky Things, and the Chemical Infrastructure of Global Health'.
70 Matlho et al., 'HIV Prevalence and Related Behaviours of Older People', 22.
71 Haacker, Bärnighausen, and Atun, 'HIV and the Growing Health Burden from Noncommunicable Diseases'.
72 Dahl, 'The Drama of De-Orphaning'.

Bibliography

'AIDS Organizations Grill Tlou for "Disturbing' Remarks"', *Sunday Standard*, 11 December 2006, www.sundaystandard.info/aids-organizations-grill-tlou-%E2%80%9Cdisturbing%E2%80%9D-remarks, accessed 3 April 2019.
Baer, Hans A., Merrill Singer, and Ida Susser. *Medical Anthropology and the World System: A Critical Perspective*. Westport, CT: Bergin & Garvey, 2003.
Bainame, Kenabetsho, Denise Burnette, and Sheila Shaibu. 'Socio-demographic Correlates of Older Adults' Living Arrangements in Botswana', *Botswana Notes and Records*, 46 (2014): 106–20.
Bassett, Mary T. 'Keeping the M in MTCT: Women, Mothers, and HIV Prevention', *American Journal of Public Health*, 91 (2001): 701.
Biehl, João. *Will to Live: AIDS Therapies and the Politics of Survival*. Princeton, NJ: Princeton University Press, 2009.
Boutayeb, Abdesslam. 'The Double Burden of Communicable and Non–communicable Diseases in Developing Countries', *Transactions of the Royal Society of Tropical Medicine and Hygiene*, 100 (3) (2006): 191–9.
Brada, Betsey Behr. '"Not Here": Making the Spaces and Subjects of "Global Health" in Botswana', *Culture, Medicine & Psychiatry*, 35 (2) (2011): 285–312.
Brada, Betsey Behr. 'How to Do Things to Children with Words: Language, Ritual, and Apocalypse in Paediatric HIV Treatment in Botswana', *American Ethnologist*, 40 (3) (2013): 437–51.
Brada, Betsey Behr. 'The Contingency of Humanitarianism: Moral Authority in an African HIV Clinic', *American Anthropologist*, 118 (2016): 755–71.
Brada, Betsey Behr. 'Between Discipline and Empowerment: Temporal Ambivalence at a Sleepaway Camp for HIV–Positive Children in Botswana', *Anthropological Quarterly*, 92 (1) (2019):173–202.
Brown, Hannah. 'Global Health Partnerships, Governance, and Sovereign Responsibility in Western Kenya', *American Ethnologist*, 42 (2) (2015): 340–55.
Bygbjerg, I. C. 'Double Burden of Noncommunicable and Infectious Diseases in Developing Countries', *Science*, 337 (6101) (2012): 1499–501.
Cappuccio, Francesco Paolo and Michelle Avril Miller. 'Cardiovascular Disease and Hypertension in Sub-Saharan Africa: Burden, Risk and Interventions', *Internal and Emergency Medicine*, 11 (3) (2016): 299–305.
Casper, Monica J. *The Making of the Unborn Patient: A Social Anatomy of Fetal Surgery*. New Brunswick, NJ: Rutgers University Press, 1998.
Comaroff, John L. and Jean Comaroff. 'On Personhood: An Anthropological Perspective from Africa', *Social Identities*, 7 (2) (2001): 267–83.
Crane, Johanna. *Scrambling for Africa: AIDS, Expertise, and the Rise of American Global Health Science*. Ithaca, NY: Cornell University Press, 2013.
Creek, T. L. et al. 'Successful Introduction of Routine Opt-Out HIV Testing in Antenatal Care in Botswana', *Journal of Acquired Immunodeficiency Syndromes*, 45 (1) (2007): 102–7.
Dahl, Bianca. 'The "Failures of Culture": Christianity, Kinship, and Moral Discourses about Orphans during Botswana's AIDS Crisis', *Africa Today*, 56 (1) (2009): 23–43.
Dahl, Bianca. 'Beyond the Blame Paradigm: Rethinking Witchcraft Gossip and Stigma around HIV-Positive Children in Southeastern Botswana', *African Historical Review*, 44 (1) (2012): 53–79.
Dahl, Bianca. '"Too Fat to Be an Orphan": The Moral Semiotics of Food Aid in Botswana', *Cultural Anthropology*, 29 (4) (2014): 626–47.

Dahl, Bianca. 'The Drama of De-Orphaning: Botswana's Old Orphans and the Rewriting of Kinship Relations', *Social Dynamics*, 42 (2) (2016): 289–303.

Darkoh, Ernest. 'Statement of Dr. Ernest Darkoh, M.D., M.P.H., M.B.A., Operations Manager, Botswana National ARV Program (MASA), Botswana Ministry of Health and African Comprehensive HIV/AIDS Partnership (ACHAP), Gaborone, Botswana.' In 'Fighting HIV/AIDS in Africa: A Progress Report'. Hearing before the Subcommittee on African Affairs of the Committee on Foreign Relations United States Senate, 7 April 2004, 38–52, www.gpo.gov/fdsys/pkgCHRG–108shrg95255/html/CHRG–108shrg95255.htm, accessed 16 April 2013.

Decoteau, Claire Laurier. *Ancestors and Antiretrovirals: The Biopolitics of HIV/AIDS in Post-Apartheid South Africa*. Chicago, IL: University of Chicago Press, 2013.

Durham, Deborah. 'Did You Bathe This Morning? Baths and Morality in Botswana'. In *Dirt, Undress, and Difference: Critical Perspectives on the Body's Surface*, edited by Adeline Masquelier. Bloomington, IN: Indiana University Press, 2005.

Echouffo-Tcheugui, Justin B. et al. 'High Blood Pressure in Sub-Saharan Africa: The Urgent Imperative for Prevention and Control', *Journal of Clinical Hypertension*, 17 (10) (2015): 751–5.

Farley, Maggie. 'At AIDS Disaster's Epicenter, Botswana Is a Model of Action,' *Los Angeles Times*, last modified 27 June 2001, http://articles.latimes.com/2001/jun/27/news/mn–15017, accessed 5 August 2016.

Fassin, Didier. 'Children as Victims: The Moral Economy of Childhood in the Times of AIDS'. In *When People Come First: Critical Studies in Global Health*, edited by João Biehl and Adriana Petryna, 109–32. Princeton, NJ: Princeton University Press, 2013.

Geissler, P. Wenzel. 'Public Secrets in Public Health: Knowing Not to Know while Making Scientific Knowledge', *American Ethnologist*, 40 (1) (2013): 13–34.

Good, Byron J. *Medicine, Rationality, and Experience*. Cambridge: Cambridge University Press, 1994.

Haacker, Markus, Till Bärnighausen, and Rifat Atun. 'HIV and the Growing Health Burden from Noncommunicable Diseases in Botswana: Modelling Study', *Journal of Global Health*, 9 (1) (2019): doi: 10.7189/jogh.09.010428.

Hamdy, Sherine. *Our Bodies Belong to God: Organ Transplants, Islam, and the Struggle for Human Dignity in Egypt*. Berkeley, CA: University of California Press, 2012.

Haraway, Donna J. 'The Virtual Speculum in the New World Order', *Feminist Review*, 55 (1) (1997): 22–72.

Hunleth, Jean. *Children as Caregivers: The Global Fight against Tuberculosis and HIV in Zambia*. New Brunswick, NJ: Rutgers University Press, 2017.

Heald, Suzette. 'It's Never as Easy as ABC: Understandings of AIDS in Botswana', *African Journal of AIDS Research*, 1 (2002): 1–11.

Ingstad, Benedicte. 'The Cultural Construction of AIDS and Its Consequences for Prevention in Botswana', *Medical Anthropology Quarterly*, 4 (1990): 28–40.

Ingstad, Benedicte. 'The Value of Grandchildren: Changing Relations between Generations in Botswana', *Africa*, 74 (2004): 62–75.

Ingstad, Benedicte et al. 'Care for the Elderly, Care by the Elderly: The Role of Elderly Women in a Changing Tswana Society', *Journal of Cross-Cultural Gerontology*, 7 (2004): 379–98.

Joint United Nations Programme on HIV/AIDS (UNAIDS). 'Epidemiological Fact Sheet on HIV/AIDS and Sexually Transmitted Diseases'. Geneva: UNAIDS, 2004.

Joint United Nations Programme on HIV/AIDS (UNAIDS). 'AIDS Epidemic Update'. Geneva: UNAIDS, 2007.

Joint United Nations Programme on HIV/AIDS (UNAIDS). '2013 Epidemiological Fact Sheet on HIV/AIDS and Sexually Transmitted Diseases'. Geneva: UNAIDS, 2013.

Joint United Nations Programme on HIV/AIDS (UNAIDS). 'The Gap Report'. Geneva: UNAIDS, 2014.

Kalofonos, Ippolytos. '"All I Eat is ARVs": The Paradox of AIDS Treatment Interventions in Central Mozambique', *Medical Anthropology Quarterly*, 24 (3) (2010): 363–80.

Keetile, Mpho, Kannan Navaneetham, and Gobopamang Letamo. 'Patterns and Determinants of Hypertension in Botswana', *Journal of Public Health*, 23 (5) (2015): 311–18.

Klaits, Frederick. *Death in a Church of Life: Moral Passion in Botswana's Time of AIDS*. Berkeley, CA: University of California Press, 2010.

Kleinman, Arthur. *Writing at the Margin: Discourse between Anthropology and Medicine*. Berkeley, CA: University of California Press, 1995.

Lambek, Michael and Jacqueline Solway. 'Just Anger: Scenarios of Indignation in Botswana and Madagascar', *Ethnos*, 66 (1) (2001): 49–72.

Letamo, Gobopamang et al. 'Prevalence and Correlates of Self-Reported Chronic Non-Communicable Diseases in Botswana: A Cross-Sectional Study', *International Health*, 9 (2017): 14.

Livingston, Julie. 'Reconfiguring Old Age: Elderly Women and Concerns over Care in Southeastern Botswana', *Medical Anthropology*, 22 (3) (2003): 205–31.

Livingston, Julie. 'Pregnant Children and Half-Dead Adults: Modern Living and the Quickening Life Cycle in Botswana', *Bulletin of the History of Medicine*, 77 (1) (2003): 133–62.

Livingston, Julie. 'AIDS as Chronic Illness: Epidemiological Transition and Health Care in South-Eastern Botswana', *African Journal of AIDS Research*, 3 (1) (2004): 15–22.

Livingston, Julie. *Debility and the Moral Imagination in Botswana*. Bloomington, IN: Indiana University Press, 2005.

Livingston, Julie. 'Productive Misunderstandings and the Dynamism of Plural Medicine in Mid-Century Bechuanaland', *Journal of Southern African Studies*, 33 (4) (2007): 801–10.

Livingston, Julie. 'Disgust, Bodily Aesthetics and the Ethic of Being Human in Botswana', *Africa*, 78 (2) (2008): 288–307.

Livingston, Julie. *Improvising Medicine: An African Oncology Ward in an Emerging Cancer Epidemic*. Durham, NC: Duke University Press, 2012.

Lock, Margaret. *Encounters with Aging: Mythologies of Menopause in Japan and North America*. Berkeley, CA: University of California Press, 1993.

Maganu, Edward. 'Access to Health Services and Its Impact on Quality of Life.' In *Poverty and Plenty: The Botswana Experience*, edited by Doreen Nteta, Janet Hermans, and Pavla Jeskova, 291–301. Gaborone: Botswana Society, 1997.

Maher, D., L. Smeeth, and J. Sekajugo. 'Health Transition in Africa: Practical Policy Proposals for Primary Care', *Bulletin of the World Health Organization*, 88 (12) (2010): 943–8.

Malinga-Musamba, Tumani. 'The Nature of Relationships between Orphans and Their Kinship Carers in Botswana', *Child and Family Social Work*, 20 (2015): 257–66.

Malkki, Liisa. *The Need to Help: The Domestic Arts of International Humanitarianism*. Durham, NC: Duke University Press, 2015.

Matlho, Kabo et al. 'HIV Prevalence and Related Behaviours of Older People in Botswana – Secondary Analysis of the Botswana AIDS Impact Survey (BAIS) IV', *African Journal of AIDS Research*, 18 (2019): 18–26.

Mendenhall, Emily. *Syndemic Suffering: Rethinking Social and Health Problems among Mexican Immigrant Women*. New York: Routledge, 2016.

Mendenhall, Emily. 'Beyond Comorbidity: A Critical Perspective of Syndemic Depression and Diabetes in Cross-Cultural Contexts', *Medical Anthropology Quarterly*, 30 (4) (2016): 462–78.

Mendenhall, Emily. 'Syndemics: A New Path for Global Health Research', *Lancet*, 389 (10072) (2017): 889–91.

Ministry of Health, Republic of Botswana. 'Botswana STEPS Survey 2007 Fact Sheet'. Geneva: World Health Organization, 2007.

Ministry of Health, Republic of Botswana. 'Collaboration Report on Developing an Integrated Response of Health Care Systems to Rapid Population Ageing using Hypertension and Stroke as Tracers to the Health Needs of the Elderly'. Geneva: World Health Organization, 2008.

Ministry of Health, Republic of Botswana. 'MOH/WHO Collaboration Report on Developing an Integrated Response of Health Care Systems to Rapid Population Ageing using Hypertension and Stroke as Tracers to the Health Needs of the Elderly'. Gaborone: Government Printers, 2011, cited in Letamo, Gobopamang et al. 'Prevalence and Correlates of Self-Reported Chronic Non-Communicable Diseases in Botswana: A Cross-Sectional Study', *International Health*, 9 (2017): 12.

Ministry of Health, Republic of Botswana, 'Botswana STEPS Survey Report on Non-Communicable Disease Risk Factors'. Gaborone: Government Printer, 2015.

Ministry of Health and Wellness, Republic of Botswana. 'Botswana National Multisectoral Strategy for the Prevention and Control of Non-Communicable Diseases 2017–2022'. Gaborone: 2017.

Mogae, Festus. 'Opening Speech'. In *Poverty and Plenty: The Botswana Experience*, edited by Doreen Nteta and Janet Hermans with Pavla Jeskova. Gaborone: The Botswana Society, 1997.

Nading, Alex. 'Local Biologies, Leaky Things, and the Chemical Infrastructure of Global Health', *Medical Anthropology*, 36 (2) (2017): 141–56.

Nguyen, Vinh-Kim. 'Government-by-Exception: Enrolment and Experimentality in Mass HIV Treatment Programmes in Africa', *Social Theory and Health*, 7 (3) (2009): 196–217.

Nguyen, Vinh-Kim. *The Republic of Therapy: Triage and Sovereignty in West Africa's Time of AIDS*. Durham, NC: Duke University Press, 2010.

Nichter, Mark. 'Comorbidity: Reconsidering the Unit of Analysis', *Medical Anthropology Quarterly*, 30 (4) (2016): 536–44.

Pfeiffer, James and Rachel Chapman. 'Anthropological Perspectives on Structural Adjustment and Public Health', *Annual Review of Anthropology*, 39 (1) (2010): 149–65.

Poku, Nana K. *AIDS in Africa: How the Poor Are Dying*. Cambridge: Polity Press, 2006.

Ramiah, Ilavenil and Michael R. Reich. 'Public–Private Partnerships and Antiretroviral Drugs for HIV/AIDS: Lessons from Botswana', *Health Affairs*, 24 (2) (2005): 545–51.

Reece, Koreen M. 'An Ordinary Crisis? Kinship in Botswana's Time of AIDS'. Ph.D. diss., University of Edinburgh, 2015.

Republic of Botswana. 'National Situation Analysis on Orphans and Vulnerable Children in Botswana'. Gaborone: Government Printer, 2008.

Reynolds, Lindsey J. '"Low-Hanging Fruit": Counting and Accounting for Children in PEPFAR-funded HIV/AIDS Programmes in South Africa', *Global Public Health*, 9 (1–2) (2014), 124–43.

Rhine, Kathryn. *The Unseen Things: Women, Secrecy, and HIV in Northern Nigeria*. Bloomington, IN: Indiana University Press, 2016.

Rosenfield, Allan and Emily Figdor. 'Where is the M in MTCT? The Broader Issues in Mother-to-Child Transmission of HIV', *American Journal of Public Health*, 91 (5) (2001): 703.

Rouse, Carolyn. '"If She's a Vegetable, We'll Be Her Garden": Embodiment, Transcendence, and Citations of Competing Cultural Metaphors in the Case of a Dying Child', *American Ethnologist*, 31 (4) (2004): 514–29.

Savoie, Hillary. 'PTSD Helps Parents Keep Their Medically Fragile Children Alive – But At What Cost?' *Romper*, last modified 6 December 2018, accessed 5 April 2019, https://www.romper.com/p/ptsd-helps-parents-keep-their-medically-fragile-children-alive-but-at-what-cost-13222452.

Schapera, Isaac. *Married Life in an African Tribe*. London: Faber and Faber, 1940.

Schoepf, Brooke Grundfest. 'International AIDS Research in Anthropology: Taking a Critical Perspective on the Crisis', *Annual Review of Anthropology*, 30 (1) (2001): 335–61.

Seedat, Y. K. 'Recommendations for Hypertension in Sub-Saharan Africa', *Cardiovascular Journal of South Africa*, 15 (4) (2004): 157–8.

Shaibu, Sheila. 'Experiences of Grandmothers Caring for Orphan Grandchildren in Botswana', *Journal of Nursing Scholarship*, 45 (2013): 363–70.

Singer, Merrill. 'A Dose of Drugs, a Touch of Violence, a Case of AIDS: Conceptualizing the SAVA Syndemic', *Free Inquiry in Creative Sociology*, 24 (1996): 99–110.

Singer, Merrill. 2009. *Introduction to Syndemics: A Critical Systems Approach to Public and Community Health*. San Francisco, CA: John Wiley & Sons, 2009.

Singer, Merrill and Scott Clair. 'Syndemics and Public Health: Reconceptualizing Disease in Bio-Social Context', *Medical Anthropology Quarterly*, 17 (4) (2003): 423–41.

Singer, Merrill et al. 'Syndemics and the Biosocial Conception of Health', *Lancet*, 389 (10072) (2017): 941–50.

Stover, John et al. 'Estimated HIV Trends and Program Effects in Botswana', *PLoS One* 3 (11) (2008): p.e3729.

Sullivan, Noelle. 'Mediating Abundance and Scarcity: Implementing an HIV/AIDS-Targeted Project within a Government Hospital in Tanzania', *Medical Anthropology*, 30 (20) (2011): 202–21.

Sullivan, Noelle. 'Enacting Spaces of Inequality: Placing Global/State Governance within a Tanzanian Hospital', *Space and Culture*, 15 (1) (2012): 57–67.

Tapela, Neo M. et al. 'Integrating Noncommunicable Disease Services into Primary Health Care, Botswana', *Bulletin of the World Health Organization*, 97 (2019):142–53.

Tlou, Sheila Dinotshe. 'Indicators of Health'. In *Poverty and Plenty: The Botswana Experience*, edited by Doreen Nteta and Janet Hermans with Pavla Jeskova. Gaborone: The Botswana Society, 1997.

United Nations Development Programme. *Botswana Human Development Report 2000: Towards an AIDS-Free Generation*. Gaborone, 2000: 60.

Upton, Rebecca L. '"Women Have No Tribe": Connecting Carework, Gender, and Migration in an Era of HIV/AIDS in Botswana', *Gender & Society*, 17 (2) (2003): 314–22.

Velkoff, Victoria A. and Paul R. Kowal. 'Population Aging in Sub-Saharan Africa: Demographic Dimensions 2006'. US Government Printing Office: Washington, DC, 2007.
Weaver, Lesley Jo. 'Transactions in Suffering: Mothers, Daughters, and Chronic Disease Comorbidities in New Delhi, India', *Medical Anthropology Quarterly*, 30 (4) (2016): 498–514.
Weaver, Lesley Jo, Ron Barrett, and Mark Nichter. 'Special Section on Comorbidity: Introduction', *Medical Anthropology Quarterly*, 30 (4) (2016): 435–41.
World Bank. 'Forever Young? Social Policies for a Changing Population in Southern Africa'. Washington, DC, 2016.
World Health Organization Regional Office for Africa. 'WHO Country Cooperation Strategy 2014–2020: Botswana'. Brazzaville, 2014.

12

Care and Cancer in Kenya

Ruth J. Prince

Introduction

It is early morning in April 2019, just after 7.00 a.m. in one of Kenya's largest urban public hospitals, in the west of the country. Nurse ('Sista') Angela and I are sitting in the room used for counselling patients in the hospital's fledging 'Cancer Care Centre', an outpatient clinic. Nurse Angela is one of the clinic's three nurses and one of only two with palliative care training in this regional Referral Hospital. She is much loved by patients and staff. Today she wants to talk to me urgently about one of her patients. Sometimes I get the impression that telling me these stories is her way of coming to terms with the difficult work she does. There is little time during the day for talking in private. During the morning, the waiting room is filled with patients, some accompanied by a relative, waiting to see the doctor on duty. During the afternoon Nurse Angela is occupied with administering chemotherapy.

'There is something that is really bothering me,' she tells me. 'It's our patient on Ward One' (a middle-aged woman with throat cancer, who is recovering from a laryngectomy and cycles of chemo, now waiting for her third. She has been on the ward for two months and cannot speak; she communicates by writing things down). 'Her condition is…' (she breaks off, emotional). 'So I was asking her, "Do you have your health insurance card?", and she just started to cry, like that.' Angela is about to continue but we are interrupted by a man, in his late 40s, who politely opens the door.

'We are not yet open,' says Angela.

'It's just a small thing, so that we can get to the laboratory early.'

She tells him to come in. He brings a small sheet of paper, a laboratory form for routine blood tests, which have to be done to assess if the patient is ready for chemotherapy. She asks for the name of his wife (the patient) and the location of their home, filling it all in neatly. Thanking her, he turns to me.

'This is a very good place,' he says, 'They have helped us so much. My wife is now walking. Nurse Angela has really helped us, she has saved my wife.'

I heard similar sentiments from many patients and also from the staff working with Nurse Angela. People would say, 'She is not just giving chemotherapy. She talks to them. She listens.'

'Listening is very important', Angela told me, 'because no one has taken time to explain to them about cancer, how to live with cancer, no one has listened to how they feel.' She continues, 'But it is only chemotherapy we are giving them. There is no follow-up, very little counselling – there is no support! And so many of our patients get lost. They just disappear! Some come back later, when their cancer is much advanced. And sometimes they disappear when they get their diagnosis. People just hear cancer and they go home. We don't know what their situation is. We only give treatment here. People come from far, and we don't know how it is in their homes.' She suspected that many do not tell relatives of their diagnosis, due to the fear and stigma surrounding cancer's association with death. Sometimes, a patient would return after months or a year of suffering at home, to seek treatment only when their cancer had severely progressed.

Our conversation is interrupted again, by a middle-aged woman whom Angela greets as an old friend, introducing her to me as Rosemary and inviting her to sit with us. Rosemary, she told me, has been pursuing cancer treatment, including a mastectomy and chemotherapy, in a private hospital 300 kilometres away, in Nairobi, financially supported by her nephews and her National Hospital Insurance Card (she is a retired civil servant). She had not known about the cancer clinic in Kisumu until she bumped into Angela, who invited her to attend the monthly cancer support group meeting, which meets in the hospital. The support group is, like the clinic, fledgling. Established by Nurse Angela and Peter, an energetic pastor with a passion for raising breast cancer awareness, it is

> attended by about 30 people, mostly women, who call themselves (with Peter's encouragement) 'cancer warriors'. Peter obtains donations of wigs and prosthetic bras from 'well-wishers' in Nairobi and among the overseas diaspora, and sometimes he has funds for tea and lunch. Some members travel from towns 100 kilometres away to attend the meetings.
>
> As I chat with Rosemary, Angela excuses herself and goes to change into her white nurses' outfit: the clinic is about to open and she, together with her colleague Nurse Alice, has a long day ahead of her. Often I find them way beyond closing hours, sitting with patients receiving chemotherapy, chatting to them and caring for them. Already at this early hour in the morning, there are 20 or more patients and their relatives waiting for the doors to open, to get their vitals checked, see the doctor, get a laboratory form, or wait in line for chemotherapy. Some patients have a National Health Insurance (NHIF) Card, which covers the cost of some chemotherapy, but rarely does it cover a full chemotherapy cycle. Many do not have insurance cover, forcing the nurses to instruct them to buy chemotherapy from private pharmacies, at a price many cannot afford. Some begin a chemotherapy course but do not finish it, others do not return.

I begin with these extracts from an ordinary day in the oncology clinic to convey the fabric of care that Nurse Angela weaves into her work, and her concerns and frustrations about its limitations, as many patients disappear after a diagnosis or during a course of treatment. Moving out of the clinic, this chapter is concerned with the itineraries of such 'disappearing' patients and their families, as they seek diagnosis, treatment and care. While I spent much time in clinics and wards, here I move beyond these spaces to examine how life situations, family relations and economic affordances, health systems and medical infrastructures enable or disrupt treatment trajectories, forms of diagnosis, and care. I show how the experience of treatment bifurcates along socioeconomic lines, with many people not being able to maintain access to treatment for financial reasons. Following the itineraries of cancer patients, and the stories they and their caregivers and relatives tell about them, I also ask how cancer is experienced as a *chronic* disease, by whom, and when. The temporality of cancer is heterogeneous. Experiences of chronicity are embedded in access to diagnosis and treatment, which remain deeply uneven and unequal, and also in forms of care. Through ethnographic research at the clinic, with the support group and in the narratives of patients and their relatives, I attend to the ways in which cancer is coming-into-being as a chronic disease, understood as prolonged, protracted or evolving, with the possibility of managing its development but rarely its cure – as well as the ways it remains invisible, unspoken, nebulous and without a coherent form.

While recent years have seen expanded capacities in cancer diagnosis and treatment in Kenya, most of this capacity is located in the country's two public hospitals with cancer wards, in Nairobi and Eldoret, and in the country's thriving – and expensive – private health sector. Cancer diagnosis and treatment are slowly becoming available in some government hospitals and clinics across the country but, where it is available, it is costly and often offered by doctors without oncological expertise.[1] The expansion of health insurance schemes has increased access, but this has been realised only very partially (for some people, and for some forms of treatment). Thus, many people cannot afford treatment, and diagnosis is often made only very late in the cancer's process. Accordingly, forms of 'living with' cancer vary immensely. Many of those we followed rarely framed their experiences of illness in terms of cancer. Their suffering was embedded in longer experiences of ill health and economic deprivation and, often, late diagnosis and lack of treatment meant that the diagnosis never has time to be installed and defined.[2] Others, usually those with financial resources, who were able to live with cancer for some time and to access chemotherapy, surgery and (more rarely) radiotherapy, came to foreground an identity as a cancer patient, but in ways that were often partial and tentative.

Since the 1990s, western Kenya has experienced one of the worst HIV/AIDS epidemics in East Africa, and HIV prevalence is still relatively high. Some cancers, such as cervical cancer, are partially associated with HIV infection. In contrast to the medical care available to people living with HIV in the region, which is dispersed through infrastructures of 'comprehensive care clinics' with generous funding from donors, cancer care receives little funding. The health system is orientated to infectious disease, and medical infrastructures for cancer diagnosis and treatment are extremely patchy. Most people with cancer must rely on families and kinship networks for financial and social support, to access treatment and for long-term care. Such relations, sometimes already precarious, may become more strained. Local initiatives around cancer care, such as the cancer support group that Nurse Angela helped to set up, offer a forum where people learn about cancer and how to live with it, share stories, and gain access to information and to occasional forms of material support. However, in contrast to the density and histories of

HIV-positive support groups in the region, cancer support groups remain rare. Indeed, in the entire hinterland of Kisumu, there exists only one support group, and it was officially established only in 2018.

An emerging literature underlines that how cancer is experienced, and how it emerges and is distinguished from other chronic diseases and life burdens, takes shape very differently in different places.[3] There is little standardised understanding or experience of the disease, nor is there standardised medicine, especially in contexts of scarcity and austerity, and where medical interventions and health systems have been structured around infectious disease.[4] Thus, while experiences of cancer in countries like Kenya are dominated by late-stage diagnosis and care, cancer in the US, with its extensive systems of screening and early treatment, is accompanied by a different set of experiences and expectations of person-tailored care.[5] But even where there is an effective, encompassing and pervasive medicalisation of cancer, supported by access to comprehensive biomedical care, cancer remains an unstable entity. Julie Livingston argues that cancer emerges as a particular object, in particular places, through particular networks and material practices of care, as well as through the availability (or not) of technologies, medicines, diagnostic tests, oncologists and other experts. In Botswana she found that the scarcity of oncology meant that a collective experience and image of the disease was largely absent: 'Lay expectations around the disease are still extremely thin, as is the vocabulary of symbols, words and images.'[6]

In Kenya, the fact that many patients with cancer are exposed both to infectious disease and to other chronic conditions complicates knowledge about cancer and capacities to act upon it. Boundaries between chronic, infectious and non-communicable diseases appear extremely porous, and do not clearly crystallise as separate conditions – whether in patients' experiences or indeed in medical practices, where access to diagnosis, oncological expertise and treatment is only slowly evolving.[7] The longer trajectory of caring for a loved one, from the beginnings of the disease until its outcome, falls on particular members of the family – a daughter, a son, a mother, an aunt – and is often done silently.[8] Unstable, precarious and stressful living conditions complicate the pursuit of treatment for patients and their families. Many families are forced to keep patients at home, waiting for treatment, while they attempt to raise resources. Often, this 'waiting' shades into the tacit abandonment of treatment, as the necessary resources do not materialise, leaving families to cope with providing some form of palliative care.[9] Other families, who are able to find the resources, often pursue treatment to the very end, beyond what would be medically effective, hoping for a good outcome.[10] This is despite the ambiguities of cancer treatment, which harm as well as heal.[11] For all families, the burden of a chronic condition and the search for treatment further weighs down the struggle to make a living, feed a family and pay school or college fees for children.

Locations, mobilities and methodology

From 2014 to 2017, I followed the stories and therapeutic itineraries of patients with chronic disease in and around the city of Kisumu, together with research assistant Biddy Odindo. This chapter draws on our engagements with 34 adult cancer patients, 23 women and 13 men, ranging in age from 19 to 80 years old.[12] About a quarter of the patients we followed belonged to what Kenyans refer to as the 'middle class' (people in formal employment, in this case mostly civil servants such as teachers and nurses) while the rest were struggling to make a living through rural smallholdings or urban informal work. While some lived in Kisumu, many lived outside the city, sometimes in rural homes several hours away by public transport. Within these groups, there was great diversity in family relations, social networks and patients' positions within them.

We interviewed and followed the patients and their caregivers, as well as other family members, visiting them at home as well as at clinics and hospital wards. We first met patients and their families at the Referral Hospital's surgical, medical and gynaecological wards and at its Cancer Care Centre, in Kisumu.[13] Until 2018, the Centre had no oncologist and was open only one day a week. It began life in 2013 offering chemotherapy to HIV-positive patients with Kaposi's sarcoma, sponsored by and linked to a US-funded research project, and gradually started offering chemotherapy, at a cost, for other cancers. We also met patients visiting the nearby 'Acacia' clinic,[14] a not-for-profit centre operating two days per week, run by a retired oncologist from Nairobi (whose relations with the hospital were fractious), which offered consultations and chemotherapy at (initially) subsidised prices. We interviewed doctors, nurses, pharmacists, radiographers, laboratory technicians, nutritionists, counsellors, community health workers and clinical officers. We were permitted access to patients' files, with patient consent and after ethical review, although in many cases these proved extremely patchy. We collected government reports and newspaper articles and attended to discussions about cancer, chronic disease and healthcare in social media.[15]

At Kisumu's Referral Hospital, medical staff encounter patients with multiple morbidities, with HIV and TB, malaria or pneumonia, hypertension, diabetes or kidney disease. Patients arrive here after a long period of uncertainty and misdiagnosis, disability and pain, usually accompanied by their caregivers (one or several members of their extended families). Until 2016, the hospital had only one pathologist, who was often absent. Even when he was replaced, and the hospital began doing regular biopsy tests, there were regular backlogs and doctors referred patients to private laboratories for quicker results. Those who could not afford private laboratories had longer waits and it was up to the patient's family to chase up laboratory results.

Research began from Kisumu's large Referral Hospital but our follow-up of patients and their caregivers took us over a geographically dispersed area, as they sought treatment in and beyond the city and, in a few cases, in Uganda and India. Despite being one of the four largest public Hospitals in Kenya, with a catchment area of 5 million people, the Referral Hospital had (and still has) no adult cancer ward, where cancer could be medicalised and socialised. While some people we met received a diagnosis at an early stage of the disease, the majority had ended up at the hospital after an extended (and often fruitless) search for diagnosis and treatment across multiple sites. However, the hospital itself had little capacity to diagnose and treat cancers, so doctors referred patients onwards, in the hope they would find treatment elsewhere. They referred patients to the outpatient Cancer Care Centre, or to the nearby Acacia clinic. Although they were aware that many people did not have the resources to make it to these places, doctors also referred patients to hospitals located several hours' journey from Kisumu – to Tenwek, an NGO Mission hospital some 300 kilometres from Kisumu, which offered operations and some cancer care, and to Kenya's largest public hospitals in Nairobi and Eldoret, which have cancer wards. (Few of the patients we followed managed to reach these destinations due to the distance involved and the cost of accommodation for themselves and their caregivers, as well as medical care.)

The pursuit of treatment thus required immense mobility and an ability to move between multiple sites, which was often expensive and difficult. Patients and their families would have to carry around piles of documents such as doctors' diagnoses, radiography and laboratory test results, treatment prescriptions, hospital discharge summaries, and national insurance cards in their attempt to pursue some continuity of treatment between such sites. Patients were almost always accompanied by a caregiver, a family member, who often took charge of these documents, as well as providing physical and emotional support, phoning relatives and church members, buying food or milk, and, when patients were admitted to hospital wards, providing bodily care.[16] Some patients always came with the same caregiver, while others were accompanied by different family members, as they tried to distribute tasks. Caregiving was embedded in gendered kinship relations, sometimes in surprising ways.[17]

Patients and their families sought diagnosis and treatment in a pluralistic therapeutic landscape which included herbal medicines, also known as 'Luo medicines' (*yadh nyaluo*), herbalists, church-based healers (known as *jolemo*, 'people who pray', in Dholuo) and *ajuoga* (healers who could divine malevolent intents through their communication with *juogi*, spirits). While some patients would not admit to seeking these forms of healing, and some adamantly refused to use them, others sought respite, diagnosis or explanations for their suffering from these sources. In particular, Luo herbal medicines, pounded at home or by a neighbour or healer, were widely used in the early stages of illness, to help with wounds, to 'add blood', to heal rashes and reduce swellings. Chinese medicines are widely available in Kenya, although their cost puts them out of reach for most people, as are globalised medical foods and supplements, which are sold by agents; some are made locally.

We conducted extensive interviews with patients and their relatives and we followed many of them inside and outside the hospital and clinics and visited them at their homes. We sought a sustained engagement throughout their struggle with the disease and sometimes beyond it. We were not able to follow all patients closely but we maintained contact with people through phone-calls and visits. In a few cases we lost contact. The research was challenging in terms of the inadequacy of care people received, the late stage in which cancer was often diagnosed, and enormity of financial contributions required. Some of the patients passed away; indeed, by 2018, 16 of the 34 patients we followed had died. As research assistant Biddy Odindo resided continuously in Kisumu during this time, her deeply caring and empathetic work ensured a continuity of contact, which greatly enriched the study, but also placed a considerable burden on her.[18]

Cancer in Kenya

Kenya has, to date, no national cancer registry (although there are plans to create one). Estimates of prevalence of different kinds of cancers, numbers of new cases per year and numbers of deaths are available at

GLOBOCAN,[19] sourced from the Nairobi Cancer Registry[20] and the Eldoret Cancer Registry, which are based on figures from the two public hospitals offering comprehensive cancer care. Elsewhere in the country, there is little capacity for collecting cancer statistics. Health information systems are orientated to collecting data on infectious diseases and maternal deaths; only in 2018 was cervical cancer inserted into the national DHIS (District Health Information System). WHO's GLOBOCAN cancer registry suggests that cancer is Kenya's third largest killer, accounting for 7 per cent of all deaths. Figures for 2018 from GLOBOCAN suggest almost 48,000 new cases in Kenya (in a population of 50 million), 32,987 cancer deaths, and 86,592 as the number of prevalent cases estimated over a five-year period.[21] The most common cancers are (in order of highest prevalence) breast, cervical, oesophagus, prostate and colorectal, which together make up 43.4 per cent of all cancers. Kaposi's sarcoma – an HIV-related cancer – is more common among men, while women have higher rates of stomach cancer.

Having grappled with the HIV/AIDS epidemic over the past 30 years, the Kenyan government is slowly turning attention to non-communicable disease.[22] While donor funding has created comprehensive infrastructure for diagnosis and treatment of HIV/AIDS, cancer remains chronically under-funded and tragically still associated with death. A cancer diagnosis has replaced the trauma of an HIV diagnosis, with patients often expressing the sentiment that they would 'rather have HIV than cancer'. Some survive HIV only to develop cancer. In 2018 there were only 35 oncologists in the country, most of them working in the private sector, and only 12 treatment centres, most of them private.[23] The Kenyan government's *National Cancer Control Strategy, 2011–16* underlines the challenge it faces in building up oncological capacity:

> Despite the fact that non-communicable diseases such as cardiovascular diseases, cancers, diabetes and chronic respiratory diseases are on the increase, the health systems in the country have traditionally concentrated on the prevention and control of communicable diseases. As a result, health and development plans have not adequately invested in the prevention and control of these diseases. The silent epidemic of non-communicable diseases now imposes a 'double burden of disease', which, unless it is addressed, will overwhelm the country in the near future.[24]

In 2006, the Cancer Incidence Report estimated that 80 per cent of cancer cases are diagnosed at advanced stages when there is little chance of cure.[25] One of the explanations given for late diagnosis – and frequent misdiagnosis – of cancer is the lack of oncological expertise in the medical profession and a health system that remains occupied with infectious diseases, as underlined in the quote above. Another reason is the difficulty of detecting cancer in its early stages, and frequent co-occurrence with infectious disease and infections. For example, cervical cancer – one of the most prevalent types in Kenya – is associated with HIV infection, as HIV-positive women are at higher risk of HPV (Human Papilloma Virus) infection due to their immune-compromised status. Called 'an AIDS-defining disease',[26] cervical cancer is nested within women's experience of HIV. Kaposi's sarcoma, caused by a herpes virus, is also an AIDS-defining disease, with HIV-positive men especially at risk of developing it. Stomach and liver cancers are linked to hepatitis B infection (HBV), which is associated with poor living conditions and poverty.

The fact that cancer emerges alongside and is partially and intimately associated with the HIV/AIDS epidemic shapes the ways cancer is experienced and acted upon. Thus, some of the patients we followed were HIV-positive and long-time 'clients' of Comprehensive Care Centres (HIV treatment and support clinics, financed largely by the US government and other donors). The global response to the HIV/AIDS epidemic has laid an infrastructure of diagnostic testing (for HIV) and treatment, a culture of counselling and patient-centred treatment, and of patient-support groups and forms of 'speaking therapy' in the region.[27] While this 'cascade of care'[28] and access to information is markedly lacking for other diseases, including cancer, it has put into circulation a language of rights to health and healthcare.

An emerging cancer epidemic and a bifurcated landscape of care

In 2012, Julie Livingston wrote that cancer in Africa has largely been invisible due to public health imaginaries, and the focus on infectious diseases and epidemic crises.[29] In the years since her book was published, cancer has risen to public prominence in Kenya. Cancer is visible now, with media reports describing a 'cancer epidemic' in the country and regular newspaper articles on cancer statistics and the experiences of cancer patients, the state of radiotherapy equipment in public hospitals, and the medical travel of Kenyan patients seeking cancer treatment in India.[30] Newspapers regularly run health supplements with information and advice on so-called 'lifestyle' diseases. In October 2019, Kenya's

Citizen TV aired a two-part series called 'Cancer Country', which traversed over five counties collecting the stories of cancer patients and highlighting inequalities in access to medical care. Many families find their personal experiences with cancer reflected in these public narratives. For others, however, cancer remains obscure and unknown.

These variable experiences of cancer are emerging amidst ongoing scarcity and austerity in the public healthcare system. Cancer diagnosis and care fall into the cracks of a public healthcare system that is largely oriented to, and receives global funding for, infectious diseases. Lack of diagnostic tools and medical expertise means that cancer is misdiagnosed and patients end up at referral hospitals at late stages of the disease. Outside of donor-funded HIV, tuberculosis and malaria programmes, a state of crisis infuses conditions of care in terms of lack of medicines and medical tools, frequent breakdown of equipment and chronic under-staffing. The scarcity and frequent breakdown of equipment are regular topics of concern in the national media, as are patients' experiences of poor care in government hospitals. In the past five years, frustration at working conditions and pay has led to frequent strikes by health workers.[31] Public hospitals stood eerily empty for weeks and even months, as patients were told to either seek care in private medical facilities or go home.

Cancer is emerging as an increasingly visible and fraught matter of concern within a highly charged and politicised terrain of healthcare.[32] The increased visibility of chronic disease has focused attention on the state of the public health system. The 'crisis of cancer care' in the country is regularly reported, alongside calls on the government to act, in letters to the editor, in reports, on social media sites and blogs.[33] Health has also become increasingly politicised against a backdrop of constitutional reform. The new 2010 Constitution introduced a devolved system of government, giving local (county) governments control over development funds, including health, making them (on paper at least) more accountable to the needs of their constituencies. The 2010 Constitution also ensconced the right to health for all citizens and the duty of the state to care for its citizens. A Cancer Prevention and Control Act was passed in 2012, and two National Cancer Control Strategy documents (2011–16 and 2017–22) have been released, focusing on prevention, screening and early detection. In 2012, the National Assembly passed a bill that sought to establish Cancer Care Centres in all the 47 counties. The government is funding the training of medical oncologists, with the support of donors. It regularly announces deals to access new medical technologies and expand cancer treatment through public–private partnerships with multinational companies.

The experience of cancer emerges within a terrain of uncertainty, scarcity and inequality, but also of new medical opportunities and aspirations, amidst expanding flows of information, and shifts in forms of and access to health insurance. The government is courting corporate investment into Kenya's growing middle-class medical markets, with an expansion of cancer treatment in private hospitals.[34] Novel opportunities for diagnosis, treatment and care – tied to expanding medical markets and new health insurances – are thus opening up for some citizens and appear within reach for others, but in deeply unequal ways.[35] Meanwhile, promises to provide better cancer care to Kenyan citizens often appear to be more political spectacle than substance. Media reports highlight that cancer patients wait for months and even years for radiotherapy at Kenyatta National Hospital, and new Cancer Care Centres have remained mostly within the private healthcare system and confined to Nairobi.[36]

Even where chemotherapy is available in public hospitals, cancer diagnosis and treatment are prohibitively expensive to the majority of Kenyans. Under the 'cost sharing' arrangement, introduced in 1989 under Structural Adjustment policies, public healthcare facilities charge patients for all forms of medical treatment and for medicines not available in the hospital pharmacies.[37] Until very recently, cancer treatment was not included in national health insurance cover (the National Hospital Insurance Fund or NHIF, a parastatal), and even when included in private health insurances, the long duration of treatment rapidly exhausts any cover. Newspapers regularly report stories of poor families being forced to sell off land and livestock to fund treatment, and of middle-class families with medical insurance getting heavily into debt.

Kenyans in formal employment are (partially) covered by the NHIF, which also has schemes for people in the informal sector. Meanwhile Kenyans salaried by private companies and NGOs often benefit from private health insurance. However, Kenyans without formal employment – the majority of the population – are largely unprotected by any health insurance as many find the NHIF's monthly premiums too high.[38] Until 2013, the NHIF only covered inpatient admittance. In 2013, it announced a new scheme to cover some outpatient treatment, including (with a cap) chemotherapy, radiotherapy and renal dialysis. However, these forms of medical care are available only at a few (urban referral) hospitals. Moreover, the cap meant that the NHIF rarely covers a full course of treatment, leaving families trying to raise large sums of money or having to pull their sick relatives out of care.

What does this shifting landscape of health care, insurance coverage and cancer treatment offer for those seeking diagnosis and treatment, for people with cancer and their families? The availability of and access to cancer diagnosis and medical treatment is heavily bifurcated in Kenya between middle-class families (who have some health insurance cover and who can draw upon assets, as well as the salaries, savings and loans of family members in formal employment), and the majority of the population (who work in the informal economy and/or practise subsistence agriculture and rarely have insurance cover). For example, an increasing number of middle-class Kenyans have travelled to India to get cancer diagnosis and treatment. Some have been funded by the NHIF; others have paid themselves, raising money from extended family, church members, colleagues and friends, selling off assets and applying for loans. Middle-class families also pursue expensive private medical care within Kenya, often getting heavily into debt. Those who are unable to access these opportunities are dependent on the public healthcare available, but cancer treatment is expensive here, too, and is often beyond their means. Experiences of cancer involve endless referrals from one public institution to another, and long waiting times for treatment, which is often inaccessible, interrupted or terminated because it is too expensive. For families without financial means, the costs of seeking medical care for a relative with cancer are often devastating.

Cancer may no longer be invisible in Kenya, but oncology (knowledge, treatment and palliative care) remains extremely fragmented outside high-end private hospitals and the two public referral hospitals with oncological expertise. This situation becomes clearer if one anchors research on the process of diagnosis and treatment not in a particular place – a ward or a hospital – but in the trajectories of patients and their families. Below, I illustrate this through the itineraries of three patients, as narrated in the stories that they and their caregivers told.

A family's pursuit of care

Mama Onyango was one of the first patients we met, on a Thursday in March 2014 at the Referral Hospital's Cancer Care Centre. Aged about 60, she was a widow with four adult children and lived at her husband's rural home in Nyakach, South Nyanza (about 30 kilometres from Kisumu city). She was weak and could not walk well, and was supported into a seat in the waiting room by her two adult sons, Francis and Onyango. It was their first time at the Clinic. We did not talk much that day as Mama Onyango was in pain. I have pieced together the following narrative from conversations with Mama Onyango and her two sons over several encounters, visits and phone calls, conducted by Biddy and myself. Onyango (aged 29) was her main caregiver and he spoke most of the time.

Mama Onyango's husband died in 1998 while working in town as a security guard, leaving her to raise her four sons alone, in their rural home. To make a living during this difficult time, she brewed and sold *chang'aa* (an alcoholic beverage) to feed the family and pay school fees. It was a tough business. Brewing *chang'aa* is illegal. Although she maintained she did not drink *chang'aa* herself, she had to hide her activities and often had to bribe the police. Later, she gave up brewing *chang'aa* and sold vegetables instead. She also became born again and 'gave my life to Christ'. She began feeling ill in January 2011 (more than three years before our first meeting). She told us that she started feeling a lot of pain in her left breast, which became swollen, so she bought painkillers from the small village shop. She thought the swelling was *yamo* (a Dholuo term referring to any bodily swelling or rashes) and bought some ointment from the chemist to rub on it as well as applying *yiende nyaluo* (Luo herbal/pot medicines, the brewing of which is often done by older women at home). As the pain continued, her family decided to bring her to the nearest hospital, a Catholic Mission Hospital, where she was treated for 'malaria' and sent home. This treatment brought little relief and after some weeks, her sons took her back to the hospital, where the doctor told them to take her to Kisumu's Referral Hospital (about 60 kilometres away). After a family consultation back at the rural home, it was decided that Francis's wife should take her there. At the Referral Hospital's outpatient clinic, she was examined, tested for malaria and typhoid, given malaria treatment and prescribed antibiotics. Mama Onyango did not know what diagnosis was made, but Francis' wife recalled that the doctor told them it could be pneumonia.

After this visit to Kisumu's Referral Hospital, the pain persisted and Mama Onyango could not sleep well. The illness got worse and this worried the family 'so much'. On the advice of a friend, they brought her to Star Hospital in Kisumu (a small private health facility with inpatient beds catering for families without health insurance or large incomes) where, in October 2011, she was admitted and diagnosed with pneumonia again. However, her condition worsened and the doctor told the family to take her back to the Referral Hospital. Having no funds for another hospital stay, they brought her home instead, to allow them time for the siblings to raise money from loans and contributions from Mama Onyango's church members. In late November 2011, they managed to take her to the hospital, where she was admitted for some days. There a biopsy was taken, almost by chance it seems, during a nation-wide cancer screening week.[39] When Onyango went to pick up the result, he was told that she had cancer of the breast and that she should go to Tenwek Mission Hospital (about 300 kilometres away) for her breast to be removed.

It took two weeks to raise money to get to Tenwek. The family decided that Onyango, the youngest son, who was attending college, should accompany his mother. (The work of care – *tich rito* – normally falls upon a female relative, but Mama Onyango had no daughters and no living sister. Francis's wife had three small children and had recently given birth, making it difficult for her to leave the house.) The Mission hospital admitted Mama Onyango, and the operation was done. Onyango took care of her during the two-month stay on the ward, relieved occasionally by Francis's wife. He reckoned that the hospital stay cost the family over 100,000 shillings (1000 euros) on accommodation, transport, food, medicines, tests and the hospital bill. They had no National Health Insurance Card, but Francis applied for one. Francis also applied for a loan: at the time he worked as a mechanic in the informal (*juakali*) sector, earning between 1,000 and 2,000 shillings (10–20 euros) per day, but he was the only family member with such an income. The siblings also raised contributions from family, friends, colleagues and church members, but the burden of the costs fell on Francis.

After discharge, Mama Onyango was instructed to return for clinical appointments every fortnight. This cost the family over 20,000 shillings (200 euros) each month for transport, accommodation, food, tests and medicines. Onyango recalled the first time they travelled back for a clinic appointment:

> Two of us had to accompany mother because she could not walk and so we had to look for a place to sleep for the two days. After leaving home at seven in the morning, we arrived at the hospital in the evening at five. They could not admit mother that day, so we just found a lodging place and for two rooms we paid 2,400 shillings.[40] We then went for supper, since the whole day we had not eaten anything, and this meal cost us 150 shillings per plate. Then we also bought mother milk at 50 shillings as she could not eat solid food, and even milk she could just sip a little by little and she struggled swallowing…

These journeys to Tenwek for check-ups 'became so challenging for the family', according to Onyango, and so they stopped taking her and she remained in the home for almost a year. During that time, she recalled, the pain was manageable, but by the end of 2013, it had become 'too much'. The family decided to bring their mother to Nightingale, another small private hospital in Kisumu, catering to patients with precarious incomes, where she was given morphine. The doctor told them she had a growth in the neck and advised her sons to take her to Kenyatta National Hospital in Nairobi for an operation. They took her home to plan what to do next.

Some weeks later, in March 2014, the family again brought Mama Onyango to Nightingale and she stayed on the ward for a week, receiving morphine. It was during this visit that a nurse advised them to take Mama Onyango to the Referral Hospital's Cancer Care Centre, to get some advice, and this is where we met her, together with Onyango and Francis, for the first time. They explained that when Mama Onyango was in pain, they brought her to the ward at Nightingale, because at least there she could get morphine. Francis told us that they were planning to take their mother to Kenyatta National Hospital in Nairobi for the operation, but they were still trying to raise the money. Two family members would have to accompany their mother to Nairobi, he said, as she was too weak to stand alone. The family had already spent a lot of money and they did not know what to do next.

During a later conversation, Onyango told us his mother's illness had forced him to drop out of college. Taking care of a very ill person is exhausting and emotionally draining, he said. 'Most of the time it is myself who stays with mother at the hospital every day, even if it is for two weeks or more.' On the hospital wards, 'relatives must do everything for their patients.' He could not sleep on the ward and had to find his own lodging, which cost a lot and also made him anxious: 'Most of the time when I am away from mother my heart is not at peace and I keep worrying how mama is.' Being the main caregiver involved 'moving with mother all the time' and this placed a deep emotional strain on him. 'Anytime I see mother in a lot of pain I feel so stressed.' He continued, 'And when you do not have money to buy the drugs, you cannot get any treatment and that is very challenging.' Francis's income was unstable, another brother was a drunkard, and they often had to seek help from relatives, friends and church members, with variable success. Their mother's sickness had gravely affected the family income, as she could not continue her small business of selling vegetables.

A week after our first meeting in March 2014, Biddy phoned up Onyango and found that he was with his mother in Nairobi, waiting for admittance to Kenyatta National Hospital (KNH). The family had managed to raise money, although only enough for Onyango to accompany her. They had travelled there by bus, even though Mama Onyango was in pain, because they could not afford the hospital ambulance (which cost 25,000 shillings, 250–300 euros). Arriving at KNH in the afternoon, they were told to return the next day as there were many patients waiting in the queue. A relative advised them to find lodgings in Kibera, one of Nairobi's large informal settlements, where they found a room for 1500 shillings (15 euros). Since his mother had travelled for a long time, they took a taxi (which cost another 15 euros). Early the following morning, they took another taxi and arrived at the hospital by eight, by which time the queue was already long, with many very sick patients; 'some were even sleeping on the floor as they were waiting to be admitted'. The doctor told them that although Mama Onyango was very sick, they could not admit her because the beds were already full, and she should come back a week later. The idea of having to stay in Nairobi for one week, with so little money, was 'very tough', Onyango said. He tried calling his relatives in Nairobi to see if they could accommodate them but 'people are not comfortable, even your relatives, when there is sickness'. They had no money for food but members of his mother's church notified fellow worshippers in the neighbourhood, who brought Onyango meals, while he bought milk for his mother. On the phone, Onyango sounded optimistic: 'I have left everything to God.' He repeated that the sickness of the mother has affected them 'so much', both financially and emotionally. He felt burdened but 'other members of the family are not ready to sacrifice their time'. He often had to skip a meal because they could not afford it but, as a Christian, he was used to praying and fasting, he said.

Onyango stayed with his mother for three weeks in Nairobi, waiting for a place in the surgical ward for the operation. We kept in regular touch. Every day, they would get to hospital by eight in the morning and wait the whole day in the queue until the evening without seeing the doctor or a nurse. The cycle repeated itself for several days. They eventually saw a doctor, who told him that his mother was too weak and could not be operated. By this time, they had spent more than 50,000 shillings (500 euros) just waiting, and after consulting Onyango's brothers, they decided to give up and travel back home, as the family was running out of money. They planned to raise money to bring Mama Onyango back for the operation.

Two weeks after returning home, the family brought Mama Onyango to Kisumu for another admission, as she was in 'too much pain'. Onyango told us they wanted her to 'just get pain killers that can relieve her of pain' and that the family was trying to raise 300,000 shillings to enable her go back to Nairobi to get the operation at KNH. This situation continued over the next few months, with Mama Onyango staying home with occasional admittance to hospital for pain relief. Onyango later recalled that they 'just could not cope with the degree of pain she was suffering'. The family 'did not know what to do'. In March 2015, Mama Onyango died, in her home.

As is customary in western Kenya, at the funeral, family members gave speeches about Mama Onyango's life, her illness and her death, positioning responsibilities and highlighting their tireless efforts to pursue care. Such narratives position *tich rito*, the 'work of care', as a constellation of economic, physical and emotional efforts, which are often unevenly distributed among family members, supported, to a greater or lesser extent, by others, whose efforts are listed and absences noted. Francis recalled the long trajectory of his mother's illness, her efforts to keep the family together and the pain she felt on learning that the family had to take Onyango out of college. Onyango explained that, in the weeks before she passed away, the family tried to get their mother admitted to the local sub-district hospital, just to get IV fluids and morphine, but as time went on the finances became drained and also the support from relatives, friends and church members dried up. Their mother died at home, and, Onyango recalled, 'There was nothing more we could do.' He recalled the times he had spent with his mother on the wards, in all the different hospitals they went to, over the months and years. He recalled the family's efforts to raise money and hopes to take her back to Nairobi. 'Most sick people in this country are dying due to lack of money', he said, as 'treatment is only available to people who are rich' and to 'those who can afford taking their people to private hospitals'.

Giving up treatment: the limits of care

Jessica was a widow with three small children and only 22 years old when we met her in June 2014, at the Acacia Clinic, where her aunt (FZ) had brought her. She agreed to an interview about her illness and we arranged that next time she came to Kisumu, we would meet, exchanging phone numbers with Jessica's aunt. At this next meeting, Jessica explained that her illness had begun in 2013, with a 'constant itching in the neck'. Later, there was a swelling, which became worse and she 'could not walk well'. At the time she was staying with her children at her husband's rural home in South Nyanza, and 'there was no-one to take care of me'.[41] She just bought some ointment and painkillers at the local shop and she used some 'pot (herbal) medicines'.

The swelling became infected. By November 2013, it was bad. She had difficulties sleeping and could not eat solids; she was 'only drinking porridge and water'. Having no one to accompany her, she left her children with her mother-in-law and took a motorbike taxi to the nearest sub-district hospital, where she was told that she had tuberculosis and referred to the nearest county hospital at Homa Bay (40 kilometres away) for further tests. As she had no support from her in-laws, she decided to travel with her children to her natal home and 'look for some money' from her paternal grandmother and other relatives (her own parents had died), to 'help me go to the hospital'. In January 2014, her paternal grandmother accompanied her to Homa Bay Hospital, where she was told she had tuberculosis and again referred, this time to Kisumu Referral Hospital, 100 kilometres away.

Jessica's grandmother discussed the matter with her paternal aunt and they agreed that instead of going to the hospital in Kisumu, Jessica should travel to another hospital, in Kericho County (about three hours from her grandmother's home), because her aunt lived nearby. She could stay with her aunt. In March, with money sent by her aunt for the journey, Jessica travelled to her aunt's home, leaving her children with her grandmother. She thus reached Kericho Hospital only in March 2014. Here, she recalled, a doctor examined her and told her to go to a private laboratory for a biopsy, which her aunt's son (FZS) paid for (her aunt showed us the paper print-out). When she returned to get the result, she was informed that she had 'cancer' (the print-out indicated lymphoma) and the doctor wrote her a referral letter for Kenyatta National Hospital (KNH) in Nairobi, to get chemotherapy and radiotherapy. (One should note that at this time, the waiting list for cancer patients at KNH was over one year.) She was in a lot of pain at this time. Since the family could not afford to take her to Nairobi, they returned to her aunt's home.

After consultation, the family decided to take her to the Referral Hospital in Kisumu, as it was nearer and they had relatives there. However, it took them six weeks to raise enough money for Jessica to travel to Kisumu with her paternal aunt. They stayed with the aunt's son, who worked as a *juakali* (informal) mechanic. According to the aunt, at the hospital's outpatient clinic, a doctor read the referral letter and told her to take Jessica to the Acacia Clinic, where the retired oncologist saw patients on Tuesdays, and chemotherapy was available at a subsidised price (at the time, 2,000 shillings per dose – later, the price rose). It was here that we first met Jessica in June 2014. Jessica's aunt brought her there, and her son paid for the registration and consultation with the doctor, who confirmed the diagnosis and advised the family to bring Jessica for a six-dose cycle of chemotherapy.

Jessica stayed with her aunt and cousin in Kisumu. When the family had raised money for the first dose of chemotherapy, her aunt took her to the Acacia Clinic, where she sat in the room set aside for chemotherapy patients while the nurse placed a canister in her vein for the chemotherapy, IV fluid and anti-vomiting medicine. After this, Jessica returned to Kisumu hospice for another five visits, between July and September 2014. However, she received chemotherapy only three times, because they did not have enough money and once because they came on the wrong day. Instead, she was given intravenous morphine. During this time, we tried to call Jessica's aunt and cousin with no success; nobody picked up the phone. In November, Biddy travelled to Jessica's aunt's home. She found that Jessica had passed away. As she had lost her phone, her aunt could not inform us. They had stopped taking her to Acacia; near the end, they took her to the nearest sub-district hospital for IV fluids and morphine. Jessica died in her aunt's home, leaving three small children with her grandmother.

Jessica spoke about her illness, the growth on her neck, her pain. She spoke of her relations, about her strained relations with her in-laws, the support of her grandmother and aunt, her worries about her children. The word 'cancer' only took shape after the biopsy, and the diagnosis did not open up a clear treatment trajectory, although it gave a name to what had been, up to this point, an undefined, painful growth. After being referred from one hospital to another, and moving between relatives, Jessica and her aunt finally ended up at Acacia clinic, where they hoped to get some relief. Her story underlines the importance of the natal family for young women. When men die of HIV/AIDS, their widows are often blamed. We do not know whether Jessica was HIV-positive, but she indicated that her husband had died of AIDS. HIV and TB infection often co-exist, but not always. When Jessica fell ill, she received little support from her husband's family. Her parents had died, and her own (younger) siblings dispersed among family members, so it was her paternal grandmother, and particularly her paternal aunt whom she could rely on. However, the burden of paying for Jessica's chemotherapy and clinical check-ups fell on her cousin, a *juakali* mechanic earning an irregular income. He and his mother struggled to raise money but could not complete the chemotherapy. We do not know if they decided to stop because they did not expect Jessica to live long. A few of the patients we followed complained bitterly about being abandoned by their relatives as they were not expected to live long or to thrive on treatment – 'they see me as a dead body'. But such cases were rare, and complicated. Like so many families with limited means, Jessica fell out of treatment, while the family were 'looking for money'.

'Treatment is only available to people who have money'

Gilbert was in his mid-60s when we met him in October 2015 at the Acacia Clinic. A retired civil servant with nine adult children, all college educated and most of them in employment, he lived in his town house in Kisumu while his wife looked after their rural home.

He told us that his illness began in August 2014 with a frequent need to urinate. After watching a TV programme about prostate cancer, his wife told him to go to the hospital and get a test. He began by visiting the retired oncologist at the Acacia Clinic, who told him to get a Prostate Specific Antigen (PSA) test and a biopsy test at a private laboratory in the city. These tests were costly (7,000 shillings, 70–80 euros), but Gilbert's sons sent money. At a second appointment, the retired oncologist told him to repeat these tests and get a CT scan from another private laboratory. By this time, the family had spent more than 30,000 shillings (over 300 euros). When the results confirmed prostate cancer, the oncologist – seeing that the family was 'financially able' – then referred him to Kenyatta National Hospital (KNH), the country's main public hospital, in Nairobi, for more tests to determine the stage of the cancer.

Gilbert travelled to Nairobi the next day, where he stayed with one of his sons and saw an oncologist at Kenyatta National Hospital, who referred him to more private laboratories for another biopsy, a MRI scan and more X-rays. These results suggested that the cancer had not spread, and he was placed on the waiting list for radiotherapy at KNH (which was, at the time, the only public hospital in the country offering radiotherapy, at a modest price of 500 shillings per session). As the waiting list was very long (almost 12 months), and the cancer had not spread, the family decided that he should follow the advice of a family friend and try out a Chinese medical clinic, which offered Chinese medicine. From September 2014 to March 2015, Gilbert made, as he recalled, about 14 visits to a Chinese General Clinic, where he received regular consultations with a Chinese doctor and received Chinese herbal treatment at the cost of 50,000 shillings (500 euros).

At this point, the ambiguous results of more tests and an MRI scan made the family worried and anxious, and Gilbert's children decided he could not wait any longer for radiotherapy at the public hospital. His oldest son arranged for a family friend, a doctor working at the private Aga Khan Hospital in Nairobi, to see his father (for a reduced price due to the family connection). Gilbert then underwent 41 sessions of radiotherapy at the private hospital from July to October 2015. This was an exhausting time; the radiotherapy made him sick and weak and it was very expensive (costing over 500,000 shillings/5,000 euros). The children organised a *harambee* (collective fund-raiser) to raise money for the treatment (a common practice, especially among the middle classes). Gilbert and his wife also sold the rental property they had invested in, after years of saving. Further scans and a PSA test suggested that the treatment had been successful and Gilbert returned to Kisumu, to the house he had built during his working years, from where he attended regular check-ups with the retired oncologist. It was here, at the Acacia Clinic, in October 2015, that we met him for the first time and later interviewed him. He told us he felt well, the treatment had been successful, but it had cost the family heavily; his sons and daughters had all contributed but he had been forced to sell the property he had bought as security for old age, and they were still spending a lot of money on medicines.

Gilbert's successful treatment is an example of the possibilities of medical diagnosis and treatment available to those who have some financial means. While not wealthy, he, his wife and their nine adult children had resources enough – through properties they had invested in over years, through salaries and access to loans – to sustain the litany of tests, scans, medicines and radiotherapy treatment they pursued. Consequently, Gilbert was able to attain not only early diagnosis but also various forms of cancer treatment, which included expensive treatment with Chinese medicine and 41 sessions of radiotherapy at a private hospital. By the end of 2015, Gilbert calculated that they had spent well over 800,000 shillings (8000 euros) in medical costs, none of which he could use his NIHF card for, and he added that the actual cost could be well over two million shillings, if transport, food, accommodation and other costs were included. As of January 2018, Gilbert was doing well and still attending clinical reviews.

A cancer diagnosis informed Gilbert's knowledge of his disease as soon as it became symptomatic, and cancer took shape amidst the multiple tests, scans and consultations that followed, as well as his and his family's research on the internet, and consultations with friends. Unlike Jessica and Mama Onyango, Gilbert described himself as a 'cancer survivor' and emphasised his vigilance, in pursuing regular clinical appointments. Gilbert's story also illustrates how middle-class patients, if they have financial means, are sent to many different private clinics, laboratories and hospitals in their search for treatment, spending a lot of money in the process. Indeed, Gilbert's treatment trajectory underlines the huge financial cost of pursuing diagnosis and treatment. Only a small proportion of this cost was covered by his NHIF card, despite the years he had paid for it, and this was a matter of some bitterness to him. Even though the NHIF began covering some chemotherapy and radiotherapy in 2015, this cover was only valid for public hospitals, which had long waiting lists.

Malignant stories: disjuncture, chronicity and the work of care

These extended cases give insights into the social, emotional, economic and medical contexts in which patients and their families experience cancer and pursue treatment and care. Cancer pushes at the boundaries of the social and it places a heavy burden on families and family relations. Our material locates the lengthy progress of illness, the search for diagnosis and treatment and the giving of care in the lives of patients and their families, in their livelihoods and relations, as illness, pain, disfigurement and anxiety emerge amidst other misfortunes, burdens and aspirations.

In Onyango's account of his mother's illness and in the narratives of Jessica and her aunt, the medical details fade into the background. More prominent are the social relations and networks that enable, and also constrain, care: the concerns about raising money, about mobility, transport and accommodation, about strained livelihoods, the struggle to make a living, to pursue treatment and to maintain care. In many cases, cancer itself does not clearly stand out as a discrete disease. With chronic conditions, there is often no singular beginning; these diseases 'creep up' rather than 'break out',[42] and diagnosis is often only reached (if at all) when the disease is far advanced. Most of the patients and families we knew spent little time discussing diagnoses. Gilbert's extensive knowledge about his disease and the way he described it was exceptional. Instead, people talked about pain, disability, the search for relief and treatment, the struggle to find money and the burden on their relatives. In some cases, patients and families were already grappling with chronic illness; some were HIV-positive, some had already experienced periods of serious illness. Like HIV, a cancer diagnosis was not always 'disclosed', or only to a select few. Lessons learned from decades of experience with HIV and exposure to HIV-advocacy and 'speaking therapy' are not easily being transferred to the management of cancer. People are learning to talk of 'cancer', but there remains much silence, secrecy and stigma surrounding a disease whose name, for many, spells an unavoidable malignant outcome and possible economic catastrophe. The huge economic burden placed on families alongside knowledge of poor treatment outcomes also creates moral ambiguity and anguish as families must make difficult decisions about care.

These cancer trajectories also expose – in particular, malignant ways – socioeconomic fault-lines and inequalities within Kenya, which intersect with scarce public healthcare and an expanding private healthcare sector to produce highly divergent outcomes. The three cases illustrate the fractured availability of medical expertise, diagnosis and treatment along lines of socioeconomic status and class. These fractures lie not only between the wealthy elite (who fly overseas for medical treatment) and ordinary citizens, but also between the middle classes and those without formal employment. Cancer treatment extends indefinitely, sucking up more and more resources. While a chronic disease placed huge financial pressure on middle-class families such as Gilbert's, who were forced to sell land and property to fund extended periods of treatment, these families are able to pursue diagnosis and access medical care. Families like Jessica's simply could not afford the necessary interventions, and, after receiving a late diagnosis, their patients quickly dropped out of treatment. As Nurse Angela lamented:

> Sometimes I try to phone a patient and there is no answer, I get the relative and he tells she died months back, or when I meet a relative in the street and ask about a patient I am told the same story.

These bifurcated itineraries shape the chronicity of cancer – the ways in which it is experienced in time or emerges as a disease. But these divergences gloss over commonalities in experience across socioeconomic differences. Many of the families we followed encountered dead ends across uneven landscapes of public and private medical care. They were referred for a MRI scan here or an operation there, for chemotherapy here or radiotherapy there, yet long waiting lists and the huge costs of treatment, or the limitations of their health insurance cover, often curtailed such possibilities of care.[43]

Navigating a fragmented terrain of cancer treatment, families shoulder both the burden of care and responsibility for the termination or continuation of treatment. In a context of therapeutic disjuncture, it is the family who must connect the dots. Patients and their families are expected to pursue treatment possibilities to the very end. While nurses like Nurse Angela experience patients interrupting treatment and 'disappearing', by contrast, families strive to continue care – and thus caring – for as long as they can. The practice of care is rooted not only in daily forms of body care – helping a mother to walk, securing food, milk and water, sitting with her and attending to her bodily needs – but also in the process of trying, of not losing hope, pursuing treatment until the very end, rather than 'giving up'. Thus, rarely did anyone tell us that treatment had terminated or that it was coming to an end. Instead they said, 'We are still looking for money' for the next step. In this way, they strive to keep the possibility of life and health – and the continuity of care – on the near horizon.

Notes

1 See Farmer et al., 'Expansion of Cancer Care and Control'.
2 See Chabrol, 'La Long Éclipse'; Whyte, 'Chronicity and Control'.
3 Livingston, *Improvising Medicine*; Mulemi,'Technologies of Hope'; Mathews, Burke, and Kampriani (eds.), *Anthropologies of Cancer in Transnational Worlds*; Mika, 'Fifty Years of Creativity, Crisis, and Cancer'; Reubi, Herrick, and Brown, 'The Politics of Non-Communicable Diseases'; Caduff and Van Hollen, 'Cancer and the Global South'; Mika, 'Cytotoxic'; Djordjevic, 'Pluripotent Trajectories'; Frieden, Graber, and M'zoughi, 'Les Maladies Chroniques dans les Suds'; Nédélec, 'Chronicité(s) et Cancers Gynécologiques'; Manderson, 'Editorial'; Manderson, 'Afterword'.
4 Burke and Mathews, 'Returning to Earth'.
5 Mulemi, 'Technologies of Hope'; Jain, *How Cancer Becomes Us*; Gibbon, 'Anticipating Prevention'; Mulemi, 'Cancer Crisis in Kenya'.
6 Livingston, *Improvising Medicine*, 54.
7 Whyte, 'Knowing Hypertension and Diabetes'.
8 Luxardo, 'As God is my Witness...'; Nelson, 'Cancer, Stress, and Ironies of Cancer Understanding'.
9 Mulemi, 'Patients' Perspectives on Hospitalisation'; Yates-Doerr, 'Counting Bodies?'.
10 Mulemi, 'Patients' Perspectives on Hospitalisation'.
11 Mulemi, 'Cancer Crisis and Treatment Ambiguity in Kenya'.
12 Nine of the 34 were 18–34 years old, eight were 35–49 years old, sixteen were 50–64 years old, and four were 65 years and above. Thirty-one patients received diagnosis for breast (5), cervix (6), prostate (3), penis (3), oesophagus (6), abdominal (4), lymphomas (2), lung (1) and skin (1) cancer. The other three passed away before their suspected cancer was confirmed.
13 This meant that we missed stories and experiences of cancer which never made it to the hospital or these clinics.
14 Pseudonyms are used.
15 We enrolled patients into the study only after a long process of explaining the research and obtaining their informed consent. Research was funded by the Norwegian Research Council with a FRISAM (Humanities and Social Science) fellowship (grant no. 213670) and conducted in collaboration with Dr Phelgona Otieno, KEMRI CRC. Research and ethical approval were granted by the Kenya Medical Research Institute's Scientific Steering Committee (SSC), and Ethics Review Committee (ERC) (KEMRI/RES/7/3/1), and by the Jaramogi Oginga Odinga Teaching and Referral Hospital's Ethical Review Committee, (ERC.1B./VOL.1/318). Dr Phelgona Otieno provided invaluable advice and support. I am also especially grateful to Dr Benson Mulemi, Philister Madiega, Professor Erick Nyambedha and Maulyn Akech. Biddy Otieno provided invaluable research assistance. Special thanks to Phelgona Otieno and Philister Madiega for their warm hospitality, and to the Mill Hill fathers, Kisumu.

16 See Brown, 'Hospital Domestics'.
17 While it is normally women who shoulder the burden of caregiving, we observed cases of male caregivers, too; younger, even teenage, brothers or sons are sometimes taken out of education to take care of a sibling or older family member.
18 This work is deeply indebted to Biddy's commitment to patients and their families, often through deeply distressing situations.
19 GLOBOCAN is created by the Global Cancer Observatory (GCO), set up by the WHO; it is a web-based platform presenting global cancer statistics.
20 The Eldoret Registry was established in 1998, followed by the Nairobi Cancer Registry, established in 2001, https://afcrn.org/membership/membership-list/85-nairobi-kenya, accessed 8 July 2019; Mutuma and Rugutt-Korir, 'Nairobi Cancer Registry'.
21 Bray et al., 'Global Cancer Statistics 2018'. Notes that these statistics only account for reported cases and do not account for cancer cases that remain undiagnosed.
22 However, Kenya has a longer history of cancer research and oncology, which remains largely invisible. See Iliffe, *East African Doctors*; Ombongi, 'The Historical Interfaces'; Mueller, 'Cancer in the Tropics'.
23 World Health Organization, Global Cancer Observatory, GLOBOCAN, https://gco.iarc.fr/today/data/factsheets/populations/404-kenya-fact-sheets.pdf.
24 Government of Kenya, *National Cancer Control Strategy, 2011–2016*, 9.
25 Nairobi Cancer Registry, 'Cancer Incidence Report 2000–2002, 2006'.
26 UNAIDS, www.unaids.org/en/cervical_cancer.
27 See Prince, 'The Moral Economy of Survival in Kenya'; Whyte (ed.), *Second Chances*.
28 Chabrol, 'La Long Éclipse', 22.
29 Livingston, *Improvising Medicine*.
30 For example, Chao, 'No Respite for Poor Patients'; Mahugu, 'Why Kenyans Opt for Treatment in India'; Kajilwa, 'NHIF to Foot Bills of Cancer Patients'.
31 See, for example, BBC News, 'Kenya Doctors' Strike'.
32 BBC News, 'Kenya Survivors'; Nyawira, 'Why Many Kenyans are Dying of Cancer'.
33 For example, Mathiu, 'There is No Excuse'; Kubania, 'Pain, Fading Hope as Therapy Stopped'; Kairu, 'Sole Cancer Machine Down, Again'.
34 Landon, 'An Investor's Plan to Transplant Private Health Care'.
35 For example, Kenya's National Hospital Insurance Fund, which insures all civil servants and most formal-sector workers, reported on its twitter feed in 2018 that 10,000 Kenyans sought treatment in India, 70 per cent of them for cancer. See also *Agile Global Health* blog, 'NHIF Visit to Agile Global Health's India Network Sparks Big Plans'.
36 For example, Njugunah, 'India Medical Centre Invests Sh650 Million'. The exception is Moi Teaching and Referral Hospital in Eldoret, which expanded its cancer care with the establishment in 2016 of a specialised centre, funded by donors.
37 The government has recently introduced a pilot 'Universal Health Coverage' programme, which has scrapped user fees for the duration of one year, in 4 of the 47 counties, including Kisumu, and promises to extend this to the whole country by 2022.
38 See Muinde, 'Health Insurance for the Poor'.
39 There was a cancer-screening month in Kisumu, during which the private Aga Khan Hospital conducted biopsies on patients free of charge, who were referred by doctors from government hospitals.
40 Approximately US$25–30.
41 Meaning, no-one who loved her enough to take care of her.
42 Whyte, 'Chronicity and Control', 68–9.
43 Sanz's concept of 'therapeutic disjunctures' helps to illuminate these temporalities. She explores how inequalities in access to treatment – which manifest in delays, interruptions, stops and starts, and an experience of 'moving in circles' – materialise in bodies and treatment outcomes among cancer patients in Colombia, creating bifurcated forms of care, and leading to the rapid decline of some bodies while enabling the prolonged life of others (Sanz,'Out-of-Sync Cancer Care').

Bibliography

Agile Global Health blog. 'NHIF Visit to Agile Global Health's India Network Sparks Big Plans' (15 March 2017), https://agileglobalhealth.com/nhif-visit-ak-global-healths-india-network-sparks-big-plans/, accessed 10 July 2019.

BBC News. 'Kenya Doctors' Strike: The Cancer Patient and the Medic', 17 February 2017, www.bbc.com/news/world-africa-38979953.

BBC News. 'Kenya Survivors: Cancer is "National Disaster"', 1 August 2019, www.bbc.com/news/world-africa-49191685.

Bray, F. et al. 'Global Cancer Statistics 2018: GLOBOCAN Estimates of Incidence and Mortality Worldwide for 36 Cancers in 185 Countries', *Cancer Journal for Clinicians*, 68 (6) (2018): 394–424.

Brown, H. 'Hospital Domestics: Care Work in a Kenyan Hospital', *Space and Culture*, 15 (1) (2012): 18–30.

Burke, N. J. and H. F. Mathews. 'Returning to Earth: Setting a Global Agenda for the Anthropology of Cancer'. *Medical Anthropology*, 36 (3) (2017): 179–86.

Caduff, Carlo and Cecilia C. Van Hollen. 'Cancer and the Global South', *BioSocieties*, 14 (4) (2019): 489–95.

Chabrol, F. 'La Long Éclipse des Hépatites Virales en Afrique', *Emulations – Revue de Sciences Sociales*, 27 (2019): 15–31.

Chao, S. 'No Respite for Poor Patients despite the New Guidelines', *Business Daily*, 3 December 2013, https://www.businessdailyafrica.com/news/No-respite-for-poor-patients-despite-the-new-guidelines/539546-2097274-8ys7siz/index.html.

Djordjevic, D. 'Pluripotent Trajectories: Public Oncology in Rwanda', *Biosocieties*, 14 (4) (2019): 553–70.

Farmer, Paul et al. 'Expansion of Cancer Care and Control in Countries of Low and Middle Income: A Call to Action', *Lancet*, 376 (9747) (2010): 1186–93.

Frieden, M. C., N. Graber, and M. M'zoughi. 'Les Maladies Chroniques dans les Suds: Expériences, Savoirs et Politiques aux Marges de la Santé Globale', *Emulations – Revue de Sciences Sociales*, 27 (2019): 7–14.

Gibbon, S. 'Anticipating Prevention: Constituting Clinical Need, Rights and Resources in Brazilian Cancer Genetics'. In *Anthropologies of Cancer in Transnational Worlds*, edited by H. F. Mathews, N. J. Burke, and E. Kampriani, Chapter 3. New York: Routledge, 2015.

Global Cancer Observatory, GLOBOCAN, WHO, https://gco.iarc.fr/today/data/factsheets/populations/404-kenya-fact-sheets.pdf, accessed 8 July 2019.

Government of Kenya. *National Cancer Control Strategy, 2011–2016*.

Iliffe, J. *East African Doctors: A History of the Medical Profession*. Cambridge: Cambridge University Press, 1998.

Jain, L. S. *How Cancer Becomes Us*. Berkeley, CA: University of California Press, 2013.

Kairu, P. 'Sole Cancer Machine Down, Again', *The Daily Nation*, 2 September 2015, www.nation.co.ke/news/Radiotherapy-Machine-KNH-Cancer-Patients/1056-2856168-format-xhtml-15hvl5lz/index.html.

Kajilwa, G. 'NHIF to Foot Bills of Cancer Patients in Full,' *The Standard*, 13 February 2019, www.standardmedia.co.ke/health/article/2001312856/nhif-to-foot-bills-of-cancer-patients-in-full.

Kubania, J. 'Pain, Fading Hope as Therapy Stopped', *The Daily Nation*, 19 March 2015, www.nation.co.ke/news/Pain-fading-hope-as-therapy-stopped/-/1056/2659862/-/dibj5xz/-/index.html.

Landon, Thomas Jr. 'An Investor's Plan to Transplant Private Health Care in Africa', *New York Times*, 8 October 2016, www.nytimes.com/2016/10/09/business/dealbook/an-investors-plan-to-transplant-private-health-care-in-africa.html.

Livingston, Julie. *Improvising Medicine: An African Oncology Ward in an Emerging Cancer Epidemic*. Durham, NC: Duke University Press, 2012.

Luxardo, N. '"As God is my Witness...": What is Said, What is Silenced in Informal Cancer Caregivers' Narratives'. In *Anthropologies of Cancer in Transnational Worlds*, edited by H. F. Mathews, N. J. Burke, and E. Kampriani, 193–211. New York: Routledge, 2015.

Mahugu, J. 'Why Kenyans Opt for Treatment in India', *The Standard*, 3 June 2018, www.standardmedia.co.ke/health/article/2001282717/why-kenyans-opt-for-treatment-in-india.

Manderson, L. 'Editorial: New Perspectives in Anthropology on Cancer Control, Disease and Palliative Care'. *Anthropology & Medicine*, 6 (3) (1999): 317–21.

Manderson, L. 'Afterword: Cancer Enigmas and Agendas'. In *Anthropologies of Cancer in Transnational Worlds*, edited by H. F. Mathews, N. J. Burke, and E. Kampriani, 241–54. New York: Routledge, 2015.

Mathews, H. F. and N. J. Burke. 'Introduction: Mapping the Landscape of Transnational Cancer Ethnography'. In *Anthropologies of Cancer in Transnational Worlds*, edited by H. F. Mathews, N. J. Burke, and E. Kampriani, 1–36. New York: Routledge, 2015.

Mathiu, M. 'There is No Excuse for the Negligence of Cancer Treatment in this Country', *The Daily Nation*, 19 March 2015, www.nation.co.ke/oped/Opinion/There-is-no-excuse-for-the-negligence-of-cancer-treatment/-/440808/2659712/-/11d8fsg/-/index.html.

Mika, Marissa. 'Fifty Years of Creativity, Crisis, and Cancer in Uganda', *Canadian Journal of African Studies / Revue Canadienne des Études Africaines*, 50 (3) (2016): 395–413.

Mika, Marissa. 'Cytotoxic: Notes on Chemotherapy at the Lymphoma Treatment Center, Uganda Cancer Institute, Kampala', *Biosocieties*, 14 (4) (2019): 573–82.

Mueller, L. M. 'Cancer in the Tropics: Geographical Pathology and the Formation of Cancer Epidemiology', *BioSocieties*, 14 (2019): 512–28.

Muinde, J. V. 'Health Insurance for the Poor: Insights from the Kenyan Coast', *Somatosphere*, 11 May 2020 (part of the series on 'Health for All? Critical Perspectives on Universal Health Coverage), http://somatosphere.net/2020/health-insurance-poor-kenya.html/.

Mulemi, B. A. 'Patients' Perspectives on Hospitalisation: Experiences from a Cancer Ward in Kenya', *Anthropology & Medicine*, 15 (2) (2008): 117–31.

Mulemi, B. A. 'Cancer Crisis in Kenya: Rapid Ethnographic Vie', *Global Medicine*, 11 (2010): 1–2.

Mulemi, B. A. 'Technologies of Hope. Managing Cancer in a Kenyan Hospital'. In *Making and Unmaking Public Health in Africa: Ethnographic and Historical Perspectives*, edited by R. J. Prince and R. Marsland, 162–86. Athens, OH: Ohio University Press, 2013.

Mulemi, B. A. 'Cancer Crisis and Treatment Ambiguity in Kenya'. In *Anthropologies of Cancer in Transnational Worlds*, edited by H. H. Mathews, N. J. Burke, and E. Kampriani, 156–76. New York: Routledge, 2015.

Mutuma, G. Z. and A. Rugutt-Korir. *Nairobi Cancer Registry: Cancer Incidence Report, 2000–2002*. Nairobi: Kenya Medical Research Institute, 2006.

Nairobi Cancer Registry. 'Cancer Incidence Report 2000–2002, 2006', KEMRI (Kenya Medical Research Institute), Nairobi, Kenya.

Nédélec, É. 'Chronicité(s) et Cancers Gynécologiques: Enjeux Thérapeutiques et Relationnels à Abidjan', *Emulations – Revue de Sciences Sociales*, 27 (2019): 33–45.

Nelson, L. C. 'Cancer, Stress, and Ironies of Cancer Understanding in South Korea', *Medical Anthropology*, 36 (1) (2017): 19–31.

Njugunah, M. 'India Medical Centre Invests Sh650 Million in Nairobi Cancer Hospital', *Capital Business*, 26 July 2017, www.capitalfm.co.ke/business/2017/07/india-medical-centre-invests-sh650mn-in-nairobi-cancer-hospital/.

Nyawira, 'Why Many Kenyans Are Dying of Cancer', *The Star*, 1 August 2019, www.the-star.co.ke/news/big-read/2019-08-01-why-many-kenyans-are-dying-of-cancer/.

Ombongi, K. S. 'The Historical Interfaces between the State and Medical Science in Africa: Kenya's Case'. In *Evidence, Ethos and Experiment: The Anthropology and History of Medical Research in Africa*, edited by P. W. Geissler and C. Molyneux. New York: Berghahn Books, 2011.

Prince, Ruth J. 'HIV and the Moral Economy of Survival in Kenya', *Medical Anthropology Quarterly*, 26 (4) (2012): 534–56.

Reubi, David, Clare Herrick, and Tim Brown. 'The Politics of Non-Communicable Diseases in the Global South'. *Health and Place*, 39 (2016): 179–87.

Sanz, C. 'Out-of-Sync Cancer Care: Health Insurance Companies, Biomedical Practices, and Clinical Time in Colombia', *Medical Anthropology*, 36 (3) (2017): 187–201.

UNAIDS, www.unaids.org/en/cervical_cancer, accessed 8 July 2019.

Whyte, S. R. 'Chronicity and Control: Framing 'Non-Communicable' Diseases in Africa', *Anthropology & Medicine*, 19 (1) (2012): 64–74.

Whyte, S. R. (ed.). *Second Chances: Surviving AIDS in Uganda*. Durham, NC: Duke University Press, 2014.

Whyte, S. R. 'Knowing Hypertension and Diabetes: Conditions of Treatability in Uganda', *Health and Place*, 39 (2016): 219–25.

World Health Organization. 'Global Cancer Observatory (GCO)', last modified 2019, https://gco.iarc.fr/, accessed 8 July 2019.

Yates-Doerr, Emily. 'Counting Bodies? On Future Engagements with Science Studies in Medical Anthropology', *Anthropology & Medicine*, 24 (2) (2017): 142–58.

Permissions

All chapters in this book were first published by UCL Press; hereby published with permission under the Creative Commons Attribution License or equivalent. Every chapter published in this book has been scrutinized by our experts. Their significance has been extensively debated. The topics covered herein carry significant information for a comprehensive understanding. They may even be implemented as practical applications or may be referred to as a beginning point for further studies.

The contributors of this book come from diverse backgrounds, making this book a truly international effort. We would like to thank all the contributing authors for lending their expertise to make the book truly unique. They have played a crucial role in the development of this book. Without their invaluable contributions this book wouldn't have been possible. They have made vital efforts to compile up to date information on the varied aspects of this subject to make this book a valuable addition to the collection of many professionals and students.

This book was conceptualized with the vision of imparting up-to-date and integrated information in this field. To ensure the same, a matchless editorial board was set up. Every individual on the board went through rigorous rounds of assessment to prove their worth. After which they invested a large part of their time researching and compiling the most relevant data for our readers.

The editorial board has been involved in producing this book since its inception. They have spent rigorous hours researching and exploring the diverse topics which have resulted in the successful publishing of this book. They have passed on their knowledge of decades through this book. To expedite this challenging task, the publisher supported the team at every step. A small team of assistant editors was also appointed to further simplify the editing procedure and attain best results for the readers.

Apart from the editorial board, the designing team has also invested a significant amount of their time in understanding the subject and creating the most relevant covers. They scrutinized every image to scout for the most suitable representation of the subject and create an appropriate cover for the book.

The publishing team has been an ardent support to the editorial, designing and production team. Their endless efforts to recruit the best for this project, has resulted in the accomplishment of this book. They are a veteran in the field of academics and their pool of knowledge is as vast as their experience in printing. Their expertise and guidance has proved useful at every step. Their uncompromising quality standards have made this book an exceptional effort. Their encouragement from time to time has been an inspiration for everyone.

The publisher and the editorial board hope that this book will prove to be a valuable piece of knowledge for students, practitioners and scholars across the globe.

Index